Encyclopedia of
Sexually Transmitted Diseases

Encyclopedia of Sexually Transmitted Diseases

ELAINE A. MOORE
with LISA MARIE MOORE

Illustrations by Marvin G. Miller

McFarland & Company, Inc., Publishers
Jefferson, North Carolina, and London

The present work is a reprint of the illustrated case bound edition of Encyclopedia of Sexually Transmitted Diseases, *first published in 2005 by McFarland.*

LIBRARY OF CONGRESS CATALOGUING-IN-PUBLICATION DATA

Moore, Elaine A., 1948–
Encyclopedia of sexually transmitted diseases / Elaine A. Moore ;
with Lisa Marie Moore ; illustrations by Marvin G. Miller.
p.   cm.
Includes bibliographical references and index.

ISBN 978-0-7864-4317-8
softcover : 50# alkaline paper ∞

1. Sexually transmitted diseases— Encyclopedias.
I. Moore, Lisa Marie, 1973–
II. Title.
RC200.1.M66   2008   616.95'1'003 — dc22   2004018309

British Library cataloguing data are available

On the cover: *background* Human papillomavirus (HPV) seen in Pap smear
(Kerry Linenberger and Cindy Forbeck); *Left and center detail:* tissue changes
in lymph node from an AIDS patient (Public Health Imaging Library, CDC);
Right detail: Neisseria Gonorrhoeae gram stain — rectal smear (Joe Miller, CDC)

Manufactured in the United States of America

*McFarland & Company, Inc., Publishers
Box 611, Jefferson, North Carolina 28640
www.mcfarlandpub.com*

To Brett,
with gratitude for your computer support

Table of Contents

Preface

Despite its romantic undertones, sacred aura, and roots that frequently lie in passion, the very nature of sexual intimacy allows for the insidious transmission of microbial organisms. In most instances, this transmission is uneventful. Most bacteria that normally inhabit the genital organs are harmless and serve a protective function.

Unfortunately, however, there are more than 30 different organisms that are pathogenic — that is, they cause infection and disease when they secretly find their way from one person to another. The diseases that result from venereal or genital contact, including anal, oral, and vaginal sex, are known as sexually transmitted diseases (STDs). STDs represent five of the ten most commonly reported infections today. Combined, STDs represent 87 percent of all reported infections. Progression of certain STDs can have serious consequences, including pelvic inflammatory disease, sterility and death; yet, in their early stages, many STDs do not cause any symptoms.

While the term STD has been widely used only in the last few decades, venereal disease epidemics date as far back as the first century. Descriptions of *Chlamydia trachomatis*, the infectious agent responsible for ophthalmia neonatorum, chlamydial infections, and lymphogranuloma venereum, are recorded as early as A.D. 60.

While early physicians did not have the means to study this infectious agent microscopically or treat it effectively, they had little doubt about its mode of transmission.

And while all STDs can be transmitted through sex, not all infections caused by the organisms responsible for STDs are sexually transmitted. Even the classic venereal diseases such as syphilis and gonorrhea can be transmitted through other means, including childbirth. And while certain STDs, such as HIV/AIDS or chlamydial infection, have a rightful place on any list of STDs, there is considerable debate among infectious disease specialists whether certain other diseases, such as hepatitis A or scabies, belong on the list. Abiding by the true definition of sexually transmitted diseases, in this book we have included all infectious diseases that may be acquired sexually. In addition we describe the opportunistic infections and neoplasms that may occur in persons with AIDS.

The STDs described in this book include a number of STDs that may also be transmitted by other means besides sex and include the following potential modes of transmission: blood-to-blood contact, infected blood products, contaminated needles and medical equipment, contaminated tattoo dyes and medicines, and exposure to other bodily fluids, such as saliva and breast milk. And as we have

1

noted, in some STDs infection can also occur during childbirth as the baby is exposed to the cervical canal during vaginal delivery. Babies can even become infected during their time in the uterus if the amniotic fluid becomes infected.

STDs are usually caused by infections with viruses and bacteria, although certain diseases such as pubic lice are caused by parasites, and microorganisms known as fungi are responsible for yeast infections. Symptoms in STDs are highly variable, with several STDs causing no or a few mild symptoms until the disease has significantly progressed or complications occur.

While some STDs, such as herpes, are generally confined to specific parts of the body, others, such as syphilis and AIDS, are systemic, that is, they disseminate throughout the body, potentially affecting all bodily organs and systems. Some STDs, such as the human papilloma virus and human herpesvirus-8, can induce cellular changes in infected cells that can lead to specific cancers. All STDs can be prevented, but not all STDs can be cured. The Herpes simplex virus and the HIV virus cannot be eradicated. While herpes is associated with recurring symptoms and long latent periods, this virus persists for life.

In some STDs, such as gonorrhea and AIDS, infective organisms can mutate and develop new strains that are resistant to the very antibiotics and anti-retroviral agents once used to treat them. For HIV/AIDS, there are treatments that halt the disease process by inhibiting viral replication, but there is no cure.

Regarding the terminology used in this text, we would like to note the following:

- Each specific STD is caused by a specific microorganism. Under the etiology information included for each disease, we list the genus and species of the responsible organism. For instance, *Trichomonas vaginalis* is the genus and species of the parasite that causes trichomoniasis. In subsequent mention of the organism, we follow traditional biological nomenclature in referring to the organism as *T. vaginalis.*

- We refer to the Centers for Disease Control and Prevention division of the U.S. Department of Health and Human Services as the CDC.

- We use the symbol < for "less than" and > for "greater than."

- The prefix "extra" refers to "away." For example, the word "extrapulmonary" refers to organs that are "away from" or "other than" pulmonary organs (lungs).

- The terms "immunosuppressed" or "immunocompetent" are used to describe a suppressed or weakened immune system caused by a decreased number of immune system cells.

Historically, the five major venereal diseases include gonorrhea, syphilis, chancroid, granuloma inguinale and lymphogranuloma venerum. Over the years, the list of STDs has grown to include scabies, genital warts, herpes, human papilloma virus (HPV), cervicitis, pubic lice, trichomoniasis, genital candidiasis, molluscum contagiosum, urethritis, cytomegalovirus CMV), chlamydial infections, hepatitis, and AIDS, a disease caused by the human immunodeficiency virus (HIV).

For each specific STD, we describe the etiology, epidemiology or prevalence, symptoms, complications, diagnosis, treatment, and risk factors; we include special considerations in pregnancy and precautions when relevant. For some diseases we also include historical information and alternative medical treatment options. In addition we have included lengthy sections describing the history of STDs, the history of syphilis and the history of HIV/AIDS. Although 500 years separate the emergence of syphilis and AIDS, the reader will note many similarities between these disorders from both a medical and sociological standpoint.

STDs are among the most common communicable diseases. Today, it is well known that STDs can affect people from all walks of life. And despite improved methods of diagnosis and treatment, the incidence of many STDs has risen in recent years. In the United States, the incidence of STDs increased steadily from the 1950s through the 1970s and then stabilized in the 1980s. At the end of the 1980s, the number of people with STDs, especially syphilis and gonorrhea, began to rise again.

In various sections of our book, we describe the sociological impact of STDs, including employment issues and legal rights. Society has traditionally viewed people infected with STDs in an unfavorable light, punishing those who harbor disease and rewarding those perceived as innocent victims. The reader will find that societal views have influenced government policy, and in some ways government policy works to shape societal views.

Our goal in writing this book is to inform readers by describing the pathological, biochemical, historical, epidemiological, legal, and sociological aspects of STDs. In addition we describe risk factors, preventive measures, insurance concerns, employment issues, treatment options, local and federal health services, STDs in the prison population, and special concerns in pregnancy and in newborns and children.

To offer insight into how STDs are transmitted and how they are sometimes able to persist despite treatment, we explain the differences between bacteria and viruses, and we describe drug resistance, DNA sequencing and gene mutations. We also describe the relationship between certain STDs and various cancers. In particular, we describe how several strains of the human papilloma virus (HPV) can cause squamous intraepithelial lesions (SIL) and cervical cancer, and we describe how the thin-prep Pap test combined with NAT testing can be used to diagnose infection as well as cellular abnormalities.

In an effort to show how the disease process in the viral STDs develops slowly over time, we describe viral load, retroviral replication, immune system function and the effects of HIV and HPV on the body's cells. We also cover conditions such as urethritis, pelvic inflammatory disease, epidymitis, and cervicitis, conditions that develop as a consequence of several different STDs.

In addition, we examine the goals of current STD/HIV research, and we describe clinical trials, including those employing vaccines and alternative medical treatments.

Because many of the topics are related, we have included cross-references in certain entries, allowing readers the opportunity to further explore specific subjects. We have also included references at the end of many sections.

Near the back of the book is a listing of resources, including hotline numbers, clinical trial information, government resources and Internet web sites.

Acknowledgments

We would like to thank the STD division of the Centers for Disease Control and Prevention in Atlanta for sharing their educational resources. We are indebted to Marvin G. Miller for his illustrations, which so clearly depict the microscopic world of STDs. We also owe special thanks to René Baker-Troscher for assisting us with proofreading and offering creative advice. And we cannot forget Lorri Genack, cytology supervisor, and Jim Ferguson, microbiology supervisor, at the Memorial Hospital Laboratory in Colorado Springs for their technical contributions.

We would like to extend a special note of gratitude to Rick and Brett Moore for their patience, help, and encouragement.

Disclaimer

Intended to educate and empower patients, *Encyclopedia of Sexually Transmitted Diseases* is not intended as a substitute for medical treatment. Individuals at risk for STDs or who have symptoms that could be caused by STDs should contact their health care providers. We would especially like to emphasize the value of preventive methods and safe sex and to remind our readers that early diagnosis and prompt treatment are essential for avoiding disease progression and reducing complications that threaten fertility, neonatal health and, in some instances, life itself.

THE ENCYCLOPEDIA

Abacivir

Abacivir (Ziagen, Trizivir, ABC) is a nucleoside reverse transcriptase inhibitor (NRTI) approved as an antiretroviral agent in the treatment of HIV infection. Its experimental code used in clinical trials is 1592U89. Abacavir is generally well tolerated and has a lower association with mitochondrial toxicity compared to other NRTIs. However, abacavir causes a hypersensitivity syndrome (HSR) in about 2–6 percent of patients. This syndrome usually occurs within the first six weeks of treatment.

HSR may cause itching and rash, but these symptoms do not always occur. Some individuals with HSR may develop fever and malaise or gastrointestinal symptoms, such as nausea, vomiting, diarrhea, and abdominal pain. Rarely, liver function tests are elevated.

Some researchers believe there is a genetic component to this reaction and have found that people who develop HSR are more likely to have the HLA B57 antigen, which influences and modulates the immune response. Patients using ABC should be cautioned about HSR but not frightened. Patients who have had a previous HSR to ABC should not use this drug again. Patients should notify their physicians immediately if they develop two or more of the following new symptoms: fever, shortness of breath, cough, sore throat, rash, itching, gastrointestinal symptoms, fatigue or general malaise after starting ABC.

Abscess

An abscess is an isolated accumulation of pus associated with a localized infection. Abscesses may cause tissue destruction, pain and swelling; severe abscesses may result in systemic disease and may require surgical drainage.

Acquired immune deficiency syndrome (AIDS)

Summary of This Entry

Etiology
Epidemiology
  SPECIAL PROBLEMS IN WOMEN
Symptoms
  ACUTE RETROVIRAL SYNDROME
  CLINICAL LATENCY
  DIARRHEA
  ACUTE INFLAMMATORY DEMYELINATING POLYNEURO-
    PATHY (AIDP)
  OSTEOPOROSIS AND OSTEOPENIA
  NEUROLOGICAL SYMPTOMS
  EYE SYMPTOMS
  SYMPTOMS IN NEONATAL AND PEDIATRIC AIDS
  AIDS DEVELOPMENT
  CLASSIFICATIONS OF AIDS
  TIMEFRAME
Diagnosis
  PROBLEMS WITH HIV ANTIBODY TESTS
  VIRAL LOAD
  NEONATAL TESTING
  CD4+ T CELL COUNTS
  AIDS DEFINING ILLNESSES
Treatment
  REVERSE TRANSCRIPTASE INHIBITORS
    Nucleoside/Nucleotide Reverse Transcriptase
    Inhibitors (NRTIs)
    Non-nucleoside Reverse Transcriptase Inhibitors
    (NNRTIs)

(continued)

See also AIDS Clinical Trials Group; AIDS dementia complex; AIDS Drug Assistance Program; AIDS history; AIDS Quilt; AIDS-related complex; AIDS-related primary central nervous system lymphoma; AIDS Vaccine Evaluation Group; AIDS Vaccine Evaluation Units; AIDS vaccines

Acquired immune deficiency syndrome (AIDS) represents the end stage of infection with the human immunodeficiency viruses types 1 and 2 (HIV-1, HIV-2). AIDS is one of the most recent STDs to emerge. It is the fourth largest cause of death globally and the leading cause of death in Africa. The first cases of AIDS were seen in the United States in June 1981 although it was several more years before the viral cause of this disease was determined.

AIDS damages the immune system as the

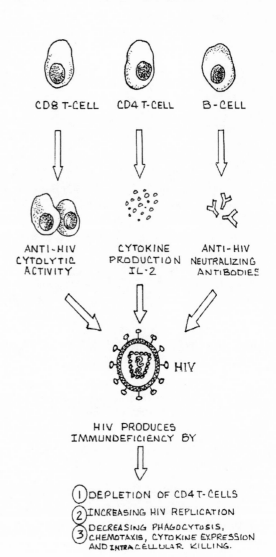

HIV infection (Marvin G. Miller).

HIV virus infects and destroys CD4+ T lymphocytes and to a lesser extent CD4+ monocytes and macrophages. These white blood cells normally protect against infection and help suppress abnormal cell growth. The immune system and its ability to control infections and malignant proliferative disorders are progressively destroyed in AIDS. Opportunistic infections and neoplastic growths are the usual causes of death in patients with AIDS. The specific infections and tumors seen in AIDS are rarely seen outside of the AIDS populations. These are conditions that a healthy immune system would easily overcome.

With the introduction of effective antiretroviral therapies, the clinical picture in AIDS is changing, with treated patients exhibiting symptoms that differ from those seen in untreated patients. Conditions once occasionally seen in AIDS, such as dementia, are more often seen today because therapeutic agents are unable to halt viral replication that occurs in the central nervous system. Certain cancers that were once rarely seen are now seen more often as treatment extends the lifespan in AIDS.

Etiology

Acquired immune deficiency syndrome is an infectious disease caused by the HIV-1 virus, types 1 and 2. HIV-1, which is responsible for the AIDS epidemic in the United States, is found throughout the world, whereas HIV-2 is still found predominately in West Africa. In the United States, most infections are caused by HIV-1, group M, subtype or clade B. The HIV virus is lymphotropic, that is, it has a predilection for lymphocytes and other white blood cells with protein molecules on their surface membrane known as CD4+ surface markers. In untreated infection, CD4+ T lymphocytes decline by approximately 50 to 100 cells/mm^3 annually. Normally, people have 500–1500 CD4+ T lymphocytes/mm^3. AIDS develops when CD4+ T cell counts fall below 200 CD4+ T lymphocytes/mm^3.

Both HIV types 1 and 2 are members of the *Lentivirinae* genus of the *Retroviridae* family. HIV-1 was first cloned and identified in France in 1983, and HIV-2 was discovered in 1986. Like other retroviruses, HIV has a single-stranded RNA genome and replicates through a process known as reverse transcription. In reverse transcription, the enzyme reverse transcriptase present in retroviruses is essential for viral replication within the host cells that it infects. HIV is new to the 20th century and seems likely to have emerged from cross-species infection from chimpanzees in Africa. Unlike other retroviruses, HIV has evolved by developing accessory genes that help facilitate its replication.

The HIV-1 virion (infectious particle) has the shape of a sphere and is about 110 nm in diameter. The core of the virion is composed of nucleoproteins complexed with two identical copies of single-stranded RNA along with the enzyme reverse transcriptase. The core is surrounded by a lipid envelope. Two genes, *gag* and *env*, encode structural glycoproteins, and the *pol* gene encodes enzymatic proteins necessary for reverse transcription, integration and the proteolyic processing of viral proteins. HIV-1 also has complex regulatory systems directed by accessory genes.

After exposure, HIV enters host cells through fusion of the virus envelope with the target or host cell's outer surface or membrane. Initial entry involves a high-affinity binding of HIV's surface envelope protein gp120 with the cellular receptor, CD4+, which is present on the surface of a subset of helper T lymphocytes and also on a select group of other white blood cells known as monocytes and macrophages.

HIV is able to mutate rapidly, and it is able to make its surface components difficult to access by neutralizing antibodies. HIV is also able to hide within monocytes and macrophages, thereby establishing proviral latency. HIV is also able to remove cell-surface receptors and destroy immune effectors. All of these factors make HIV difficult to eradicate and sometimes difficult to treat effectively.

A study by the National Institutes of Health published in *Science Daily* in December 2002, showed that it is possible for an individual to become infected with two closely related strains of HIV. The case studied involved a person whose HIV was kept in check for many months during structured treatment interruptions. How-

FIGURE 1. Proportion of AIDS cases* among men aged ≥13 years who have sex with men (MSM), by race/ethnicity and year of diagnosis—United States, 1989–1998

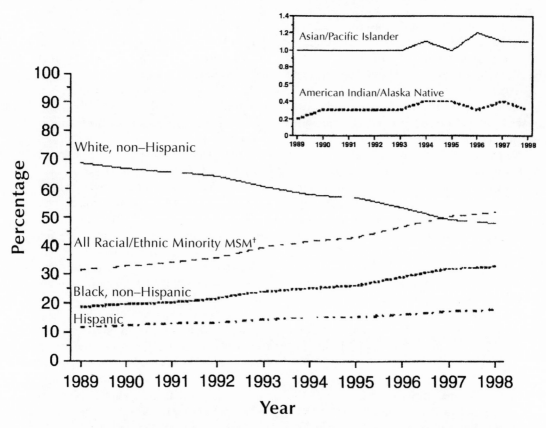

*Estimated number of AIDS diagnoses adjusted for delays in reporting of AIDS cases and anticipated redistribution of cases initially reported with no identified risk; data reported to CDC through June 1999.
†Defined as non–Hispanic black, Hispanic, American Indian/Alaska Native, and Asian/Pacific Islander MSM.

AIDS cases among MSM by race/ethnicity (Dr. Demetri Vacalis, CDC).

ever, nearly a year later, the patient's viral load suddenly rose despite several more attempts to interrupt therapy. Further studies showed a second strain of HIV with a nucleotide sequence that differed by about 12 percent. See the entries on **HIV, HIV-1, Lentiviruses, Retroviruses,** and **Retrovirus replication** in this book for a more comprehensive description of HIV and its ability to replicate and cause infection.

Epidemiology

The HIV virus is passed from one person to another through sexual contact, saliva, childbirth, breast milk, and blood-to-blood contact, including blood transfusions, organ transplants, contaminated medical equipment, injection drug use, body piercings, and tattoos. The HIV virus can exist in blood found on contaminated needles and syringes for up to four weeks, although it can be killed by treatment with bleach solutions. The HIV virus is not transmitted through casual contact. The Options Project, a CDC sponsored study, found that the risk of becoming infected with HIV through unprotected oral sex is lower than in anal or vaginal sex but still significant. The Options Project found that 7.8 percent of recently infected men who have sex with men in San Francisco were probably infected through oral sex.

Since June 1981, when the epidemic began, until July 2002, more than 460,000 people in the United States died of AIDS. Largely due to efforts of AIDS awareness and prevention programs, HIV infections in the U.S. were reduced from a high of 150,000 infections per year in the early 1980s to 40,000 new cases annually by the early 1990s. By the mid–1990s, AIDS-related deaths begin to decline significantly, primarily as the result of new drug therapies that inhibit viral replication.

However, preliminary CDC reports from January 2003 show that a lack of compliance with prevention measures is responsible for an increase in newly diagnosed cases of both HIV infection and syphilis, especially in large cities. The rate of HIV infection among intravenous drug users has also increased. By June 2002, 36 percent of AIDS cases in the United States reported to the CDC had occurred among intravenous drug users, their sexual partners, and children. Infection in up to two-thirds of children with AIDS is reported to be directly or indirectly connected to intravenous drug use. The global problem remains at crisis levels, and researchers project that by 2010 HIV/AIDS will reduce average life expectancy in some southern African countries to around 30 years.

As of December 2002, about 900,000 people in the United States and 42 million people worldwide were living with HIV infections. In 2002 alone, approximately five million new infections were expected, 45,000 of which were anticipated in North America. The CDC reports that the epidemic is growing most rapidly among minority populations and is one of the leading causes of death for African-American males aged 25 to 44 years. AIDS is six times more prevalent in African-Americans and three times more prevalent in Hispanics when compared to the rate of AIDS in whites. Among Latinos, AIDS is the fourth leading cause of death of those aged 25 to

44 years, and half of those deaths were caused by injections with contaminated needles. Among children with AIDS, 40 percent occur as a result of mothers infected by intravenous drug use. Of these, 17 percent of maternal infections occurred in women who had sex with intravenous drug users.

Incarcerated women are three times as likely as incarcerated men to be living with AIDS. In the general population, three times as many men as women are infected with AIDS. Approximately 75 percent of the two million people in prisons and jails are Latino or African-American. African-Americans are almost eight times more likely to be incarcerated in local jails than their Caucasian counterparts. Women of color represent 60 percent of the female incarcerated population. The CDC reports that Latino and African-American women of childbearing age now constitute 75 percent of female AIDS cases.

• SPECIAL PROBLEMS IN WOMEN—The number and proportion of women who have HIV in the United States have been gradually increasing. In 1997, 27.1 percent of cases of AIDS reported to the CDC occurred in women, compared to seven percent in 1985. HIV infection is the third leading cause of death for women ages 25 to 44 years. In 1997, 60.1 percent of women with AIDS in the U.S. were African-American, 19.7 percent were Hispanic and 19 percent were white. Heterosexual transmission has surpassed injection drug use as the primary route for women acquiring HIV infection in the U.S.

Factors influencing male to female transmission include advanced disease in the infected partner; anal receptive intercourse; genital ulcers; lack of condom use; and lack of antiretroviral therapy in the infected source. Factors influencing female to male transmission include advanced disease in the infected partner; genital ulcers; sexual intercourse during menses; and lack of condom use. The efficiency of male-to-female transmission of HIV has been estimated to be 2.3 times greater than female to male transmission.

Women with HIV infection are more likely to have gynecologic symptoms. Up to 50 percent of women infected with HIV develop recurrent candidial vaginitis, which often precedes oral or esophageal candidiasis. About 18 percent of women infected with HIV also develop recurrent genital herpes simplex virus infections, which can be more severe or refractory to treatment. HIV infected women are also five times more likely to have abnormal Pap smears, and their risk for developing HPV infection and cervical cancer is higher compared to women who are not infected with HIV.

Symptoms

Symptoms of HIV infection vary. Some people do not notice any symptoms while others experience fever, sore throat, weight loss, myalgia (muscle pain), and swollen lymph glands shortly after infection. Fever and myalgia are the most common symptoms. Other less frequently observed signs and symptoms include headache, cervical lymphadenopathy, diffuse rash that mimics a drug rash or measles, and ulcerations of the oral or genital region. Some patients present with a cluster of symptoms, such as fever, headache, light sensitivity, and stiff neck, symptoms resembling those of aseptic meningitis. The median duration

of symptoms is 14 days. These symptoms generally fade within a few weeks and may be mistaken for influenza. Several reports show that the severity of early symptoms corresponds to the clinical course of the disease.

Although most patients seek medical assistance, HIV infection is rarely diagnosed in early or acute infection because tests for HIV antibodies are negative at this time. Plasma HIV RNA levels, however, are very high at this time, and patients with acute infection are thought to be highly infectious. Tests for HIV RNA or proviral DNA can be used to diagnose early infection, but they are seldom used as diagnostic tools. When HIV is suspected and tests for HIV RNA are not readily available, repeat HIV antibody tests should be ordered at three and six-month intervals. When acute infection is suspected or confirmed, experts recommend initiating an aggressive anti-retroviral treatment regimen even in the absence of supporting laboratory data.

The early symptoms of HIV infection are often referred to as acute retroviral syndrome, which is described later in this section. Early symptoms of HIV infection are also described later in this book in entries concerning HIV disease. Symptoms in neonates and children are included later in this section under the heading **Neonatal infection** and also in a separate entry, **Pediatric AIDS.**

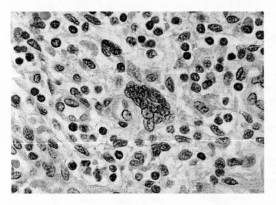 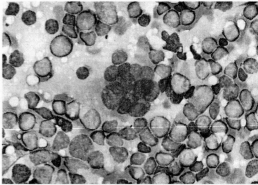

Left: Tissue changes in lymph nodes from an AIDS patient. *Right:* Tissue section changes in lymph node of an AIDS patient (Public Health Imaging Library, CDC).

During the course of infection, various symptoms and syndromes including symptoms of arthritis may also occur in AIDS. These symptoms are related to common and opportunistic infections, as a result of treatment, and as separate syndromes related to viral infection or immune system destruction. Symptoms and syndromes commonly seen in early AIDS in both adults and children such as diarrhea are described in this entry on symptoms; specific opportunistic infections and neoplasms (such as **Coccidiomycosis** and **Kaposi's sarcoma**); conditions of **Peripheral neuropathy**; **Esophagitis**; **Mononeuritis multiplex** (MM); **Wasting syndrome**; **Lipodystrophy**; and others are listed and described in separate entries.

Other common HIV-related symptoms and conditions, such as sinusitis, skin conditions, bacteremia and co-existing syphilis, are included later in this entry under the heading *Complications*. Symptoms associated with treatment are included in this entry under the heading *Treatment* and in separate sections describing treatment.

• ACUTE RETROVIRAL SYNDROME—In approximately 40–80 percent of all cases, a transient, typical flu-like illness known as acute retroviral syndrome has been reported as occurring a few days to a few weeks following high-risk exposure or infection. Acute retroviral syndrome is sometimes called primary HIV infection. It is not known what factors determine the severity of acute retroviral syndrome, but it is suspected that the size of the inoculum (initial viral exposure), the virulence of the infecting strain, and the patient's immune status could be involved. One case series of transfusion-associated cases found that severe early symptoms were more frequent among those infected by individuals with late-stage disease.

Considered a sign of early infection, this syndrome is characterized by clinical signs of immune activation and dysfunction in multiple bodily symptoms. Patients frequently seek medical attention due to a condition resembling influenza or infectious mononucleosis with fever, sore throat, generalized lymph node enlargement or pain (lymphadenopathy), oral ulcers, night sweats, arthralgia (joint pain), myalgia (muscle pain or weakness), fatigue, rash, and/or weight loss. The rash, which is known as a maculopapular rash, consists of multiple reddened papules with occasional blisters, which affect the face, neck and trunk more than the limbs, although the palms and soles may be affected. Lesions may also occur in the mouth and on the genital mucosa.

Occasionally, diarrhea, pancreatitis, mild liver test abnormalities, bacterial sepsis, low platelet count, epiglottitis (inflammation of the cartilage behind the tongue, causing difficulty swallowing), pulmonary dysfunction, or self-limiting neurological disorders such as stiff neck, headache, disordered consciousness, meningitis, encephalitis, muscle disorders, and polyneuropathy may occur. Symptoms in early HIV infection often resemble those of infectious mononucleosis or meningitis.

Opportunistic infections typically seen only in advanced immunodeficiency, such as esophageal candida (yeast) infection, may also be seen. Pulmonary symptoms may occur although they are more likely to be seen in intravenous drug users. Symptoms associated with early HIV infection typically resolve within five to 10 days and rarely longer than 14 days, although there have been reports of symptoms lasting up to 90 days.

HIV antibody tests, which are the diagnostic tests most often used, are negative at this time, making diagnosis difficult. Blood tests for HIV RNA, branched chain DNA or p24 antigen, however, are positive at this time although they are not routinely ordered. During acute HIV-1 infection, the CD4+ T cell count drops rapidly although it later rises during the latent period.

The goal of antiretroviral therapy in acute HIV infection is to reduce the number of infected cells, thereby preserving

HIV-specific immune responses. The first pilot studies in patients who were treated during acute HIV-1 infection show that the HIV-1 specific immune response could be boosted in these patients. Patients were then able to produce neutralizing antibodies capable of destroying HIV. Most patients treated for early infection were subsequently able to discontinue therapy and experienced at least temporary control of viral replications, with viral load occasionally remaining below 5,000 copies/ml for more than three years. However, some patients experienced increased viral loads and had to resume therapy. The long-term effects of initiating early antiretroviral therapy have not yet been demonstrated. Experts advise that patients with early infection should be treated in controlled clinical trials. If this is not possible, the option of first-line therapies should be discussed and the toxic effects of antiretroviral therapy should be addressed.

• CLINICAL LATENCY—Within days or weeks of initial acute infection, the blood contains millions of viral copies of HIV. In addition, the blood and tissues contain numerous HIV-infected cells. The turnover of productively infected CD4+ T lymphocytes is also high with half of the normal CD4+ T cell population eliminated within the first day. However, within a few weeks, viral levels in the blood drop rapidly, and symptoms resolve. The early acute stage of HIV infection is followed by a long stage of disease-free clinical latency.

In the latent period, people infected with HIV usually have no or very few symptoms although they are capable of transmitting the virus to others. Tests for HIV antibodies may remain negative for up to six months following infection. However, HIV viral production is very active and this can be demonstrated by the presence of viral particles in the blood (using tests for HIV RNA or HIV proviral DNA). Eventually, the progressive immune system destruction caused by the HIV virus causes clinical disease progression.

Studies show that HIV-1 infection causes the producing of neutralizing antibodies directed against HIV-1's envelope protein. However, the virus evolves rapidly enough to avoid detection by the antibodies. In monitoring the level of an enveloped gene of HIV-1 in infected individuals, researchers found that the epitope (the part of the protein usually identifiable to antibodies) does not change, but the sugar molecules that surround the envelope protein do evolve, possibly for the purpose of protecting the protein from being recognized and targeted by neutralizing antibodies.

• DIARRHEA—During early HIV infection, diarrhea, a condition of uncontrolled, loose, and frequent bowel movements, may occur. Severe or prolonged diarrhea can lead to weight loss, wasting and malnutrition. Diarrhea can be life-threatening when the body is deprived of nutrients such as potassium that are essential for heart function.

Diarrhea in AIDS can have many causes, including enteric infection (enterocolitis) with cytomegalovirus, *Salmonella* species, *Shigella flexneri*, *Campylobacter jejuni*, *Clostridium difficile*, *Mycobacterium avium* complex and the parasites Cryptosporidium, Microsporidia, and Giardia lamblia. Infectious agents that cause diarrhea in otherwise healthy people may cause severe, prolonged, or recurrent diarrhea in HIV/AIDS. The source of diarrhea should be determined by stool culture or tests for ova and parasites so that appropriate treatment can be prescribed. Prolonged periods of diarrhea contribute to malabsorption of nutrients, electrolyte imbalances, and wasting syndrome. *See also* **Healthy Life Choices Project**.

• ACUTE INFLAMMATORY DEMYELINATING POLYNEUROPATHY (AIDP)—Another syndrome seen in early infection is acute inflammatory demyelinating polyneuropathy (AIDP), which is also known as Guillain-Barré Syndrome. AIDP is an autoimmune condition that often develops in normal people after viral infection or vaccinations. It is a rapidly progressing, potentially fatal condition characterized by myelin (protective sheath covering nerve fibers) inflammation, mild sensory loss, and severe motor loss or paralysis. Chronic idiopathic demyelinating polyneuropathy (CIPD) is described in a separate entry.

• OSTEOPOROSIS AND OSTEOPENIA— Both of these disorders are characterized by severely low bone mineral density (BMD) compared to people of the same sex and age. A T-score (deviation from the average person of the same sex and age) between –1 and –2.5 in the absence of fracture indicates osteopenia. A T-score of –2.5 or lower indicates osteoporosis. Reports indicate that individuals with HIV disease are at risk for both osteopenia and osteoporosis. While HAART has been implicated, studies have yielded conflicting supporting data.

• NEUROLOGICAL SYMPTOMS—After HIV enters the blood stream, it is able to move into the central nervous system (CNS). HIV enters the CNS early after infection, establishes a viral reservoir, and remains largely inaccessible to antiretroviral therapies, which are unable to cross the blood-brain barrier. In certain individuals, slowly evolving symptoms of cognitive impairment (difficulty with reason and logic) emerge in approximately 10 percent of persons with HIV infection. Less severe symptoms of cognitive dysfunction occur in about 50 percent of persons infected with HIV.

Imaging and tissue studies show that macrophage cells and microglial cells in the brain become infected with HIV and release soluble factors that contribute to the destruction of central nervous system cells known as neurons. Productive viral replication occurs within the brain, and the number of infected macrophage cells correlates with the degree of frank dementia. The relationship between the viral load (level of HIV RNA) in the blood and neurologic symptoms remains controversial with different researchers finding different correlations. Most studies show that there is no clear correlation between the blood viral load and the development of AIDS dementia complex.

Researchers also suspect that even in patients using highly active antiretroviral therapy (HAART), a number of CD4+ T cells harbor the HIV virus and are latently infected shortly after the acute retroviral syndrome. Therapies are being investigated that would cross the blood-brain barrier and prevent viral replication within the central nervous system. See the entry **AIDS dementia complex (ADC) HIV-associated cognitive motor complex.**

• EYE SYMPTOMS—The HIV virus may also cause ocular findings in persons who have developed other opportunistic infections. Clinical ocular findings are seen in more than 70 percent of persons with AIDS. The most common cause is cytomegalovirus (CMV) infection, which causes retinitis, necrosis of retinal tissue, and retinal detachment. Although CMV can affect the brain, lungs and gastrointestinal system, it primarily targets the eyes and can cause blindness. Typically, CMV retinitis occurs late in AIDS infection, when CD4+ counts fall to 50 or less. Studies show that up to 37 percent of persons with AIDS are likely to develop CMV retinitis.

Ocular symptoms commonly seen in persons with CMV infection include retinal changes that cause visual deficits causing the appearance of cotton-wool spots (caused by ganglions on nerve fibers), decreased visual function, decreased color vision, optical microaneurysms, and retinal hemorrhages.

Conjunctivitis, which may progress to conjunctival intraepithelial neoplasia, may also occur as a result of *Molluscum contagiosum* and *Cryptococcus neoformans* infections, and it may occur in persons with Kaposi's sarcoma. Corneal infection, causing dry eyes and keratitis, may be caused by microsporidiosis, herpes simplex virus, varicella-zoster virus, *Histoplasma capsulatum*, CMV, and other organisms.

Retinal and uveal tract ocular infection may be caused by *Toxoplasma gondii*, *Pneumocystis jiroveci*, *Cryptococcus neoformans*, *Treponema pallidum*, *Candida* species, *Mycobacterium tuberculosis*, *Mycobacterium avium* complex, *aspergillus fumigatus*, or they may occur in primary intraocular lymphoma.

Optic neuropathy may occur as a result of infection with CMV, *Histoplasma capsulatum*, *Treponema pallidum*, and *Cryptococcus neoformans*. Orbital infections may be caused by *Pseudomonas aeruginosa*, *Staphylococcus aureus*, *Aspergillus fumigatus*, *Rhizopus arrhizus*, *Toxoplasma gondii*, and *Pneumocystis jiroveci*.

Some drugs such as rifabutin used in the treatment of *Mycobacterium avium* in AIDS patients may also cause uveitis. Children infected with HIV may also develop loss of retinal pigment and retinal lesions.

• SYMPTOMS IN NEONATAL AND PEDIATRIC AIDS—In all lentiviral infections, the young are more prone to disease development and often exhibit symptoms that are not seen in adults. For instance, acute HIV encephalitis and a condition of lentiviral lymphoid interstitial pneumonitis (LIP) are common in children, but are rarely seen in adults. Neonatal HIV infection is described later in this entry. **Pediatric AIDS** is also described in a separate entry.

• AIDS DEVELOPMENT—Clinical illness in HIV infection results from the progressive decline of CD4+ T lymphocytes and also the immune system dysfunction associated with viral replication. Besides infecting and destroying CD4+ cells, HIV interferes with the production of other immune cells, and infects and impairs immune cells within the thymus and bone marrow.

In untreated individuals, the CD4+ T lymphocyte count declines by approximately 50 to 100 cells/mm3 annually. Following acute HIV infection, high blood levels of HIV RNA decline to a stable level (viral set point) of approximately 10,000 to 1,000,000 copies of HIV-1 RNA/ml. This represents equilibrium between virus production and clearance. HIV disseminates widely throughout the body, following acute infection, and in some areas of the body, such as the central nervous system, viral replication is more extensive. Antibodies that form against HIV can have a neutralizing effect and may help in controlling viral replication and contribute to viral set points.

This relentless production of HIV proteins caused by viral replication in infected cells and the elimination of host CD4+ cells over many years finally leads to immune system destruction and AIDS. During this process leading to overt AIDS, infected people may experience fever, sweating, fatigue, rapid weight loss, body wasting syndrome (cachexia), malignancies, swollen lymph glands, and frequent herpes outbreaks. AIDS is defined as a CD4+ T cell count less than 200 cells/mm^3 or the presence of an AIDS defining illness.

• CLASSIFICATIONS OF AIDS—In the early years of the epidemic, the Centers for Disease Control and Prevention (CDC) attempted to classify the various stages of AIDS, using terms such as asymptomatic seropositive (positive HIV antibody test, absence of symptoms), lymphadenopathy-associated syndrome (characterized by swollen lymph nodes), and "lesser AIDS." By 1987 these classifications had been revised. In 1987 AIDS was classified into four categories: 1) acute infection; 2) asymptomatic infection; 3) persistent lymphadenopathy; and 4) other disease, depending on the group of HIV-1 present. Around this time, the Walter Reed Hospital was characterizing AIDS as occurring in nine separate stages. Today, these classifications and stages have been replaced with the terms HIV infection (HIV disease) and AIDS.

• TIMEFRAME—The median time to AIDS development in untreated adults ranges from a few months to 17 years (median 10 years) following infection and is similar in both homosexual men and in drug addicts. In the absence of treatment, almost all persons infected with HIV go on to develop AIDS. Incubation time varies, and about five to 10 percent of infected people are "rapid progressors," developing AIDS within the first three years following infection. "Non-progressors," on the other hand are free of symptoms as long as seven to 20 years after infection. Data from large prospective cohort studies suggest that about 13 percent of HIV-positive homosexual men will remain AIDS free for 20 years after seroconversion (development of HIV antibodies).

Prompt diagnosis and treatment is important because treatments are available that slow the decline of immune system function. Use of these therapies is associated with substantial declines in HIV-associated morbidity and mortality. Early diagnosis enables health care workers to counsel patients, refer them to various support services and help prevent HIV transmission to others.

In 1993, the CDC revised its definitions of AIDS to include all HIV-infected people who have fewer than 200 CD4+ T lymphocytes (T cells). The definition also includes people infected with HIV who have one or more of 26 clinical conditions known as AIDS-defining illnesses, primarily opportunistic infections and rare neoplasms. These conditions, which are rarely seen in people with healthy immune systems, are known to affect people with advanced HIV disease.

Diagnosis

AIDS is diagnosed when HIV infection is confirmed and certain specific requirements are met. The CDC describes AIDS as a condition occurring in HIV-infected persons who either have a CD4+ T lymphocyte count less than 200 cells/mm^3 or the presence of one or more AIDS-defining illnesses. AIDS-defining illnesses, which are described later in this entry, are opportunistic infections and neoplasms that do not usually occur in people with healthy immune systems. Most of these disorders were rarely seen before the emergence of AIDS. In fact, the unusual prevalence of certain disorders, such as *Pneumocystis jiroveci* pneumonia (PCP) and Kaposi's sarcoma, was the first sign that the United States had encountered a new infectious disease epidemic.

HIV infection is usually diagnosed by screening tests for HIV-1 and HIV-2 antibodies. Tests that measure both antibody subtypes are called HIV-1/2 antibody tests. In the U.S. informed consent must be given before an HIV test can be performed, and in some states written consent is required. Before giving their consent, patients must be informed of the nature of the test along with its restrictions, including the fact that a positive screening test does not mean that a person has or will develop HIV infection. Also, a negative screening test does not mean that an individual is not infected with HIV.

The CDC announced an initiative in April 2003 aimed at reducing the number of new HIV infections in the U.S. by increasing voluntary testing and enhancing prevention for persons living with HIV. In several U.S. cities, recent outbreaks of primary and secondary syphilis among men who have sex with men and among heterosexuals have created concern that HIV incidence is also increasing. The CDC reports that many HIV infected persons do not get tested until late in their infection, and many of these persons do not return for their results. Of the 18,000 positive HIV CDC-funded test results in 2001, 31 percent of those infected did not return to learn their test results. A recent FDA ruling, allowing CLIA labs to now perform rapid HIV tests in outpatient clinics, is designed to help patients receive their results quickly. The new initiative includes making HIV testing a routine part of medical care; counseling those who are HIV infected to help prevent new infections; and further decreasing perinatal transmission.

The majority of HIV infection in the United States, Europe and Africa is caused by the HIV-1 subgroup of the human immunodeficiency virus. HIV-2 infection is primarily seen in West Africa. However, because isolated cases of HIV-2 infection may occur in the United States, newer tests measure the presence of both antibodies. The CDC advises that HIV-2 infection should be suspected in persons who have epidemiologic risk factors, including sex partners from West Africa or persons who received blood transfusions or non-sterile injections in a West African country.

Enzyme immunoassay (EIA) screening tests are most often used for HIV antibody detection in blood. Rapid tests and home based screening tests provide faster results than traditional antibody tests, but they are more subject to error.

Any positive or reactive screening tests for HIV antibodies must be confirmed by additional tests, such as the Western blot or a method known as an immunofluorescence assay (IFA). Using the Western blot, HIV antibody is detectable in at least 95 percent of HIV-infected patients within three months after initial infection. Antibody tests cannot detect recent infection because antibodies do not develop for several weeks to months after initial exposure. Urine HIV tests were approved in 2003, including Calypte Biomedical's HIV-1 Urine Western Blot test and its HIV-1 urine EIA test.

Patients can be infected with HIV and be infectious without seroconverting, that is, they begin producing detectable HIV antibodies and also later in the disease as their immune system fails. In these cases, nucleic acid testing (NAT) methods can be used to detect HIV RNA, HIV proviral DNA, or uncomplexed p24 antigen. Positive results with these tests demonstrate the presence of HIV proteins in blood specimens. The CDC recommends that health-care providers be aware of symptoms of acute retroviral syndrome. When this syndrome is suspected, individuals should be tested with nucleic acid testing techniques (such as viral load) to detect HIV infection.

These tests have been used in research studies, including the Multicenter AIDS Cohort Study, to show signs of recent infection, but they are very laborious and expensive. However, except for cohort studies of patients with high risk for infection, the short duration when these proteins are positive prohibits the routine use of these tests as diagnostic screening tools. Although they are not FDA approved for routine use, they are used for special circumstances such as neonatal infection and blood donor screening.

• PROBLEMS WITH HIV ANTIBODY TESTS—Besides not detecting early infection, HIV antibody screening cannot distinguish recent from long-term infections. Because patients may be infected for years before they develop AIDS and seek diagnostic treatment, the statistics regarding new infections may be inaccurate.

To compile accurate statistics, provide early treatment and counseling, and to identify high-risk groups for vaccine trials, it is advantageous to be able to differentiate recent from long-term infection. The Multicenter AIDS Cohort Study and the BMA cohort study in Thailand accomplish this by performing repeat testing on high-risk people who initially are HIV-negative. By testing these individuals often, researchers can detect new infections and provide important information on incidence estimates. However, recruitment bias and loss to follow-up prevent these studies from accurately determining the rate of new infections.

A 1998 study by Janssen, et al., showed that using a commercially available antibody test and using various dilutions of serum may help in diagnosing recent infection. Researchers used a less-sensitive commercial EIA method that is non-reactive in early infection and tested various dilutions of serum, increasing the test sensitivity. This approach is termed as the "serologic testing algorithm for recent HIV seroconversion," or STARHS method, and is primarily used in research.

It is also known that various antibodies to different HIV proteins are produced at different times. In early infection, antibodies to anti-*gag* (p24) and anti-*env* (p41) are observed, while later in infection, anti-*pol* responses develop. The basic problem with the early diagnostic tests for HIV manufactured by Abbott, compared to the HIV test manufactured in France, was its failure to test for the early antibodies directed against p24 and p41. Tests today measure antibodies to all HIV proteins.

The Western blot used to confirm an EIA antibody-screening test has a positive predictive value greater than 99.9 percent. The Western blot detects serum antibodies directed against specific HIV proteins of varying molecular weights, including antibodies to core protein (p17, p24, and the precursor p55), polymerase protein (p31, p51, and p66), and envelope protein (gp41, gp120/160). A positive test requires the presence of antibodies to two of the following: p24, gp41, or gp120/160.

Experimental methodologies to measure different HIV antibodies are used in research. As HIV infection progresses, antibodies to gp120 develop, and as AIDS develops, antibodies to p24 decline. Tests are also being developed to measure the binding ability of various antibodies, because it has been noted that this binding ability (measured as affinity/avidity) increases as HIV infection progresses. Recently introduced but not yet available IgG-capture EIA methods using gp41 sequences are able to detect HIV antibodies for longer periods (up to two years) following infection.

• VIRAL LOAD—HIV RNA testing, branched DNA testing, and p24 antigen, although not FDA approved for diagnostic use, are excellent tests for determining recent infection, including the period from exposure to seroconversion (antibody production). HIV-1 RNA (viral load testing) is often used to monitor antiretroviral therapy, and assays for CD4+ lymphocytes are performed to determine progression from HIV infection into AIDS. Viral load is also used to determine the efficacy of investigational therapies and determine if accelerated approval is indicated. Until tests for viral load were developed in 1996, investigators had no way of evaluating the efficacy of antiviral therapy. Roche Molecular Systems offers a national patient assistance program to help uninsured patients who need viral load testing. Information is available by calling 1-888-TEST-PCR.

• NEONATAL TESTING—Because maternal HIV antibodies may cross the placental membrane, HIV antibodies may be seen in neonates who do not have HIV infection. The CDC recommends that a definitive determination of HIV infection for infants less than 18 months should be based on laboratory evidence of HIV (viral antigens, RNA or DNA) in blood or tissues by culture, NAT, or antigen detection. The most commonly used test for neonatal infection is a qualitative HIV-1 DNA assay using polymerase chain reaction (PCR) amplification. Newer NAT tests for HIV RNA are also commonly used.

• CD4+ T CELL COUNTS—HIV destroys white blood cells known as T lymphocytes that contain surface markers known as cluster designation 4 (CD4+ T cells). The severity of HIV infection and the response to therapy can be determined by measuring CD4+ T cell counts. A CD4+ T cell count lower than 200 cells/mm^3 is also used to diagnose the progression of HIV infection into AIDS.

Diagnostic tests for HIV infection and timeframes for antibody conversion are also described in the following entries: **Branched DNA assay (bDNA test); CD4+ T lymphocytes (CD4+ cells); HIV blood tests; HIV-1; HIV home tests; HIV-1 RNA; Human immunodeficiency virus (HIV); P24 antigen test; Rapid HIV tests; Seroconversion; Seroconversion window; Western blot test;** and **Viral load.**

• AIDS DEFINING ILLNESSES—When HIV infected individuals experience extensive immune system destruction (evidenced by a CD4 count of less than 200 cells/mm^3), opportunistic infections and neoplasms may occur. AIDS-defining illnesses are specific conditions, primarily opportunistic infections and malignancies that are included in the CDC's criteria for a diagnosis of AIDS. A CD4+ T cell count less than 200 cells/mm^3 of blood or the presence of certain conditions, primarily opportunistic infections, brain and nerve diseases, certain cancers, and HIV wasting syndrome, signals the progression of HIV infection into AIDS in adults or adolescents 13 years old or older. In children younger than 13 years, the definition of AIDS is similar to that in adolescents and adults, except that lymphoid interstitial pneumonitis and recurrent bacterial infections are included in the list of AIDS-defining conditions for children. The list is regularly updated and is likely to increase as new disorders associated with HIV infection emerge.

The 2002 CDC guidelines list the following conditions as AIDS-defining illnesses:

AIDS dementia complex
Anal dysplasia/cancer
Aspergillosis
Candidiasis, esophageal
Candidiasis of bronchi, trachea, or lungs
Cervical cancer, invasive
Coccidiomycosis, disseminated or pulmonary
Cryptococcosis, extrapulmonary or cryptococcal meningitis
Cryptosporidiosis, chronic, intestinal greater than one month duration
Cytomegalovirus (CMV) infection, other than liver, spleen or lymph nodes
CMV retinitis with loss of vision
Encephalopathy, HIV related
Herpes Simplex Virus, types 1 and 2 causing chronic ulcers longer than one month duration or that causes bronchitis, pneumonitis or esophagitis
Human papilloma virus
Histoplasmosis, disseminated or extra-pulmonary
Isosporiasis, chronic intestinal, greater than one month duration
Kaposi's sarcoma
Lymphoma, Burkitt's or equivalent form; primary, of brain
Microsporidiosis
Molluscum contagiosum
Mycobacterium avium complex or *M. kansasii*, disseminated or extrapulmonary
Peripheral neuropathy
Pneumocystis jiroveci pneumonia
Pneumonia, bacterial and recurrent
Progressive multifocal leukoencephalopathy (PML)
Salmonella septicemia, recurrent
Toxoplasmosis of brain
Wasting syndrome due to HIV

Treatment

Treatment for HIV/AIDS includes counseling as well as pharmaceutical intervention. The CDC recommends that persons who test positive for HIV should be counseled, either on site or through referral, about the behavioral, psychosocial, and medical implications of HIV infection. Providers should assess patients for immediate care and support needs and direct patients to available resources for emtional and medical support, substance abuse counseling and prevention management.

Primary medical treatment for HIV infection includes an arsenal of antiretroviral agents intended to halt different steps of the retroviral life cycle, including viral entry into host cells. These treatments work by stopping replication of viral genes or stopping the production of viral proteins, thereby reducing viral load and restoring immune function. Other approaches of combating HIV infection have been proposed, but only anti–HIV therapy has been proved to slow disease progression and extend life. The objectives of anti–HIV therapy should be to prolong life and improve quality of life for the long-term; suppress virus to below the limit of detection (below 50 copies HIV RNA) or as low as possible for as long as possible; and to minimize drug toxicity.

When used in combination, antiretroviral drugs are more successful at reducing viral load (levels of HIV RNA) and restoring CD4+ T cell levels. When tests for viral load were introduced in 1996, researchers were able to understand fully the efficacy of certain treatment regimens as well as the concept of drug failure. Drug failure primarily occurs when certain mutated strains of HIV develop resistance to specific therapies.

The primary antiretroviral agents used for HIV include reverse transcriptase inhibitors; protease inhibitors; entry inhibitors; and integrase inhibitors. Several types of antiretroviral drugs are prescribed together in a protocol known as highly active antiretroviral therapy (HAART). In addition, adjuvant drugs are often prescribed to facilitate treatment by helping to reduce the side effects associated with antiretroviral drugs. Current guidelines recommend initiating antiretroviral therapy with at least three drugs, usually using a nucleoside combination plus a protease inhibitor or NNRTI, although other combinations, including three NRTIs, may be used.

Several factors are considered when selecting an antiretroviral combination, including the patient's unique medical history and lifestyle, HIV treatment history, viral load, CD4+ T lymphocyte count, and laboratory results. Other considerations include drug potency, dosage requirements, possible adverse events, and drug resistance in a given population. Tests for drug resistance (genotype/phenotype) can also be performed before starting treatment. Several studies have shown that people who used therapies based on resistance testing had longer lasting responses to anti–HIV regimens compared to people who did not have this information available. Experts also emphasize the importance of following the recommended dosage regimen. Lowering the dose of an antiretroviral therapy is often responsible for the development of drug resistance.

Treatment may also be interrupted in a protocol known as structured treatment interruption (STI). In STI, antiretroviral therapies are frequently given during the early, acute stage of infection, but halted after the immune system has had time to adapt to the virus. Often, STI works well enough to keep HIV suppressed with treatment.

Types of drugs and specific drugs used as HIV treatments are described in the following sections and they are also described later in this book in these and other related entries: **Genotype (genotypic) assay; Highly active antiretroviral therapy (HAART); Nucleoside/nucleotide reverse transcriptase inhibitors (NRTIs); Non-nucleoside reverse transcriptase inhibitors (NNRTIs); Onconase; Phenotype assay; Protease inhibitors; Structured treatment interruption (STI); and Zidovudine.** Information on available therapies and viral load testing is also available through Project Inform, by calling 1-800-822-7422 or visiting its website, http://www.projinf.org/fs/HIVDiagnostictest.html VL.

• REVERSE TRANSCRIPTASE INHIBITORS—Reverse transcriptase inhibitors, the first drugs approved for treating HIV, include nucleoside and nucleotide analog reverse transcriptase inhibitors (NRTIs) and also non-nucleoside analog reverse transcriptase inhibitors (NNRTIs). These agents work by inhibiting the action of the enzyme reverse transcriptase, a viral enzyme needed by HIV to infect host cells successfully.

When HIV infects a host cell, it copies its own genetic code into the host cell's DNA. This causes the cell to be programmed to create new copies of HIV. HIV's genetic material is in the form of RNA. In order for HIV to infect host cells, this RNA must first be converted into HIV with the help of the enzyme reverse transcriptase. NRTIs or "nukes" prevent healthy T cells in the body from becoming infected with HIV. Reverse transcriptase inhibitors act as chain terminators when incorporated into proviral DNA. All of the NRTIs are nucleoside inhibitors except for tenofovir (Viread), which is a nucleotide reverse transcriptase inhibitor.

Nucleoside/Nucleotide Reverse Transcriptase Inhibitors (NRTIs). The first treatment approved for HIV infection, azidothymidine (AZT, zidovudine, ZDV, Retrovir), is a nucleoside reverse transcriptase inhibitor drug, which had been developed years earlier and tested, unsuccessfully, as an anticancer drug.

NRTIs contain flawed versions of the building blocks (nucleotides) used by reverse transcriptase to convert RNA to DNA. When reverse transcriptase uses these faulty building blocks, new DNA cannot be produced correctly. In turn, HIV's genetic material cannot be incorporated into the healthy genetic material of the cell, preventing the cell from producing new virus. Nucleotide analogues differ from nucleoside analogues although they work in the same way. Nucleoside analogues must undergo chemical changes in which they combine with phosphorus to work inside the body. Nucleotide analogues bypass this metabolic step and are already chemically activated.

Early in the epidemic, it looked as though AZT might be sufficient to slow viral reproduction and halt progression of the disease. However, it soon became apparent that HIV was able to mutate and form strains that were resistant to AZT.

Consequently, other NRTIs were developed and include lamivudine (3TC, Epivir); didanosine (ddl, BMY-40900, Videx and Videx EC delayed release capsules); tenofovir disoproxil fumarate (tenofovir DF, TDF, Bis (POC) PMPA, Viread); abacavir (ABC, 1592U89, Ziagen); stavudine (d4T, Zerit, BMY-27857); and the experimental drugs emtricitabine (Coviracil, FTC) and amdoxovir (DAPD). Fixed combination NRTIs include Trizivir, which contains abacavir, zidovudine and lamivudine, and Combivir, which contains zidovudine and lamivudine.

Abacavir may cause a hypersensitivity reaction, which is described earlier in this book under the listing for Abacavir. Zidovudine should not be combined with stavudine or with ribavirin. Stavudine increases the risk of white blood cell toxicity and ribavirin antagonizes the antiviral activity of zidovudine.

Non-nucleoside Reverse Transcriptase Inhibitors (NNRTIs). The NNRTIs are polycyclic compounds that bind to reverse transcriptase and interfere with its function. Although they actively inhibit HIV-1, these drugs lack activity against HIV-2. These enzymes are substrates of isoenzymes of cytochrome P450 (CYP450), and are potential enzyme inducers and inhibitors. Therefore, these drugs have the potential for drug-drug interaction when combined with many other classes of drugs used to treat multiple medical conditions. Nonnucleoside inhibitors include nevirapine (Viramune), efavirenz (Sustiva), and delaviridine (Rescriptor). Allergies to NNRTIs are fairly common and cause a reversible, systemic reaction that initially causes fever and a red, itchy rash mainly over the trunks and arms. Symptoms usually occur in the second or third week of therapy and resolve soon thereafter. Antihistamines may be used in persistent allergy.

New NNRTIs under development include capravirine and TMC-125. Capravirine may not be released because of reports of vasculitis (blood vessel inflammation) occurring in subjects in clinical trials. The true test of capravirine will be its effectiveness in patients who have developed resistance to other NNRTIs. Early reports show that TMC-125 is an effective inhibitor of HIV. After seven days of study, subjects in clinical trials had an impressive viral load decrease of about two logs and an average CD4+ cell count increase of 100 cells/mm^3.

• PROTEASE INHIBITORS—Protease inhibitors bind within the cleavage domain of the protease enzyme, blocking its ability to produce proteins. Like the NNRTIs, protease inhibitors are substrates, inducers and inhibitors of CYP450 isoenzymes. Ritonavir, the most potent inhibitor of CYP450 in this class, is often combined with other protease inhibitors to improve the pharmacokinetic actions of the companion drug, reduce drug dosages, or eliminate the food restrictions required of indinavir. However, this pharmacokinetic boosting may increase the incidence of adverse events.

Protease inhibitors include saquinavir (Invirase, Fortovase), ritonavir (Norvir), indinavir (Crixivan), nelfinavir (Viracept), amprenavir (Agenerase) and lipinavir/ritonavir fixed dose (Kaletra). Side effects include gastrointestinal symptoms, such as diarrhea, nausea, and abdominal discomfort, elevated liver enzymes, and headaches; long-term treatment may cause lipodystrophy, elevated lipid levels, and reduced glucose tolerance. Most protease inhibitors should not be taken with rifampicin, triazolam, ergotamines, lovastatin, and St. John's wort. Protease inhibitors are best when taken with meals.

New protease inhibitors soon to be released include tipranavir, a drug reported to remain active against HIV strains that are resistant to most protease inhibitors and atazanavir. In clinical studies lower doses of tipranavir caused greater reductions in viral load. The most common side effects included diarrhea, nausea, headache, dizziness, fatigue and abnormal dreams. Atazanavir was officially released in 2003, although it was released earlier in a large expanded access program. Atazanavir offers the convenience of once-daily dosing, and it did not cause elevated blood lipid levels in clinical trials. Patients switched from nelfinavir to atazanavir also experienced reductions in their blood lipid levels.

Studies show that the p-glycoprotein (p-GP) responsible for making many cancer drugs ineffective may also block the effects of protease inhibitors in women with HIV infection, especially during the luteal phase of the menstrual cycle when p-GP levels in the vagina are highest. In infected women, the vagina serves as a reservoir for HIV.

• TRANSCRIPTASE INHIBITORS (NARTIS AND NTARTIS)—The first drug of this class, emtricitabine (Coviracil, FTC), is reported to resemble closely the NRTI lamivudine (3TC). In early studies, people using emtricitabine alone experienced an average two log reduction in viral load after two weeks. This drug is currently being tested in clinical trials and approval is expected if FTC performs well in drug resistance trials. Another drug under investigation, DAPD, has proved to reduce viral load by an average of 1.5 logs in two weeks. How people respond to higher doses will determine if the drug has a place in the antiretroviral arsenal.

• ENTRY INHIBITORS—Entry inhibitors are the newest drugs being studied in clinical trials. In March 2003, the fusion inhibitor Fuzeon was the first drug of this class to receive FDA approval for the treatment of HIV. Entry inhibitors work by preventing HIV from entering host cells. HIV enters host cells by binding to the CD4 receptor, a surface molecule found on certain white blood cells, binding to co-receptors of CD4+ cells, and by fusing with the host cell. Entry inhibitors are drugs that inhibit attachment, act as antagonists to co-receptors, or inhibit fusion of HIV to the host cell.

Fusion Inhibitors. In order for HIV to bind to CD4+ cells, the proteins on HIV's outer coat must bind to the proteins on the surface of the CD4+ cells. Fusion inhibitors work by inhibiting specific HIV surface proteins, such as gp41 or gp120.

The first fusion inhibitor to receive FDA approval, enfuvirtide (Fuzeon or T-20), manufactured by Roche, was introduced in March 2003 and targets the gp41 protein on HIV's surface. Fuzeon is a relatively large peptide, comprising of 36 amino acids, and, like insulin, it must be given by subcutaneous injection. In phase III clinical trials in North America and Brazil, Fuzeon was shown to reduce viral loads by

1.70 log compared to 0.76 log in the control group.

Fuzeon, used in combination with other anti–HIV agents, is indicated for the treatment of HIV infection in treatment-experienced patients, rather than as a first line therapy. Its primary usefulness appears as a salvage therapy to replace other agents in a HAART protocol that have failed. Possible side effects of enfuvirtide include injection site reactions (itching, swelling, redness, pain, skin hardening, bumps), pneumonia, vomiting, chills, rigors, hypotension, elevated liver enzymes, and allergic reactions. Side effects usually occur within the first week of treatment and can recur as the drug is continued. In studies, patients using enfuvirtide developed bacterial pneumonia more often than patients not using this drug. It was unclear if this was related to Fuzeon or to other risk factors. Other fusion inhibitors under investigation include T-1249, which also targets the gp41 protein. Developed by Roche, T-1249 may offer more promise than T-20, based on the early results of PhaseI/II clinical trials.

Attachment Inhibitors. BMS-806, developed by Bristol-Myers Squibb, is an early attachment inhibitor that inhibits the attachment step by binding to HIV's gp120 protein and preventing it from grabbing on the CD4+ cells. Still undergoing clinical trials, BMS-806 has been shown to react differently with different HIV isolates, indicating potential rapid development of resistance.

Another attachment inhibitor, Pro-542 is a soluble antibody-like fusion protein that also works by binding to gp120. Phase I studies have shown good tolerance and a decrease in viral load after a single infusion. However, this compound must be infused, which is a significant drawback. TNX-355, produced by Tanox, is a monoclonal antibody (genetically engineered antibody) that inhibits HIV by binding to host CD4 receptors.

Co-receptor Antagonists. Co-receptor antagonists are also undergoing clinical trials. One of the most promising compounds, SCH-C or Schering C from Schering Plough, is a CCR5-receptor antagonist that can be taken orally. Side effects, which were primarily seen with high doses, include heart arrhythmias. Small pilot studies have shown a significant decrease in viral load. However, mutant strains with resistance to CCR5-antagonists have already emerged. Other compounds under investigation include SCH-D, Pro-140, and AMD-3100.

Peptide-T is an entry inhibitor developed by Candace Pert and Michael Ruff, professors at Georgetown University Medical Center. Peptide-T works by adhering to the CCR5 receptor site of T lymphocytes, preventing HIV from entering healthy cells. In clinical trials at St. Francis Hospital in San Francisco, Peptide-T has shown no signs of drug resistance, and it has not been associated with adverse side effects. In Phase I and II trials, clinically and statistically significant improvements in neurocognitive function have been demonstrated in HIV-infected patients. More information can be found on this compound, including clinical trials, at Pert's website, http://www.tinm.org.

• INTEGRASE INHIBITORS—Integrase is one of the three key enzymes encoded by the HIV *pol* gene. After HIV enters a host cell, it must splice its genetic material into human DNA in the cell nucleus in order to replicate or reproduce. Integrase is involved in this integration of viral DNA into the host genome. Integrase inhibitors differ from entry inhibitors in that they do not prevent entry of virus into the cell. Integrase is the last of HIV's three enzymes to be targeted as a drug therapy.

Early studies showed initial promising data and the drugs in this class have low toxicity, but resistance has been demonstrated. Integrase inhibitors, primarily diketobutanoic (diketo) acids, under investigation include S-1360, L-870812, and L-870810. S-1360 (GW810781) is furthest along in clinical trials and has been shown to work well in combination with other drugs.

• HIGHLY ACTIVE ANTIRETROVIRAL THERAPY (HAART)—HAART refers to the use of a combination of antiretroviral therapies. Federal recommendations on combination therapy include using either: efavirenz (Sustiva); indinavir (Crixivan); nelfinavir (Viracept); ritonavir and indinavir; ritonavir/lopinavir; or saquinavir SGC/HGC and ritonavir along with either zidovudine and didanosine; stavudine and didanosine; zidovudine and lamivudine; or stavudine and lamivudine. Alternative regimens including using saquinavir SGC; ritonavir; nevirapine; abacavir; amprenavir; delavirdine; or nelfinavir and saquinavir SGC along with either didanosine and lamivudine; or zidovudine and zalcitabine.

HAART is a highly effective treatment and is known to reduce quickly viral load and restore immune function. On HAART, patients experience an initial rapid decrease in viral load, followed by a slower reduction. A decrease to levels below the level of detection should occur within 3–4 months or 4–5 months in patients with high initial viral load counts. Increases in CD4+ T lymphocyte count vary, and immune reconstitution is reported to be slower and not as appreciable in older patients.

Although the majority of patients are able to tolerate HAART, side effects can prevent its use. Furthermore, in the event of drug resistance to one drug included in the protocol, patients will experience drug failure. Side effects include lipodystrophy, insulin resistance, hyperglycemia, elevated lipid levels and associated cardiac symptoms. In addition, 2–18 percent of patients on HAART develop severe liver toxicity and liver failure. Liver toxicity is primarily related to the use of nevirapine and the protease inhibitors.

The immune restoration that occurs with HAART can cause an exacerbation of symptoms related to infections that were previously treated. Studies show that cryptococcosis may recur during immune restoration even when patients are receiving fluconazole therapy.

• CHANGING DRUG REGIMENS—The patient's development of clinical disease while receiving antiretroviral therapy constitutes drug failure. Federal guidelines recommend that people switch or add new therapies 1) when there is less than a 0.5–0.75 log reduction in viral load after four weeks or less than one log after eight weeks of starting therapy, although response may be prolonged in people with initial low CD4+ counts and high viral loads; 2) when HIV levels remain detectable after 4–6 months of starting anti–HIV therapy; 3) when detectable HIV levels occur after being undetectable; 4) when there are persistent decreases in CD4+ T cell counts; 5) when new symptoms of HIV disease emerge; and 6) when a threefold or greater increase in HIV levels occurs compared to the lowest viral load levels. Conditions of influenza or receiving vaccines can raise HIV levels temporarily, but levels usually fall within 2–4 months. Prior to making changes to a regimen, any changes such as infections or vaccines, should be taken into consideration.

Slight increases in viral load known as "blips" do not indicate that therapy has failed. When viral load reaches undetectable levels, these blips can occur, especially in patients on protease inhibitors. Data from the CDC's HIV Outpatient Study show that patients with blips generally return to having undetectable levels even when therapy is not changed.

• ANTIRETROVIRAL DRUG RESISTANCE— The HIV virus can mutate and form strains resistant to specific drug therapies. Once a therapy has failed to prevent viral replication, future therapeutic options with currently available drugs are also limited. Laboratory tests can be used to show whether a person's HIV is likely to be suppressed or resisted by each of the various antiretroviral drugs. Genotype assays look for genetic mutations that have been linked to drug resistance, and phenotype assays assess which drugs can stop HIV growth in a lab setting. For NNRTIs and several NRTIs, such as lamivudine, a single mutation can cause a high degree of drug resistance. For this reason, these drugs are best used as part of a highly effective treatment regimen (HAART).

• ANTIRETROVIRAL THERAPY IN PREGNANCY—Combination antiretroviral therapy is recommended during pregnancy and is not associated with preterm labor. Untreated HIV infection, however, is associated with a high rate of preterm labor. Patients using protease inhibitors should be monitored closely for symptoms of hyperglycemia. The use of nucleoside analog drugs is associated with mitochondrial toxicity and may cause symptoms of neuropathy, myopathy, cardiomyopathy, pancreatitis, liver problems and lactic acidosis. Symptoms generally resolve when nucleoside analog drugs are withdrawn. Also, the CDC recommends that d4T and ddI be used cautiously during pregnancy because of their association with lactic acidosis.

Before one prescribes antiretroviral therapy, pregnant women should be evaluated for the degree of existing immunodeficiency with a CD4+ count and their risk for disease progression with an HIV-RNA test (viral load). Other factors to consider are gestational age, prior use of antiretroviral therapies, and supportive care needs. Pregnant women should also be advised of the benefits of zidovudine therapy to reduce neonatal HIV transmission. Patients should also be counseled and advised of risk factors for perinatal transmission, including cigarette smoking, illicit drug use and unprotected sexual intercourse with multiple partners during pregnancy. In addition, the CDC recommends that infected women in the U.S. refrain from breastfeeding their infants to avoid postnatal transmission of HIV to their infants through breast milk. Combination therapies should follow the same

guidelines used in non-pregnant patients.

• SIDE EFFECTS OF ANTIRETROVIRAL TREATMENT—Side effects of antiretroviral drugs usually occur within the first two to four weeks of starting a new drug regimen although some effects, such as liver toxicity, may occur after several months of treatment and hypersensitivity to abacavir may occur within the first 12 weeks of treatment. Up to 40 percent of patients using the NNRTI efavirenz experience transient central nervous system effects including, dizziness, insomnia, nightmares, and mood changes during the first few days or weeks of treatment. Anemia may occur with long-term use of NRTIs, particularly zidovudine. Occasionally neutropenia (low count of neutrophilic white blood cells) may also develop.

Gastrointestinal (GI) disturbances are the most common symptoms and are related to all antiretroviral therapies. Symptoms include abdominal discomfort or pain, nausea, diarrhea, vomiting, loss of appetite, heartburn, and constipation. Symptoms usually resolve after 3–4 weeks. If prolonged, GI side effects can lead to dehydration, malnutrition and wasting, and poor drug absorption. Most antiretroviral drugs can be taken with meals with the exception of didanosine, indinavir, and rifampin. Taking medications on an empty stomach is most likely to cause gastrointestinal symptoms. Saltine crackers, ginger, cola drinks, peppermint tea and chamomile tea may be used to help reduce symptoms of nausea. In severe nausea, pharmaceutical preparations, including cimetidine, ranitidine, and dimenhydrinate, may be prescribed.

Diarrhea associated with protease inhibitors can often be helped with the use of oat bran tablets or psyllium capsules taken together with antiretroviral therapy. The protease inhibitor indinavir may cause kidney problems related to a buildup of indinavir crystals in urine. Symptoms include acute back pain, flank pain, and abdominal pain, which may radiate to the groin. Prophylactic treatment includes increased fluid consumption, and symptoms can be relieved with nonsteroidal anti-inflammatory drugs.

Mitochondrial toxicity is associated with the use of NRTIs, and liver toxicity is associated with the use of NNRTIs and protease inhibitors. Patients with HIV and hepatitis are at the highest risk for developing liver toxicity, and symptoms may occur at any time during the course of treatment. Mitochondrial toxicity may lead to pancreatitis, a condition that may be fatal and is caused mainly by didanosine and occasionally stavudine plus didanosine. The addition of hydroxyurea causes a high risk of pancreatitis.

Lactic acidosis is a rare life-threatening condition that may occur in patients treated with stavudine and didanosine. Although 15 percent of patients treated with NRTIs will experience increased lactic acid levels, only rarely does lactic acidosis develop. Risk factors include obesity, female sex, and pregnancy. Symptoms of lactic acidosis include fatigue, nausea, vomiting, abdominal pain, weight loss, and shortness of breath. Blood tests for lactic acid are used to confirm the diagnosis.

Lipodystrophy, a condition of fat redistribution may develop in the early stages of AIDS and is not related to disease progression. It is more commonly related to the use of anti-retroviral agents. A condition of lipoatrophy, which refers to facial wasting related to subcutaneous fat loss in the cheeks and temples, may also occur in patients with manageable HIV infection. Human growth hormone used in the treatment of lipodystrophy and AIDS wasting syndrome is associated with carpal tunnel syndrome, a condition of nerve impairment affecting the nerves of the wrist.

Peripheral neuropathy is also linked to the use of NRTIs, particularly zalcitabine, didanosine and stavudine. **Lipodystrophy** and **Peripheral neuropathy** are described in separate entries.

- MICROBICIDES—Topical microbicides are being investigated for their benefits in HIV prevention. Approximately 50–60 different compounds are in various stages of development. Several different microbicides are being evaluated in clinical trials, and roughly 4,000 high-risk women have already participated in clinical trials for microbicides, significantly more than have been tested with AIDS vaccines. According to the Alliance for Microbicide Development, 38 biotech companies, 28 not-for-profit groups, and seven public-sector agencies are investigating microbicides. Microbicides work by killing or inactivating infectious pathogens; blocking fusion into host cells; inhibiting post-fusion activity; or enhancing naturally occurring vaginal defense mechanisms.

Microbicides are used as vaginal gels, creams, or as a slow-release vaginal ring. These agents kill or inactivate HIV and other STD pathogens, including compounds that disrupt lipid cell membranes (surfactants or detergents), increase membrane porosity (peroxides/peroxidases and antimicrobial peptides), cause agglutination (monoclonal antibodies), maintain an acid vaginal pH (acidic buffers), or coat cells (lipids). A few plant extracts have been identified that kill or inactivate pathogens, probably through one or more of these mechanisms. Cyanovirin-N is a protein isolated from cultures of freshwater blue-green algae or produced by recombinant DNA techniques. The U.S. National Cancer Institute discovered that Cyanovirin binds irreversibly to the HIV gp120 surface protein, and shows promise as a microbicide.

The compound B69 developed by researchers at the New York Blood Center has been found to block the CD4 receptor on HIV target cells. The New York Blood Center is also evaluating cellulose acetate phthalate (CAP or B195), a compound that binds to gp120 and other HIV receptors on target cells. Gilead Sciences is also testing the NRTI tenofovir (Viread) as a topical gel. In this formulation tenofovir was shown to prevent simian immune deficiency (SIV) infection in macaques. Trials with nonoxynol-9 (N-9) spermicidal gel were abandoned in Cameroon, Thailand, and South Africa after studies showed than N-9 can increase the risk of HIV because its use is associated with genital lesions and vaginal tears.

Carraguard gel, Emmelle, Pro-2000, and Ushercell are all sulfated or sulfonated polymers currently being evaluated in Phase III effectiveness trials. Carraguard gel is made of carrageenan derived from seaweed and has been found to block infection with HIV, herpes simples virus type 2, human papillomavirus, and *Neisseria gonorrhoeae* in in-vitro and animal systems. Clinical trials with Carraguard in Chiang-Rai, Thailand retained more than 90 percent of participants. Trials in South Africa also reported high retention. Informed consent forms were used that did not directly involve the consent of male partners. Phase III Carraguard trials will also include women as young as 16, primarily those who have already given birth since their parents will know that they are sexually active.

• CELLULAR FACTOR INHIBITORS—Hydroxyurea (Droxia, Litalir) is an old chemotherapeutic agent with relatively low toxicity sometimes used in the treatment of chronic myelogenous leukemia. Hydroxyurea inhibits DNA synthesis. Used in combination with didanosine, hydroxyurea was shown in 1994 to reduce HIV replication. Despite similar results in other small studies, hydroxyurea was implicated in causing polyneuropathy in a substantial number of patients. In another study in which hydroxyurea was combined with didanosine, three deaths occurred related to pancreatitis. The CDC does not recommend using hydroxyurea as a treatment for HIV infection.

Mycophenylate (Cell-Cept), a drug long used to prevent rejection of kidney transplants, has been used in studies to reduce lymphocyte proliferation, thereby reducing the number of cells that can be targeted and infected with HIV. Small studies have shown a reduction in viral load, but these reports need to be confirmed with randomized trials. Researchers suspect that mycophenylate will work best when paired with an antiviral, such as abacavir, that produces false building blocks. Mycophenylate is currently being studied in clinical trials with advanced-stage patients who have failed all other drug therapies. Cell-Cept should not be used with AZT or d4T since it is likely to impair the activity of those drugs.

HE-2000, produced by Hollis Eden, is currently under investigation in clinical trials. It is said to work by starving HIV of the essential proteins it needs for survival. HE-2000 is given directly into muscles by injection. In trials with SIV-infected chimps, HE-2000 showed good results. Whether it does as well in humans remains to be seen.

• ADJUVANT THERAPIES—Adjuvant therapies refer to the use of medications that either reduce symptoms related to primary therapy, such as antiemetics prescribed for nausea. Adjuvant therapy also refers to drugs used to enhance primary treatment.

Cytokines. Interleukin-2 (IL-2, aldesleukin, Proleukin) is a cytokine produced by the immune system during the immune response to stimulate immune cell production. IL-2 is currently being investigated in combination with antiretroviral therapies to help boost CD4+ and CD8+ T lymphocyte cell counts. IL-2 is usually administered subcutaneously (injected through skin) over five days in cycles 6–8 weeks apart. Side effects include fever, chills, and severe flu-like symptoms. Interferon has also been used in clinical trials but is primarily used as a salvage therapy. Granulocyte stimulating factors have been used successfully in patients with CMV retinitis although the mechanisms have been unclear.

Cannabinoids and Marijuana. The synthetic cannabinoid, dronabinol (Marinol), is FDA approved and sometimes prescribed to alleviate symptoms of nausea and stimulate appetite in patients with wasting syndrome.

Marijuana is illegal under federal law, although some cities like San Francisco have local laws permitting physicians to prescribe marijuana for some medical conditions, including HIV wasting syndrome. The safety of using marijuana in HIV infection has not been established. Studies from the Multicenter AIDS Cohort Study evaluating outcomes in 1,662 HIV-infected users of psychoactive drugs (marijuana, cocaine, LSD) found that none of the drugs were linked to a higher rate of HIV disease progression or decreases in CD4+ cell counts. However, increased lung infections including asthma and aspergillosis, are associated with the use of marijuana. Long-term studies are needed before the safety of marijuana in HIV infection can be established.

Cyclosporin A (Sandimmun). Cyclosporin A is used to slow the immune system down, in an attempt to reduce viral replication in people with normal CD4+ counts.

Onconase. Onconase described in a separate entry, is a new cancer drug with antiviral properties that has shown success in clinical trials for HIV-1.

• EXPERIMENTAL THERAPIES—Experimental therapies include a number of new antiretroviral compounds that are currently undergoing clinical trials. Promising therapies include the NNRTIs TMC 125, DPC 083, capravine (AG1549), and emivirine (EMV, MKC-442, Coactinon), and the NRTIs amdoxovir (DAPD) and alovudine FLT (MIV-301). New protease inhibitors under investigation include atazanivir (BMS-008), tipranavir, and mozenavir. Researchers at MIT have discovered a form of RNA (siRNA) that is capable of inhibiting HIV replication in human-derived cell lines by silencing genes that are essential to HIV infection. In a collaborative effort with the National Cancer Institute, MIT is attempting to develop HIV therapies using this form of RNA.

Zinc finger inhibitors are under investigation for their ability to interfere with the packaging of RNA into new virions. Disruption of the nucleocapsid leads to the production of a dysfunctional, ineffective virus. Azodicarbonamide (ADA), which is under development by Hibriphar in Belgium, is the most advanced zinc finger inhibitor under development. Results of Phase I/II trials show moderate activity against HIV. The compound GPG-NH2, which interferes with the assembly of HIV's p24 protein, is also under investigation in Sweden.

The compound AXD-455, under development in Germany, works by blocking the enzyme eIF-5A that transports viral genetic material from the host cell nucleus to the main body of the cell for processing and assembly. The compound PA-457, under development by Panacos, is a betulinic acid derivative that appears to inhibit HIV assembly and budding. Laboratory studies show that it is effective against three strains of HIV. Drugs that show significant benefits, particularly reduction of viral load, may be granted accelerated approval.

Drugs that are no longer being pursued as a treatment for HIV due to toxicity or disappointing effectiveness include: dOTC (BCH-10652); DPC-681; DPC-684; DPC-961; emivirine (Coactinon, MKC-442); GW420867X; L-756,423 (MK-944); lodenosine (Fdda); mozenavir (DMP-450); and TMC-126.

• ALTERNATIVE MEDICINE—Alternative medicine plays an important role in the treatment of AIDS. The focus of alternative medicine is on lifestyle changes and therapies such as antioxidant vitamins and other supplements that help strengthen the immune system. In December 2002, subjects infected with HIV were being recruited by the National Center for Complementary and Alternative Medicine

(NCCAM) for clinical trials involving the use of Reiki in advanced AIDS, stress management approaches to improve psychosocial functioning, immune restoration by alpha lipoic acid, treatment with massage for depression in end stage AIDS, the use of acupressure to help heal infections, Acupuncture and moxibustion for chronic diarrhea related to HIV infections, and garlic to lower lipid levels related to HAART therapy.

In the *Perricone Prescription* (New York: HarperCollins, 2002), Dr. Nicholas Perricone describes successfully treating an HIV positive patient who remains free of AIDS for extreme fatigue with N-acetyl-cysteine (NAC), using 1,000 mg twice daily, a half teaspoon of pure glutamine powder three times daily, and 250 mg alpha lipoic acid used twice daily. The NAC is an amino acid with antioxidant properties that is a precursor of the powerful antioxidant glutathione, which is not absorbed well taken orally. Dr. Perricone also prescribes a cream containing 450 mg per cubic centimeter of glutathione, which can be absorbed via topical preparations. Dr. Perricone explains that glutathione is essential whenever inflammation is present, and glutamine is necessary for successful healing of the gastrointestinal system. He also describes the spice turmeric as an AIDS therapy that blocks activation of the LTR gene in the HIV DNA, interfering with viral replication.

Writing in *Sugars That Heal*, Emil Mondoa notes that glyconutrients have been found to increase the potency of traditional AIDS drugs in humans. In particular, he describes one study in which intravenous lentinan, an extract from the shiitake mushroom, increased helper T cell counts (CD4+ counts) in AIDS patients by an average of 142 when given in combination with the drug didanosine (ddI), whereas the CD4+ count fell in the control group. An extract of maitake is also reported to be effective against Kaposi's sarcoma. However, in studies of patients with advanced AIDS, glyconutrients showed no benefits.

In Molecules of Emotion, Candace Pert, a Georgetown University neuroscientist, explains how peptides, neurotransmitters and receptors respond to emotion. She writes that there is a close correspondence between the highest, most concentrated areas of enrichment of certain neuropeptides and the location of the body's "chakras." Chakras represent the body's "energy centers" in Eastern medicine. Pert has found that the neuropeptide vasoactive intestinal peptide (VIP) is intended to bind with the CD4+ receptor that HIV targets and binds to. Pert and colleagues have synthesized peptide-T, an entry inhibitor that binds with co-receptors and blocks HIV's entry into host cells. Pert's research includes observations that patients with high levels of self-esteem are less likely to develop severe symptoms when they are infected with HIV because of changes in their neuropeptides in response to their emotions. Pert believes emotions are the key to coordinating all parts of the body into a harmonious whole and attaining optimal health. *See also* **National Center for Complementary and Alternative Medicine.**

Considerations in Pregnancy and Birth

According to early researchers about one in seven HIV positive mothers transmits HIV infection to her infant in the womb or through fluid exchanges at birth. However, reports show that pregnant women treated with a combination of anti–HIV drugs do not appear to transmit the virus to their neonates.

Two Ugandan studies, reported in *Lancet* in February 2003, demonstrated that a short course of an anti–HIV drug might cut the risk of early mother-to-child transmission by up to 50 percent in a breastfeeding population. One dose of the drug nevirapine given to mothers at the start of labor and to newborn babies within 72 hours is twice as effective at cutting transmission rates as several doses of AZT given to mothers during labor and to babies in the first week of life. Researchers calculate that a single nevirapine dose for both mother and baby costs only $400, representing 10 percent of the cheapest longer-term regimens. The researchers concluded that nevirapine therapy could have a major public health impact in developing countries, where mass use of anti–HIV drugs is not considered to be cost effective.

• BREASTFEEDING—Up to 10 percent of children who are breastfed by HIV positive mothers could become infected, according to a three-year study conducted by researchers from Johns Hopkins University. The study involved 672 Malawian infants with HIV positive mothers and showed that infants born without the virus carried a 10.3 percent risk of contracting HIV after breastfeeding. None of the mothers in the study had been given anti–HIV drugs to cut the risk of mother-to-child transmission. Researchers reported that the risk of contracting HIV appeared slightly higher in the early months after birth, but infection rates rose the longer a child was breastfed.

The risk of HIV transmission to the neonate during breastfeeding is not influenced by low levels of maternal plasma HIV-1 RNA (viral load). Rather, transmission is associated with maternal cervical HIV DNA load and genital ulcer disease.

• NEONATAL INFECTION—The risk of HIV-1 infection in neonates is highly related to the viral load of the mother, with a low maternal viral load dramatically lowering the incidence of infection. In neonates, the HIV-1 viral load increases rapidly over the first one to two months of life, followed by a slow decline over the next two years. However, viral loads of greater than 100,000 copies/ml are generally maintained during the first year of life. Without antiretroviral therapy, a high viral load in infancy that remains high at six months is highly predictive of disease progression within the first two years of life. Viral loads

greater than 100,000 copies/ml are associated with growth retardation, encephalopathy, development of opportunistic infections, and increased mortality. In maternally transmitted pediatric infection, disease progression appears to follow two distinct modes. One subgroup of children progresses rapidly to AIDS at a median age of approximately five months, and the other 20 percent of maternally transmitted pediatric AIDS patients develop AIDS at about 12 months.

In neonatal AIDS, the mean time from birth to a stage of AIDS causing severe symptoms is estimated to be 6.3 to 6.6 years. The time to death is estimated to be approximately 6.3 to 9.4 years from birth. In studies involving 2,148 perinatally infected children (infected around the time of childbirth), the mean durations of the stages of infection were 10 months for the symptom-free interim (stage N of the CDC's 1994 pediatric guidelines), four months for stage A (mild signs or symptoms), 65 months for stage B (moderate signs or symptoms), and 34 months for stage C (severe signs or symptoms). Although children with perinatally transmitted AIDS usually develop moderate symptoms by the second year of life, they may not progress for a long time. In one study, as many as one-third of those infected are estimated to remain free of AIDS by 15 years. Children started on antiretroviral therapy generally experience the same reduction in viral load as adults and have a better prognosis. For more information on neonatal HIV infection, see the section in this book on **Pediatric AIDS**.

Risk Factors

It is well known that individuals with other STDs are at increased risk for HIV infection. In addition, in a report in *Popular Science*, researchers at the Armed Forces Institute of Pathology in Washington, D.C., report that HIV is more readily transmitted to people who are also infected with *Mycoplasma genitalium*. In studies where one partner had HIV and the other did not, the second partner was likely to become HIV infected if he or she was co-infected with *M. genitalium*. The idea that mycoplasma might act as cofactors in AIDS goes back to the early 1980s when Luc Montangier, the French co-finder of the AIDS virus, also isolated Mycoplasmas from HIV positive patients. This finding explains why some women are often infected with HIV after one sexual encounter although only 15 percent of women who are steady partners of HIV-infected men acquire the virus.

Other known risk factors are anal sex, increased number of sexual partners, sexual partners from areas in which HIV is endemic, visiting commercial sex workers (particularly migrant prostitutes), genital cuts and other lesions that can facilitate HIV transmission, immune deficiency due to immunosuppressive medications or infection, intravenous drug use, unprotected sex, and sexual relations with intravenous drug users.

Precautions

Patients with AIDS with persistently low CD4+ counts are at risk for opportunistic infections and cancers. Malabsorption syndromes and diarrhea can also contribute to nutrient deficiencies that interfere with the response to therapy.

With the advent of HAART therapy and the restoration of CD4+ counts, prophylactic treatment used to prevent opportunistic infections is no longer recommended and post-infection life-long treatment is not usually needed.

Complications

Patients with AIDS are also at risk for many different opportunistic infections as well as skin disorders, sinusitis, pneumonia, enterocolitis, retinitis, bacteremia, malabsorption syndromes and neoplastic diseases. Retinitis is included in this section along with eye symptoms. **Wasting syndrome** is described in a separate entry.

• OPPORTUNISTIC INFECTIONS—Pa-tients with HIV infection are at risk for developing fungal, bacterial, viral and parasitic infections. Common fungal infections seen with HIV infection include *Pneumocystis jiroveci* pneumonia (PCP), candidiasis, histoplasmosis, aspergillosis, and coccidiomycosis. Common parasitic infections that may accompany HIV infection include toxoplasmosis, cryptosporidiosis, and microsporidiosis. Common bacterial infections seen in persons with HIV include skin infections, pneumonia, pneumonitis, bacteremia, and enteric infections. Commonly seen viral infections include herpes simplex and human papillomavirus (HPV). The circulating CD4 count is the best indicator of current susceptibility to opportunistic infection as well as prognosis.

With the introduction of effective antiretroviral treatments, the epidemiology of opportunistic infections and complications is gradually changing. For example, in the early years of the epidemic PCP was the most common infection to occur in HIV infection and affected 75–90 percent of all HIV infected persons. With improved HIV treatments and the use of prophylactic treatments for PCP, its incidence has declined. In contrast other infectious complications such as those due to cytomegalovirus and *Mycobacterium avium* complex are steadily increasing in frequency.

Eye symptoms and conditions were described earlier with symptoms. HIV-related skin disorders, bacterial pneumonia, sinusitis, and bacteremia are described later in this entry. **Opportunistic infections** and AIDS-defining illnesses, such as **Kaposi's sarcoma** and **Coccidiomycosis**, as well as several other HIV-related disorders, such as tuberculosis, are listed as separate entries.

• SINUSITIS—Both acute and chronic sinusitis are common complications of HIV infection. Symptoms may include headache, fever, congestion and cough. However, many patients only have headache or cough without more typical symptoms of bacterial sinusitis. In one study, the organisms most commonly isolated as the cause of sinusitis were viridians streptococci, *Streptococcus pneumoniae*, and *Pseudomanas aeruginosa*. Other organisms that may be responsible include *H. influenzae*, other *Haemophilus* species, and *Moraxella catarrhalis*.

Diagnosis of sinusitis is often made during a clinical examination, although CT scanning, sinus radiographs and cultures can be used and are useful in determining the causative microorganism. Treatment includes a decongestant in addition to antimicrobial therapy. Antimicrobial therapy is based on culture reports or determined on empiric grounds with first-line options including amoxicillin-valviulanate, clindamycin, cefuroxime, clarithromycin, or azithromycin.

• BACTERIAL PNEUMONIA—Patients infected with HIV are five times more likely to develop bacterial pneumonia than individuals who are HIV negative. The risk is highest in intravenous drug users with HIV infection. In one large study of pulmonary complications in HIV, tobacco smoking was found to be associated with a significantly higher risk of bacterial pneumonia in both individuals with HIV infection and those who were HIV negative. A reversal of the ratio of CD4+ T cells to CD8+ T cells, which occurs in HIV infection, contributes to the risk of developing bacterial pneumonia. Other risk factors for pneumonia in HIV infection include prior history of pneumonia, low serum albumin, not receiving the pneumonia vaccine, and low CD4+ T cell counts.

Epidemiological evidence strongly suggests that HIV-infected individuals have an increased risk of developing severe *Streptococcus pneumoniae* infection. For this reason, the CDC recommends that all HIV-infected patients receive the 23-valent pneumococcal polysaccharide vaccine early in the course of HIV infection.

The clinical course of bacterial pneumonia is similar to that seen in patients without HIV infection. There is usually an acute onset of symptoms, including fever, productive cough, dyspnea, and pleuritic chest pain. Imaging studies of the chest show local infiltrates, and sputum studies show numerous white blood cells and an overgrowth of organisms. The most common causes of bacterial pneumonia in HIV infection include *Streptococcus pneumoniae*, *Haemophilus* species, *M. catarrhalis*, *Klebsiella pneumoniae*, and *Staph. Aureus*. Rarely, bacterial pneumonia in HIV infected patients is caused by *Rhodococcus equii*. Treatment depends on the infectious agent but usually consists of vancomycin, ciprofloxacin or imipenem.

• BACTEREMIA—Bacteremia, a condition of bacteria present in the blood circulation, may frequently occur as a result of Salmonella infection and pneumonia. Bacteremia may also be associated with soft tissue and urinary tract infections. Intravenous drug use is associated with the development of *Staphylococcus aureus* bacteremia and endocarditis (infection of the heart and its valves). In bacteremia, a low CD4+ count is associated with high mortality.

Bacteremia may also occur as a result of indwelling catheters used for the management of other conditions such as the intravenous treatment of cytomegalovirus retinitis. In one study of HIV infected patients with bacteremia, 35 percent had infections related to intravenous catheters. In these instances most infections were due to *Staphylococcus aureus* and coagulase-negative species of staphylococci. Although rare, infections with gram-negative organisms, such as *Escherichia coli*, *Proteus mirabilis, and Serratia marascens*, have also been related to intravenous catheters. Until the exact causative organism is isolated by culture technique, patients are usually started on empiric therapy with vancomycin and an aminoglycoside antibiotic.

• NEOPLASTIC DISORDERS—Approximately 30–40 percent of patients with HIV infection are likely to develop Kaposi's sarcoma (KS) and or lymphomas during the course of their disease. The three malignancies considered to be AIDS-defining illnesses include Kaposi's sarcoma, peripheral and central nervous system (CNS) intermediate or high-grade B-cell non–Hodgkin's lymphoma (NHL), and invasive cervical cancer as well as other cancers associated with the human papilloma virus. Hodgkin's disease has also been increasingly described in patients with HIV infection. These malignancies are described later in entries for **Kaposi's sarcoma, Non-Hodgkin's lymphoma,** and **Human papilloma virus.**

• SKIN CHANGES AND CONDITIONS RELATED TO HIV—A number of dermatological conditions, including skin infections, inflammatory conditions, and tumors commonly occur in patients infected with HIV. Skin conditions may be the sentinel event that brings the patient to the physician.

Infectious Skin Conditions. Bacterial skin infections vary from impetigo to folliculitis to skin abscesses. Skin abscesses may also be associated with injection drug use. Recurrences of skin infections tend to occur more often than in people who are HIV negative. The most common causes of infection are *Staphylococcus aureus, Pseudomonas aureuginosa, Mycobacterium* species, and *Bartonella* species.

Infection with *Staphylococcus aureus* is common in HIV infection, especially in children. Up to 50 percent of persons with HIV are *S. aureus* carriers. Infections may be superficial, such as impetigo or folliculitis, or deep, causing abscesses, cellulitis, botryomycosis, and may be complicated by septicemia (blood infection). Treatment is generally with penicillinase-resistant penicillin, cephalosporin, and mupirocin for single lesions; for children; if streptococcus is excluded, clindomycin and ciprofloxacin can be used. Antibacterial soaps and antihistamines can be used as adjunctive therapies. For recurrences additional antibiotics such as rifampin

may be added. In deep infection, intravenous antibiotics may be needed followed by oral therapy, and surgical resection and drainage may be necessary.

In HIV-associated *Mycobacterium avium* complex, skin lesions related to disseminated disease include nodules, ulcerations, reddened lesions, pustules, abscesses, folliculitis, panniculitis (inflammation of the fat layer below the skin), and soft tissue swelling. Therapy typically consists of azithromycin or clarithromycin with ethambutol, and additional antibiotics may be added.

Mycobacterium tuberculosis infection in early HIV infection is similar to that seen in persons who are HIV negative, with most patients showing exclusively pulmonary symptoms. At later stages, cutaneous manifestations of TB include papules, vesicles, necrotic ulcerations, and subcutaneous nodules and pustules. Chronic recurrent tuberculous rectal abscesses have also been reported. Therapies used for TB are effective for the skin manifestations associated with this disease.

Viral infections commonly seen in HIV infection include Herpes simplex virus (HSV), Varicella Zoster virus (VZV), Epstein-Barr virus (EBV), Cytomegalovirus (CMV), Human papillomavirus (HPV), and Molluscum contagiosum. Herpes simplex typically occurs in HIV as a reactivation of latent virus. HSV infections typically present as small, grouped vesicles on a reddened base, which eventually forms pustules, erosions, and sometimes frank ulcers. In HIV infection, deep ulcers, wart-like erosions or mixed infections are likely.

Among HIV-infected children and adults, the manifestations of VZV infections include primary varicella (measles with or without complications of pneumonia and speech disturbances), increased incidence of herpes zoster (cold sores), and chronic infection with verrucous lesions.

Cutaneous CMV infection in patients with HIV/AIDS indicates a poor prognosis. Frequently, a non-healing ulcer in the anal region occurs that may be resistant to acyclovir treatment. Papular eruptions, purpura, nodules, ulcerations, and wart-like lesions may also occur.

Fungal skin infections in HIV infection are usually related to *Candida albicans, Tinea* species, *Histoplasma capsulatum, Cryptococcus neoformans, Coccidiodes immitis,* and *Penicillium marneffei.* Vulvovaginal (affecting the vulva and vaginal area) candidiasis frequently occurs in women early in the course of HIV infection. Tinea infections may occur in varying locations including the hair, beard, and nails. Cryptococcal infections cause skin lesions resembling those of Molluscum contagiosum and they may also form ulcers, pustules, draining sinuses, granuloma, cellulitis, and gangrenous lesions. Coccidiodes infection may cause granulomatous papules, nodules or plaques, wart-like nodules, scar-like nodules, cold abscesses, and scaling patches. *Pneumocystis jiroveci* can rarely cause skin lesions, including nodules in the auditory canal and near the ear. Patients with superficial fungal infections are more likely to develop more invasive fungal infections requiring systemic therapy.

Infestation with scabies as well as with amoeba of the *Acanthamoeba* and *Naegleria* species may also occur. These amoeba often infect the skin, nasal mucosa, sinuses, and brain. The skin lesion begin as blistering nodules that eventually develop into deep ulcerations.

For more information on infectious skin disorders in HIV see the separate entries on **Bacillary angiomatosis; Candidiasis; Cryptococcosis; Coccidiomycosis; Folliculitis; Herpes simplex virus; Histoplasmosis; Penicilliosis; Epstein-Barr virus; Cytomegalovirus; Human Papillomavirus; Molluscum contagiosum; Reiter's syndrome; Scabies;** and **Tuberculosis.**

Inflammatory Skin Conditions. Inflammatory skin conditions seen with HIV infection include psoriasis, Reiter's disease, folliculitis, sebborrheic dermatitis, generalized pruritits (itching), and HIV associated eosinophilic folliculitis. Psoriasis appears as a chronic inflammatory condition characterized by reddened papules and plaques covered by silvery, adherent scales. The nails may also be affected and develop pitting, separation from nail beds (onycholysis), and other nail deformities. An accompanying arthritis may be seen in HIV patients, which may be more resistant to treatment. In patients who are immunosuppressed, psoriasis and related conditions of eczema tend to flare.

Eosinophilic folliculitis is characterized by a chronic eruption of sterile, usually itchy papules and pustules that occur in the hair follicles. This condition generally occurs in patients with CD4+ T cells counts less than 100 cells/mm^3. Lesions typically occur in hair follicles on exposed body parts, including the face and especially the forehead. Blood counts show a marked increase in white blood cells known as eosinophils. Treatment generally consists of a combination of antihistamines, corticosteroids, itraconazole, isotretinoin, dapsone, or metronidazole.

Generalized HIV-associated pruritis is diagnosed when itching occurs without other causes. Lesions appear as excoriations, erosions, ulcers, papules, plaques, pigmentation changes and scars. HIV-associated papular eruptions may also occur and are thought to be related to hypersensitivity to insects, including mites. *See also* **Kaposi's sarcoma** and **Cutaneous lymphoma.**

• HERPES AND HIV—Genital herpes has reached epidemic scope in the last decade. The CDC reports that this is related to the fact that herpes is a chronic infection and that the virus is continually shed even when patients do not have symptoms. The clinical symptoms in herpes can also be misleading in that symptoms may be confused with "jock itch" when genital ulcers don't develop. A meta-analysis of 27 studies suggested that the risk of HIV acquisition was doubled in persons with HSV-2.

One African study found a five-fold increase in HIV infection in individuals with HSV-2. The CDC recommends short courses of acyclovir, valacyclovir or famciclovir, for instance, using acyclovir 800 mg three times daily for two days instead of the standard five-day regimen. One recent CDC study showed that all agents are effective, but valacyclovir appeared most effective. All three antiviral agents are considered safe for use in HIV infection.

• SYPHILIS IN PATIENTS WITH HIV—The CDC reports that unusual serologic responses have been observed among HIV-infected persons who have syphilis. Most reports have involved serologic titers that were higher than expected, but false-negative serologic test (RPR) results and delayed appearance of sero-reactivity have also been reported. When clinical findings suggest syphilis, but serologic tests are nonreactive or the interpretation is unclear, alternative tests, such as darkfield examination or direct fluorescent antibody staining of lesion material may be helpful for diagnosis.

HIV-positive patients with syphilis may have higher rates of treatment failure with currently recommended regimens and they may be at increased risk for neurologic complications. For primary and secondary syphilis in persons with HIV, treatment with benzathine penicillin G, 2.4 million units IM in a single dose is recommended. Some specialists recommend additional treatments at one-week intervals for three weeks. Patients with early latent syphilis should be managed and treated according to the recommendations for HIV-negative patients who have primary and secondary syphilis. HIV-infected patients who have either late latent syphilis or syphilis of unknown duration should have a cerebrospinal fluid examination before treatment.

The clinical manifestations of syphilis in patients with HIV infection are usually similar to syphilis in patients who are HIV-negative. However, florid or unusual manifestations of disease have been described in several case reports, particularly in patients with advanced HIV infection. In patients with suspected syphilis who test negative, serum should be diluted and retested and repeated using a different assay method. Alternate testing in patients with early syphilis includes a dark-field examination and direct fluorescent antibody staining for *T. pallidum* from a scraping or suspected lesions or skin biopsy.

• HEPATITIS C IN HIV INFECTION—The CDC reports that about one quarter of HIV-infected persons in the United States are also infected with the hepatitis C virus (HCV). Of importance, HCV infection progresses more rapidly to liver damage in HIV-infected persons, and HCV infection may affect the course and management of HIV infection. Co-infection with HIV and HCV is common (50–90 percent) among HIV infected injection drug users. Co-infection is also common among persons with hemophilia who received clotting factor concentrates before concentrates were effectively treated to inactivate both viruses (products used before 1987). The risk for acquiring infection through perinatal or sexual exposures is much lower for HCV than for HIV. For persons infected with HIV through sexual exposure, co-infection with HCV is no more common than among similarly aged adults in the general population (3–5 percent).

Infection with both HIV and HCV is associated with higher titers of HCV, more rapid progression to HCV-related liver disease, and an increased risk for HCV-related cirrhosis of the liver. Because of this, HCV infection was included in the 1999 "Guidelines for the Prevention of Opportunistic Infections in Persons Infected with HIV." As HAART and prophylaxis of opportunistic infections increase the life span of persons living with HIV, HCV-related liver diseases have become a major cause of hospital admissions and deaths among HIV-infected persons. Some studies have also suggested that infection with certain HCV genotypes is associated with more rapid progression to AIDS or death.

Persons with HIV and HCV infection should be given information about prevention of liver damage, undergo evaluation for chronic liver disease, and, if indicated, be considered for treatment. Persons with both infections should be advised not to drink excessive amounts of alcohol and to consult with their physicians before adding any new medicines, including over-the-counter and herbal preparations. For further information, see the CDC Divisions of HIV/AIDS Prevention's "Frequently Asked Questions and Answers About Coinfection with HIV and Hepatitis C Virus," August 2001, http://www.cdc.gov/hiv/pubs/facts/HIV-HCV_Coinfection.htm.

• TUBERCULOSIS IN HIV INFECTION— Tuberculosis (TB) is a highly contagious disease that is spread from person-to-person through the air. People with HIV are especially susceptible to TB, and worldwide, TB is the leading cause of death among people infected with HIV. Worldwide, TB is the cause of death for one out of every three people with AIDS. The CDC reports that an estimated 10–15 million Americans are infected with TB bacteria and have the potential to develop active TB in the future. About 10 percent of these people will go on to develop active TB. However, the risk is much greater for people infected with HIV and living with AIDS. Studies also show that people with HIV who develop TB experience a significant increase in viral replication.

Because HIV infection so severely weakens the immune system, people dually infected with HIV and TB have a 100 times greater risk of developing active TB disease and becoming infectious compared to people not infected with HIV. The CDC estimates that 10 to 15 percent of all TB cases and nearly 30 percent of cases among people ages 25 to 44 are occurring in HIV-infected individuals. The CDC recommends that all people infected with HIV be tested for TB, and if infected, complete preventive therapy as soon as possible to prevent TB disease. (CDC Divisions of HIV/AIDS Prevention, "The Deadly Intersection Between TB and HIV," November 1999). *See also* **ACT UP; AIDS-related primary central nervous system lymphoma;** AIDS **dementia complex; AIDS history; AIDS Quilt; AIDS vaccines; Anal sex; Antiretroviral drug resistance; Aspergillosis; Bacillary angiomatosis; Bug chasers; CD4 cell count; Central nervous system (CNS) damage in HIV; Coccidiomycosis; Cryptococcosis; Cryptosporidium; Genotype (genotypic) assay; Highly active antiretroviral therapy (HAART); Histoplasmosis and penicilliosis; HIV; HIV-1; HIV-1 RNA; HIV-2; HIV blood tests; HIV mutation; Institut Pasteur; Kaposi's sarcoma; Lentiviruses; Lipoatrophy; Lipodystrophy; Lymphadenopathy syndrome;** *Mycobacterium avium*-**complex; Non-nucleotide reverse transcriptase inhibitors (NNRTIs); Nucleoside/nucleotide analog reverse transcriptase inhibitors (NRTIs); Onconase; Pediatric** AIDS; **Peripheral neuropathy; Phenotype assay;** *Pneumocystis jiroveci* **pneumonia; Protease inhibitors; Rapid HIV test; Reiki; Opportunistic infections; Quantitative RNA (QRNA) test; Retroviruses; Retrovirus replication; Reverse transcriptase; Social Security Disability for HIV/AIDS; Ryan White Comprehensive AIDS Resources Emergency Act; SUDS test; Viral load; Viruses; White, Ryan; World** AIDS **Day.**

Armstrong, Donald, and Jonathan Cohen. *Infectious Diseases.* London: Mosby/Harcourt, 1999.

Centers for Disease Control and Prevention. *Sexually Transmitted Diseases Treatment Guidelines 2002.* Atlanta: U.S. Dept. of Health and Human Services, 2002.

CDC. *Guidelines for Preventing Opportunistic Infection Among HIV-Infected Persons-2002.* Atlanta: U.S. Dept. of Health and Human Services, 2002.

CDC MMWR Recommendations and Reports. U.S. Public Health Service Task Force: *Recommendations for Use of Antiretroviral Drugs in Pregnant HIV-1 Infected Women for Maternal Health and Interventions to Reduce Perinatal HIV-1 Transmission in the United States.* Nov 22, 2002. Atlanta: U.S. Dept. of Health and Human Services, 2002.

Dobbs, Trudy, et al. "Detecting Recent Human Im-munodeficiency Virus type 1 Infection: Why and How?" *Medical Laboratory Observer*, May 2002, 35(5):12–22.

Holmes, King K., editor. *Sexually Transmitted Diseases*. 3rd Edition. New York: McGraw-Hill, 1999.

Mondoa, Emil. *Sugars That Heal*. New York: Ballantine, 2001.

Pert, Candace. *Molecules of Emotion*. New York: Simon and Schuster, 1997.

Pomerantz, Roger, editor. *Clinics in Laboratory Medicine: Clinical HIV-1 Virology*. Philadelphia: W.B. Saunders, 2002.

Rico, M. Joyce, et al., "Guidelines of Care for Dermatologic Conditions in Patients Infected with HIV." *Journal of the American Academy of Dermatology*, Sept. 1997, 37(3): 1–28.

Schupbach, Jorg. "Human Immunodeficiency Viruses." Chapter 63 in *Manual of Clinical Microbiology*. 7th Edition. Washington DC: ASM, 1999).

Sinha, Gunjan. "What's Really Causing Gulf War Illness?" *Popular Science*, April 1999.

ACT UP

In early 1987, the AIDS Coalition to Unleash Power (ACT UP) was founded in New York City. ACT UP was committed to direct action to end the AIDS crisis. Its demands included better access to the recently introduced AZT and lower prices for AIDS drugs, public education regarding AIDS and the prohibition of AIDS-related discrimination. On March 24, 1987, ACT UP held its first mass demonstration on Wall Street. Many of the placards used in their demonstrations displayed a pink triangle on a black background, with the legend "Silence = Death," borrowed from the Silence = Death project. This motto became the symbol of AIDS activism.

One ACT UP committee used the emblem in a window display called "Let the Record Show," at the New Museum of Contemporary Art in New York. This group later reorganized as Gran Fury. Over the next few years Gran Fury produced many high profile public projects, including the art-banner announcing that "All People with AIDS are Innocent," and a poster stating the number of HIV positive babies born in New York City. *See also* **AIDS history**.

Acupressure

Acupressure is a form of traditional Chinese medicine that involves the use of pressure on the same acupoints as in acupuncture. Pressure is applied for five seconds and then relieved for five seconds. Points that exhibit pain represent "energy blockages." Acupressure is currently being investigated in NCCAM clinical trials for its use in controlling nausea and vomiting in patients with HIV/AIDS. The study is being held at Columbia University School of Nursing's Center for AIDS research in New York City. For more information contact Bernadette Capili at 212-305-4015 or bc42@columbia.edu.

Acupuncture

Acupuncture is a traditional Chinese healing technique that involves inserting very thin needles into different acupuncture points (meridians) that allegedly follow "energy flow" through the body. Acupuncture is used to improve what practitioners refer to as the flow of the body's vital energy, qi or chi. In some alternative medicine protocols, acupuncture is used to manage the pain of the peripheral neuropathy that can accompany AIDS, and to reduce addiction cravings.

The NCCAM division of the NIH is conducting clinical trials to evaluate the use of acupuncture, including moxibustion, on patients with HIV who have chronic diarrhea. For more information, contact Ann Chung at 212-305-3041 or amc103@columbia.edu.

Acute

Acute is a term used to describe symptoms or conditions that are quick or sudden in onset and generally aggressive. Acute is used in contrast to chronic. Chronic conditions are long-lasting. *See also* **Infection**.

Acute HIV infection

Acute IV infection refers to the period of rapid viral replication that occurs immediately following exposure to HIV. An estimated 80 to 90 percent of individuals with primary HIV infection develop an acute syndrome characterized by flu-like symptoms of fever, malaise, lymphadenopathy, pharyngitis, headache, myalgia, and sometimes rash. Following primary infection, seroconversion and a broad HIV-1 specific immune response occur, usually within an average of three weeks after transmission of HIV. In the early years of the epidemic, it was thought that HIV was relatively dormant during this phase. However, it is now known that during the time of primary infection, high levels of plasma HIV RNA are present. *See also* Acute retroviral syndrome in the entry on **AIDS**.

Glossary of HIV/AIDS-Related Terms, 4th edition. HIV/AIDS Treatment Information Service, Centers for Disease Control and Prevention, 2002.

Acyclovir (Zovirax)

Acyclovir is an antiviral drug used to treat herpes simplex virus types 1 and 2 (HSV-1, HSV-2) and also varicella zoster infections (chicken pox and shingles). When used in combination with AZT, acyclovir has been shown to prolong survival in some patients with AIDS. Acyclovir is also the active metabolite of the drug valacyclovir.

Adenopathy

Adenopathy is a condition involving or causing enlargement of glandular tissues, especially lymph nodes. *See also* **Lymphodenopathy Syndrome**.

Adenovirus

Adenoviruses belong to a family of double-stranded DNA viruses that are responsible for the common cold.

Adjuvant therapy

Adjuvant refers to a substance added to another substance to help enhance its effects. Adjuvant therapy is therapy that improves the outcome of a primary therapy. For instance, the drug perphenazine used to control nausea related to AZT therapy is considered an adjuvant therapy.

Adolescents with STDs

The CDC guidelines report that there are several issues that relate specifically to adolescents. The rates of many STDs are highest among adolescents. For instance, the rate of gonorrhea is highest among females aged 15 to 19 years. Clinic-based studies have demonstrated that the prevalence of human papilloma virus (HPV) infections, and possibly chlamydial infections, is also highest among adolescents. In addition, surveillance data indicate that nine percent of adolescents who have acute hepatitis B infection either have had sexual contact with a chronically infected person or multiple sex partners or their sexual preference is listed as homosexual.

Adolescents at risk for STDs include male homosexuals, sexually active heterosexuals, clients in STD clinics, and intravenous-drug users. Younger adolescents (less than 15 years) who are sexually active are at a particular risk for infection. For instance, young girls have a higher risk for chlamydial infection. Adolescents are at greatest risk for STDs because they frequently have unprotected intercourse, are biologically more susceptible to genital infection, and face multiple obstacles that prevent the utilization of health care.

With limited exceptions, all adolescents in the United States can consent to the confidential diagnosis and treatment of STDs. Medical care for STDs can be provided to adolescents without parental consent or knowledge. Furthermore, in many states adolescents can consent to HIV counseling and testing. Consent laws for vaccination differ by state. Several states consider provision of vaccine similar to treatment of STDs and provide vaccination services without parental consent. Providers of health care are advised to appreciate the importance of confidentiality and to follow policies that comply with state laws to ensure the confidentiality of STD-related services provided to adolescents.

Counseling and health education should be appropriately adapted for adolescents and their development level. Counseling should identify known risk factors.

Centers for Disease Control and Prevention. *1998 Guidelines for Treatment of Sexually Transmitted Diseases.* Atlanta: U.S. Dept. of Health and Human Services, 1997.

Adoptive immunotherapy

Adoptive immunotherapy refers to the use of a graft of immune tissue, such as bone marrow, from a healthy donor to help rebuild the immune system of an individual whose immune system has been damaged or destroyed.

Adult AIDS Clinical Trials Group (AACTG)

The Adult AIDS Clinical Trials Group is the largest HIV clinical trials organization in the world. The AACTG plays a major role in setting standards of health care for HIV infection and also opportunistic diseases related to HIV/AIDS worldwide. The AACTG is composed of, and directed by, leading clinical scientists in HIV/AIDS therapeutic research. For more information see the HIV/AIDS Bureau of the U.S. Department of Health & Human Services at http://hab.hrsa.gov/.

Adult T-cell leukemia/ lymphoma (ATL)

ATL is a form of cancer involving T-lymphocytes that is caused by the HTLV-I virus.

Etiology

The infectious agent is HTLV-1, the first human retrovirus discovered. ATL was first reported in Japan in 1977, and the virus was first isolated in 1979 from an African-American patient with cutaneous (primarily affecting the skin) T-cell leukemia. Subsequent studies in Japan and the Caribbean and among migrants from these areas unequivocally linked HTLV-I to ATL. The HTLV-I is transmitted sexually and also via intravenous drug use, contaminated blood products, and from mother-to-child, particularly during breastfeeding.

Epidemiology

ATL is found world-wide, with higher prevalence occurring in certain select geographic areas, including southern Japan, the Caribbean, and the West Indies. ATL occurs in equal frequency in men and women, although women are more likely to develop HTLV-I infection. The peak incidence of ATL occurs in the mid–50s in Japan and in the mid–40s in the West Indies. The risk of HTLV-I infection as a cause of leukemia/lymphoma is highest in people 40 to 50 years old, and the risk declines thereafter. In Jamaica and Trinidad 70 percent of all lymphoid malignancies are attributed to HTLV-1 exposure. Rarely, ATL may occur in children as young as five or six years. Among healthy carriers of HTLV-I the lifetime risk of infection is approximately one to five percent, although this figure might be low since it could underestimate patients who were infected early in life. In Jamaica and Trinidad, studies over eight years show HTLV-I involvement in all reported cases of non–Hodgkin's lymphoma.

Symptoms

ATL causes a variety of clinical signs and symptoms. In peripheral blood smears, mononuclear white blood cells may have a characteristic multi-lobed appearance causing them to be called flower cells.

Patients with ATL may have elevated blood calcium levels, bone lesions, and cutaneous, nodal, and extranodal involvement with a pleomorphic (many different forms) type of lymphoma. The skin involvement in ATL can mimic the fungal infection mycoses fungoides in the early stages.

The prognosis of patients with acute ATL and lymphoma type ATL is poor; most patients die within six months of diagnosis. Death usually occurs from involvement with rapidly growing tumor cells, bacterial sepsis and opportunistic infections.

Subtypes of ATL

Four major subtypes of ATL have been reported: an acute or prototypical type; lymphoma type; chronic type; and a smoldering type of disease. The milder, more benign forms of ATL typically evolve into the more aggressive types. The specific ATL subtypes may be endemic to different geographic regions.

Acute ATL is an aggressive mature T-cell lymphoma that shows leukemic (abnormal cell proliferation) involvement in 80 percent of cases, with an abnormal distribution of flower cells. Up to 50 percent of patients develop hypercalcemia (elevated blood calcium levels) as calcium is leached from bone, and 40 percent of patients develop skin lesions ranging from flat papular rashes to tumorous lesions. Multiple organs and lymph nodes may be involved.

Lymphoma type ATL is similar to acute ATL, but patients do not show signs of leukemia in their peripheral blood. Chronic ATL presents as T-cell chronic lymphocytic leukemia (CLL). Many of these patients also have skin lesions, although lymph nodes are not usually affected and patients do not develop hypercalcemia. The smoldering form of ATL resembles mycosis fungoides/Sezary syndrome, a condition marked by cutaneous involvement that presents as a reddened rash (erythema) or as infiltrative plaques or tumors along with distinct abscesses known as Pautrier's microabscesses.

Diagnosis

Nearly all patients with ATL develop HTLV-1 antibodies, and tests for HTLV-1 antibodies can be used to determine the presence of HTLV-1 infection. Viral particles can also be demonstrated in tumors. In the absence of HTLV-1 antibodies in suspected ATL, histologic studies can be performed to show the presence of HTLV-1 in tumor cells.

Treatment

ATL is generally refractory to most conventional and experimental chemotherapeutic agents. A multiple therapy approach using antiretroviral agents is currently being investigated.

Cleghorn, Farley, and William Blattner. "Human T-cell Lymphotropic Virus and HTLV Infection." Chapter 19 in *Sexually Transmitted Diseases*. 3rd edition. Edited by King K. Holmes, et al. New York: McGraw-Hill, 1999.

Adverse reaction

Adverse reactions, which are also known as side effects, are toxic or unpleasant reactions that occur as a result of drug treatment. Adverse reactions may range from mild rash or headache to more severe side effects such as peripheral neuropathy, bone marrow suppression, seizures, and liver or kidney failure.

Africa

In the entire world, sub–Saharan Africa is the region most affected by HIV/AIDS. At the end of 2000, 25.3 million adults and children in this region were living with HIV/AIDS, representing 70 percent of the global total. During 2000, 2.4 million AIDS deaths occurred in sub–Saharan Africa, representing 80 percent of global AIDS deaths that year. In 2000, 3.8 million people in this region became infected with HIV, representing about 72 percent of all new global HIV infections. At the end of 2000, the region's adult (ages 15–49) HIV/AIDS prevalence rate was 8.8 percent. Of the region's HIV positive adults, 55 percent were women. More than 80 percent of women worldwide living with HIV/AIDS live in sub–Saharan Africa.

In 2000, Botswana had the world's highest adult HIV prevalence rate (35.8 percent), up from 25.1 percent in 1997. According to UNAIDS, between 1988 and 1997, 94 percent of HIV transmission in Botswana was heterosexual and 6 percent was mother-to-child. According to the U.S. Census Bureau, in the absence of AIDS, life expectancy in Botswana would have risen to 66 years by 2010. In 2010, life expectancy is projected to be 39 years.

African-Americans

The CDC reports that African-American have the highest STD rate in the nation. Compared to whites, African-Americans are 27 times more likely to have gonorrhea and 16 times more likely to have syphilis. Because STDs cause physical changes including genital lesions that facilitate HIV transmission, African-Americans also have the highest rates of HIV/AIDS.

Although African-Americans make up about 12 percent of the U.S. population, they accounted for half of the new HIV cases reported in the U.S. in 2001. It is estimated that half of these infections occur among teenagers and young adults aged 25 years and younger. In 2001, 64 percent of the HIV cases reported among women occurred in African-Americans. African-Americans have accounted for nearly 35 percent of the more than 816,000 AIDS cases reported to the CDC by the end of 2001. By this time, more than 168,000 African-Americans had died from AIDS. In 2001, African-Americans accounted for about 49 percent of the more than 43,000 new AIDS cases reported among adults. AIDS is the leading cause of death among African-American women ages 25–34 and African-American men ages 35–44.

The CDC reports that certain challenges make African-Americans more susceptible to STD infections. These factors include: 1) poverty — nearly 25 percent of African-Americans live in poverty — which results in limited access to health care and higher levels of substance abuse; 2) denial, specifically a reluctance to admit homosexuality or drug abuse; 3) partners at risk, with most African-American women infected as a result of sex with men. These women may not be aware of their partners' other sex partners, drug use or bisexuality; 4) substance abuse: injection drug use is the second-leading cause of HIV infection for both African-American men and women. Needle-sharing and risky sexual behavior are both related to substance abuse; and 5) the presence of other STDs.

The CDC is committed to working with communities to slow the spread of HIV among African-Americans. Of the $744 million that the CDC received for domestic HIV/AIDS prevention in 2001, more than 40 percent supported activities targeted to reduce HIV/AIDS among African-Americans, including peer education and other programs in Indiana, New Orleans, Detroit and Chicago.

AIDS: *for main entry see* Acquired immune deficiency syndrome *(page 5); for specific topics see "AIDS…" entries on pages 40–50*

AIDS Clinical Trials Group (ACTG)

The AIDS Clinical Trials Group is a network of medical centers located throughout the United States in which federally funded clinical trials are conducted to test the safety and efficacy of experimental treatments for AIDS and HIV infection. These studies are funded by the National Institutes of Health's National Institute of Allergy and Infectious Diseases (NIAID). For more information see http://www.nih.gov/niaid.

AIDS dementia complex (ADC, HIV-associated cognitive/motor complex)

Aids dementia complex is a condition of mental impairment caused by HIV infection. Symptoms may include cognitive impairment, such as difficult concentrating and memory loss, disorientation, mood and personality changes, speech and vision difficulties, psychomotor dysfunction (lack of coordination, incontinence), and paralysis. AIDS dementia typically affects people in the later stages of HIV disease. Early stages of this syndrome are referred to as HIV-associated minor cognitive/motor disorder.

Studies show that early in infection, HIV enters the central nervous system (CNS) where it infects macrophage cells and microglial cells. These infected cells cause the release of various immune system chemicals known as cytokines. Cytokines and similar chemicals contribute to the destruction of neurons (cells which make up the central nervous system, including the brain).

Unfortunately, antiretroviral treatments are unable to cross into the central nervous system. Therefore, while antiretroviral therapies reduce viral load and preserve immune system function, they have no affect on the central nervous system effects of HIV infection. Neuronal damage and cell death are consistent pathologic findings in the brains of patients with ADC, and multiple cell model systems have demonstrated neurotoxicity caused by HIV infection of macrophages and microglial cells. Therapeutic agents that inhibit neuronal death-signaling pathways, for instance, p38 MARK inhibitors, or that stimulate cell survival pathways are being investigated for their therapeutic role in AIDS dementia complex. *See also* **Acquired immune deficiency syndrome**.

AIDS Drug Assistance Program (ADAP)

ADAP is a program administered by individual states and authorized under Title II of the CARE Act. ADAP provides FDA approved medications to low-income individuals with HIV disease who have limited or no coverage from private insurance or Medicaid. ADAP funds may also be used to purchase insurance for uninsured CARE Act clients as long as the insurance costs do not exceed the cost of drugs through ADAP and the drugs available through the insurance program at least match those offered through ADAP.

AIDS history

Information presented at the 13th International AIDS Conference in July 2000 indicates that the AIDS virus most probably first jumped from chimpanzees to humans as early as 1675, although it did not establish itself as an epidemic strain in Africa until about 1930. Dr. Anne-Mieke Vandamme of the Riga Institute in Leuven, Belgium, in collaboration with colleagues in France, Germany and Ireland, devised a technique for tracing the family tree of viruses that dated the virus to 1675.

The Simian Link

Vandamme found the separation between SIVcpz (chimpanzee simian immunodeficiency virus) and HIV-1 occurred in 1675 to 1700. Although some researchers do not agree, many experts explain that it took a new mode of transmission such as use of non-sterile needles, non-sterile blood products, and widespread promiscuous sexual behavior for the virus to become epidemic.

The link between chimpanzees had already been established. In February of 1999, researchers at the University of Alabama studied frozen chimpanzee tissue and found that the simian virus in chimpanzees was almost identical to HIV-1.

These researchers have suggested that HIV could have crossed over from chimpanzees as a result of humans killing a chimp and eating it for food. HIV-2 has been found to correspond to an SIV found in the sooty mangabey monkey (SIVsm), which is sometimes known as the green monkey, a primate indigenous to West Africa.

Studies performed at the Los Alamos National Laboratory have also confirmed that the first M-class form of HIV-1 emerged in Africa in 1930, although the oldest known HIV samples date to 1959. In 1998 researchers found HIV in a plasma sample taken in 1959 from an adult male living in what is now the Democratic Republic of Congo. HIV has also been found in tissue samples from an African-American teenager who died in St. Louis in 1969, and in tissue samples from a Norwegian sailor who died around 1976. The finding of HIV-1 in the 1959 sample suggests that HIV-1 was introduced into humans around the 1940s or early 1950s. Other scientists suggest that HIV-1 may have been introduced into humans as long as 100 years ago.

In January 2000 at the 7th Conference on Retroviruses and Opportunistic Infections, Dr. Bette Korber reported that her computer-generated viral tracings indicated that the first case of HIV infection occurred around 1930 in West Africa, with a 20-year variation. Many researchers have indicated that HIV likely crossed over to humans on more than one occasion. Several studies show that it is likely that HIV emerged in the Americas before it emerged in Africa and that HIV first appeared in the late 1970s. What is clear is that HIV first emerged in the middle of the 20th century.

Theories Regarding the Origin of AIDS

Medical experts agree that HIV can be traced to chimpanzees, but not everyone believes that HIV emerged from direct human-chimpanzee contact, either in the form of chimpanzee bites, bizarre sexual rituals, or eating chimpanzee meat and organs. One popular theory also suggests that a hunter may have nicked himself while skinning an infected monkey, but these theories all rely on speculation. However, the manner that HIV emerged and the timing indicate that HIV was probably not a natural event.

The British journalist Edward Hooper, the reporter Tom Curtis, and several prominent researchers propose that HIV can be traced to the testing of an oral polio vaccine called CHAT that had been grown in the kidney cells of chimps or African Green Monkeys in the Congo, at the Wistar Institute and in Belgium. This vaccine was administered to people in Leopold in the Belgian Congo (now Kinshasa, Zaire), Ruanda, and Urundi in the late 1950s. These areas correspond to the regions where AIDS is most pervasive. Of the 39 first reported cases of AIDS in Africa, 87 percent came from areas where CHAT was given, and 100 percent occurred within a 90-mile radius of these areas.

In this campaign headed by the scientist Hilary Koprowski, an oral polio vaccine of a lot called CHAT was administered to at least 325,000 people, and perhaps more than half a million people, in equatorial Africa from 1957 to 1960. There are no existing records that establish the source of the kidneys used to grow the virus. Hooper has found evidence showing that chimpanzee kidneys were used for some lots of the vaccine. Koprowski denies this.

Although Koprowski had reported in an interview with Curtis that there was no remaining vaccine to test, in February 2000, scientists at the Wistar Institute announced that they tested a phial of the original vaccine and that it showed no trace of either HIV or chimp DNA. However, the vials submitted for testing may have been seed lots, and if in fact they were vials of the original vaccine, it is likely that not all vials were contaminated. Critics of the Wistar report note that no vials of the vaccines produced in Belgium or the Congo were tested. Of interest, in 1959, Dr. Jonas Salk, who was researching polio vaccines at the same time, reported in the *British Medical Journal* that he had isolated but not identified an unidentified cell-killing virus in the Chat vaccine.

In his 1999 book *The River: A Journey to the Source of HIV and AIDS*, Hooper writes that he is pursuing this information so that "we might learn more about where and when the initial introduction of HIV into North American actually occurred."

In response, officials from Wistar described a person who had been infected with HIV in 1950 before the CHAT campaign. However, subsequent analysis of the blood specimen by Dr. David Ho of the Aaron Diamond Institute showed that the person in question had not been infected with HIV, but that the sample had been contaminated during the testing process with the blood of another patient who had HIV. To date there is no evidence of anyone being infected with HIV before the oral polio campaign was initiated. And while it was widely assumed that the debate over the origin of AIDS had been settled with the Wistar report showing no evidence of HIV in the specimens they tested, this matter has not yet been resolved. In 2001, the Royal Society of London investigated the claims and found that while it was possible, they did not have enough evidence to support Hooper's theory.

In November 1991, an article in *Nature* offered another hypothesis: that the disease may have sprung from scientific experiments that lasted from 1922 into the 1950s in which chimpanzee and monkey blood was directly injected into 70 human beings to see if people could carry the form of the malaria parasite that infests those primates.

In addition, there are numerous reports of researchers who have died from exposure to monkey viruses during the course of their work. In mid–1967 many researchers became ill and 7 died after being exposed to the Marburg virus, which was traced to monkeys shipped from Uganda. It has also been established that simian viruses that cross species to cause disease in man do not cause the same symptoms in primates.

The most convincing argument to date is that early trials of live Hepatitis B vaccine (1978–1980) recruited gay men from New York City. This vaccine was also given to African natives in the regions where AIDS is now endemic. This idea was first suggested by Leonard Horowitz, a Harvard physician specializing in public health. Chimpanzees were used to make the hepatitis B vaccine, and AIDS first erupted in New York City gay men in 1979 a few months after the experiment began in Manhattan. Of those gay men who volunteered for the study, as many as 20 percent were infected with HIV by 1981, and by 1984, 64 percent of the vaccine recipients had AIDS.

Also, scientists involved in the Special Virus Cancer Program had previously worked with chimp viruses. Dr. Robert Gallo, partially credited for discovering the AIDS virus, had worked in this program, where viral contamination often occurred. Eight subtypes of HIV have been found, and each one is targeted for a different group. For instance, HIV-2 is most likely to target vaginal tissue, and in Africa most cases of HIV-2 occur through heterosexual transmission. In the U.S., the subtype and clade most prominently seen targets rectal tissue. In April 2003, delegates from Amnesty International, USA met to discuss this theory. The investigation continues and reports of AIDS being associated with vaccines are held by the U.S. Department of Justice and unavailable.

If HIV had been transmitted unintentionally, it would not have been the first time a simian virus had been accidentally transmitted. In 1961, batches of Salk and Sabin vaccine given to millions worldwide were contaminated with SV40, a monkey virus that causes cancer in hamsters and is suspected of causing brain tumors in humans. As for the first HIV positive specimen dating back to 1959, a careful review of the data shows that only two HIV genes were seen, which would be considered indeterminate at best.

Factors Causing the Pandemic

Several reasons have been given for the rapid spread of HIV and the resulting pandemic, such as international travel, the blood industry, and drug use. International travel has been highlighted in the case of "Patient Zero," a Canadian flight attendant named Gaetan Dugas who traveled extensively worldwide. Analysis of several early cases of AIDS showed that the infected individuals were either direct or indirect sexual contacts of Dugas. This was one of the first clues investigators had that AIDS was caused by a single transmissible agent.

As blood transfusions became a routine part of medical practice, the blood industry emerged. To meet the demand for blood, in the U.S. donors were usually paid, and intravenous drug users frequently donated blood. This blood was sent worldwide, and in 1960 the blood industry began concentrating Factor VIII for the treatment of hemophiliacs. Rudimentary screening tests for hepatitis were performed, but blood was not screened for HIV, a virus that no one had heard of until 1983.

The availability of heroin following the Vietnam War, and other conflicts in the Middle East, led to a new generation of heroin users. The development of plastic syringes and the emergence of shooting galleries where people could buy drugs and rent equipment provided another route for disease transmission.

The Emergence of AIDS

By March 1981, the unusual occurrence of Kaposi's sarcoma was reported in at least eight young gay men in New York City. About this time, physicians began seeing increasing numbers of *Pneumocystis jiroveci* pneumonia (PCP) in California and New York. A drug technician, Sandra Ford, reported in *Newsweek* that she had noticed a high number of requests for the drug pentamidine used in the treatment of PCP. In June 1981, the CDC published a report of five men in Los Angeles with PCP. This report is often referred to as the beginning of the AIDS epidemic. A few days later, the CDC formed the Task Force on Kaposi's Sarcoma and Opportunistic Infections (KSOI).

Around this time a number of theories were introduced regarding the possible causes of these infections. Early theories included infection with cytomegalovirus and the use of amyl nitrite or butyl nitrite "poppers," which were widely used in the gay community. In July 1981, Dr. Curran of the CDC in describing this new infection reported that there was no apparent danger to non-homosexuals from contagion. By December 1981, it was clear that this was incorrect, because the first cases of PCP were reported in intravenous drug users.

The disease still did not have a name. The CDC referred to it by its symptoms, for instance "lymphadenopathy syndrome" for the swollen glands often seen in infected patients, and sometimes they referred to it as KSOI for the Task Force. The British medical journal, *Lancet*, referred to it as the "gay compromise syndrome," while newspapers began calling it the *gay disease, gay cancer* or *gay-related immune deficiency*.

By the beginning of July 1982, a total of 452 cases from 23 states had been reported to the CDC. Later in July, the disease was reported in Haitians and also hemophiliacs. By August 1982, the new disease was called AIDS or acquired immune deficiency syndrome. Doctors approved this name because it suggested that people acquired rather than inherited this condition.

By 1982, a number of AIDS voluntary organizations had emerged in the U.S. including the San Francisco AIDS Foundation, AIDS Project Los Angeles, and Gay Men's Health Crisis (GMHC). In November 1982, the first AIDS organization was set up in the UK, the Terry Higgins Trust. In December 1982, a 20-month-old child who had received multiple blood product transfusions died from infections related to AIDS. That month, the CDC also reported the first cases of possible mother-to-child transmission.

At that point there was genuine fear that anyone could acquire AIDS. Hospitals began to refuse treatment for patients suspected of having AIDS. Laboratories and medical staff increased their efforts to prevent blood exposures. Law enforcement agencies began using masks and gloves when responding to calls regarding possible AIDS suspects. Landlords begin evicting individuals with AIDS and the Social Security Administration began interviewing clients by phone rather than in person.

In early 1983, the CDC reported that AIDS could be spread heterosexually from men to women. In May 1983, researchers at the Institut Pasteur in France isolated the AIDS virus, which they called lymphadenopathy-associated virus or LAV. France applied for patent rights for a blood test and sent a sample of LAV to the National Cancer Institute. In October 1983, WHO held its annual meeting in Denmark. Here, it was reported that there had been 2,803 AIDS cases in the United States. AIDS in Central Africa was investigated in 1984 and the incidence of AIDS there strongly suggested heterosexual transmission. The CDC investigated Patient Zero that year and established a transmissible route of infection. In April 1984, Dr. Mason of the CDC reported that they had found the cause of AIDS based on the French reports. The next day, on April 23, 1984, United States Health and Human Services Secretary Margaret Heckler announced that Dr. Robert Gallo of the National Cancer Institute had isolated the AIDS virus, which he named HTLV-III, confusing it as an HTLV

virus. Heckler also announced that an AIDS vaccine would be ready in about two years. The same day, Gallo filed a patent application for his work, although it was clear that LAV and HTLV-III were the same virus. By the end of 1984, there had been 7,699 reports of AIDS and 3,665 deaths from AIDS in the United States. An additional 762 cases had been reported in Europe. In the United Kingdom there had been 108 reported cases and 46 deaths.

In March 1985, the FDA licensed the first blood test for AIDS based on Gallo's HTLV-III application. The FDA also announced that anyone with antibodies to HTLV-III in his or her blood would no longer be able to donate blood. Problems regarding patient confidentiality emerged and many individuals found that a positive HIV test could mean more than medical problems. Reports of people being infected from contaminated blood products continued until it was determined that the HTLV-III test lacked specificity and sensitivity. It was also determined that Gallo's isolate had somehow been contaminated with the French LAV strain.

Because the French waited for their blood test patent to be approved, testing of the French blood supply was delayed. French blood banking officials were fined for negligence, but the charges were later removed. The U.S. eventually agreed to share patent royalties for the early AIDS test with the French in light of the fact that the French had applied for the patent earlier and had been the first to isolate the AIDS virus. In May 1986, the International Committee on the Taxonomy of Viruses ruled that the names HTLV-III and LAV should be dropped. The AIDS virus was christened human immunodeficiency virus (HIV).

Blaming the Victim

Inaccurate statements propagated by CDC officials and fueled by the media caused many people to regard the gay population as the source or cause of AIDS, while hemophiliacs were considered victims. Still, the plight of Ryan White, who contracted AIDS through a blood transfusion, illustrates how people with AIDS were generally mistreated because of fear and misinformation. When Ryan White's heroic struggle to lead a normal life was broadcast on national network television, people's perceptions of AIDS began to change. A number of celebrities began working with AIDS voluntary organizations to raise funds and broaden research efforts. In August 1986, the U.S. government accused a hospital of discrimination for dismissing a nurse with AIDS and refusing to offer him an alternative job. In a court ruling that marked a change in the times, this job dismissal was seen as a violation of the nurse's civil rights.

The Social Context

In 1987 ACT UP was founded by the gay community in New York with demands for better AIDS services, including the availability of antiretroviral drugs, increased research efforts, increased educational efforts regarding safe sex, and humanitarian treatment for those with AIDS. In Australia, the Grim Reaper education campaign was launched, with television images of death mowing down a range of victims in a bowling alley. Although this campaign was widely criticized at the time, it proved to be very effective in bringing awareness to the AIDS crisis.

In April 1987, President Ronald Reagan made his first major speech on AIDS in which he addressed the Philadelphia College of Physicians and Surgeons and advocated a modest federal role in AIDS education, with an emphasis on sexual abstinence. About this time the World Health Organization (WHO) developed a Global AIDS strategy, which included the advice that all countries have a supportive and non-discriminatory social environment. However, on May 31, 1987, President Reagan spoke at an American Foundation for AIDS Research dinner and focused on increasing both routine and compulsory AIDS testing. The following day when Vice President George Bush opened the Third International Conference on AIDS in Washington, DC, and defended these testing proposals, the audience booed him. At a demonstration in front of the White House, police officials wearing long yellow gloves arrested demonstrators, an image displayed on the news worldwide.

In June 1987, the U.S. Public Health Service added AIDS to its list of diseases for which people could be barred entry to the United States. In July, Senator Jesse Helms proposed that this include anyone testing HIV-positive. Although this policy has been widely criticized, it continues to exist.

In July 1987, the United Kingdom expanded its syringe exchange programs, and the Ray family in Arcadia, Florida, a family with three HIV-infected hemophiliac sons, was told that their sons could no longer attend school. After the family moved to Alabama, they were still denied school admission and their home was torched and burned. In August 1987, the book *And the Band Played On*, by Randy Shilts, which documented the AIDS epidemic, was released. Although scholars have criticized certain details, the book is generally regarded as an accurate portrayal of the early years of the AIDS epidemic.

In May 1988, Surgeon General C. Everett Koop released his informational pamphlet, *Understanding AIDS*, which was widely distributed and read in the U.S. and helped the public understand that AIDS was a virus that could infect anyone. In June 1988, the Presidential Commission on the HIV Epidemic reported that the FDA arrangements for drug approval were not meeting the needs of the people with AIDS. In response, ACT UP demonstrators virtually shut down FDA headquarters in October 1988. Eight days after the demonstration, the FDA announced new regulations that accelerated drug approval for conditions lacking sufficient therapies.

In November 1988, the first syringe

exchange was started to reduce HIV transmission through drug use in New York City and San Francisco. Despite the success of these programs, Congress prohibited the use of federal funds to support needle exchange programs.

In April 1989, a Dutch man with AIDS, Hans Verhoef, was jailed in Minnesota under the federal law banning travelers with HIV from entering the United States. In June, at the Fifth International Conference on AIDS in Montreal, 250 protestors stormed the stage criticizing the U.S. travel law. Protests about the U.S. travel ban continued, and many people boycotted the 6th International AIDS Conference held in San Francisco. Of those who attended, many speakers criticized the U.S. for its travel restrictions. June Osborn, the chair of the National Commission on AIDS, called the policy misguided and irrational. The International AIDS Society (IAS) announced that no further IAS sponsored conference would be held in a country that restricted HIV-infected travelers. As a result, no major international AIDS conference has been held in the U.S. since 1990.

In early 1991, the CDC published a report confirming that an AIDS patient, Kimberly Bergalis, had been infected by her dentist, David Acer, during a dental procedure, and that two other patients had probably also been infected. Later that year, Earvin (Magic) Johnson announced that he had tested positive for HIV and was retiring from basketball. His educational efforts, especially with the young, have been influential in communicating that anyone can get AIDS. Later that year in the UK, Freddie Mercury, the lead singer of the rock group Queen, confirmed that he had AIDS. He died a day after his announcement. The red ribbon became an international symbol of AIDS awareness in 1991 after the organization Visual AIDS in New York joined with Broadway Cares, and Equity Fights AIDS to promote AIDS awareness. The red ribbon continues to signify support for people living with HIV/

AIDS. In 1992 the 8th International Conference cancelled its scheduled appearance in Boston because of the U.S. travel policy. The conference was held in Amsterdam.

Although the U.S. travel policy still exists, attitudes regarding AIDS have changed. People with AIDS are not as blatantly discriminated against, although there is a significant disparity among medical services provided to minority populations. With Healthy Project 2010, the CDC aims to provide equal health services to all people. With the introduction of effective antiretroviral therapies, the mortality associated with AIDS has declined, although it is still the leading cause of death in many minority groups.

Federal Government's Response

The federal government's response to AIDS in the 1980s was extremely inadequate to meet the growing epidemic. Representatives of both the CDC and the U.S. Department of Health & Human Services erred in reporting that the heterosexual community was not at risk and that researchers were close to finding both a cure and a vaccine to prevent AIDS. Delays and misinformation led to the development of blood tests for HIV that lacked sensitivity and specificity, to the detriment of the nation's blood supply. Even with today's highly sophisticated tests for HIV, in 2002 there were isolated instances in which people became infected with HIV as a result of contaminated blood products.

The federal government finally acknowledged the AIDS crisis and the need for comprehensive services with the Fair Housing Act of 1988 and the passage of the Ryan White CARE Act in 1990. That act now provides more than $1.9 billion of vital services for people living with HIV/AIDS, including drug treatments, primary medical care, and essential supportive services. The Americans with Disabilities Act of 1990 also helps in that it prohibits discrimination based on disability, including HIV/AIDS. The federal government also sponsors research and provides preventive and treatment services through the National Institutes of Health, the U.S. Public Health Service, and the Centers for Disease Control and Prevention.

However, critics wonder how much of the $15 billion President George W. Bush pledged over five years in 2002 targeted for Global AIDS will be paid. Many existing programs, including those providing state assistance, experienced budget cuts in 2002–2003. Furthermore, syringe exchange programs still cannot be funded with federal dollars despite studies showing they reduce the incidence of STD transmission. *See also* ACT UP; AIDS Quilt; **Syringe exchange programs; Ryan White Comprehensive AIDS Emergency Act; and White, Ryan**.

Beggars, Omar. *HIV and Molecular Immunity: Prospects for the AIDS Vaccine*. Natick, MA: Biotechnology Books, 1999.
Curtis, Tom. "The Origin of AIDS." *Rolling Stone*, March 19th, 1992.
Hooper, Edward. *The River: A Journey Back to the Source of HIV & AIDS*. New York: Penguin, 1999.
Grmek, Marko D. *History of AIDS*. Princeton, NJ: Princeton University Press, 1990.
Horowitz, Leonard. "The Origin of AIDS and HIV May Not Be What You have Learned. http://www.originofaids.com.
_____. "Hepatitis B Vaccine and the Origin of HIV/AIDS: Perspectives on a Possible Vaccine Induced Endemic." May 29, 2001, oral presentation available at http://www.whale.to/m/horo.html.
Martin, Brian, and Tom Keske. "Statistical Analysis Linking U.S. AIDS Outbreak to Hepatitis Experiments. http:www.whale.to/v/keske1.1.html; "Polio Vaccines and the Origins of AIDS," *Townsend Letter for Doctors*, Jan. 1994, No. 26: 97–100.

AIDS Quilt

In February 1987, in San Francisco, gay rights activist Cleve Jones made the first panel for the AIDS Memorial Quilt in memory of his friend Marvin Feldman. Along with Mike Smith, Jones also founded The Names Project AIDS Foundation. The project's mission is to use the AIDS Memorial Quilt to bring an end to AIDS. The project's goal is to provide a creative means for remembrance and healing.

The AIDS Quilt, which is made of 3 × 6 foot individual panels, provides a memorial to those who have died of AIDS. As of March 2003, 5,644 blocks of eight panels have been created. The quilt was first displayed in October 1987, in the National Mall in Washington, D.C., and was completely displayed for the last time in October 1996, at which time it covered the entire National Mall in Washington, D.C. The AIDS Quilt was nominated for a Nobel Peace Prize in 1989, and has raised more than $3 million toward AIDS research. Headquartered in Atlanta, the Names Project has 23 chapters in the United States and 40 affiliate chapters in other countries. For more information see http://www.aidsquilt.org or call (404) 688-5500.

AIDS-related complex (ARC)

AIDS-related complex is an older term used to describe a syndrome characterized by symptoms that typically occur in patients with early HIV infection before they develop AIDS. These symptoms include swollen lymph nodes (progressive generalized lymphadenopathy or PGL), night sweats, recurrent fever, oral hairy leukoplakia, fungus infection of the mouth and throat, and diarrhea. Patients with ARC may have HIV antibodies, chronic deficiency of white blood cells (leukopenia), or a poorly functioning lymphatic system. Symptoms associated with ARC are typically less severe than the symptoms that occur when AIDS develops and are not associated with the opportunistic infections required for a diagnosis of AIDS. *See also* **Lymphadenopathy syndrome**.

AIDS-related primary central nervous system lymphoma

Primary central nervous system lymphoma (PCNSL) is a major complication seen in the late stages of AIDS. A type of large B-cell lymphoma, PCNSL affects the central nervous system and represents a major cause of death among AIDS patients. The Epstein-Barr Virus is seen in nearly all AIDS-related PBNSL lesions, which suggests that the EBV virus may play a role in disease development. Studies so far suggest that latent EBV may be re-activated in patients with immune suppression. A relationship to HHV-8 was once suspected, but several studies have concluded that HHV-8 does not contribute to PCNSL development.

AIDS Vaccine Evaluation Group (AVEG)

Sponsored by the National Institute of Allergy and Infectious Diseases (NIAID) division of the National Institutes of Health (NIH), AVEG is a network that conducts trials of experimental HIV vaccines at research centers called AIDS Vaccine Evaluation Units (AVEU) located at research centers throughout the United States.

AIDS Vaccine Evaluation Units (AVEU)

Sponsored by the National Institute of Allergy and Infectious Diseases (NIAID) division of the National Institutes of Health (NIH), AVEU are specialized research centers that conduct trials with AIDS vaccines.

AIDS vaccines

A safe, effective preventive vaccine for AIDS has not yet been identified although there is a great deal of ongoing research in this area and a number of experimental vaccines are being tested in clinical trials. An AIDS vaccine represents the best long-term hope for the control of AIDS.

An ideal AIDS vaccine would prevent HIV infection or limit it to a transient asymptomatic (not associated with any symptoms) infection that is unlikely to be transmitted to others. The goal of completely preventing infection may be impossible to achieve, but, as in other infectious diseases, limiting and eradicating the infection may be sufficient. The ability of the HIV vaccine to rapidly mutate causing great genetic diversity within the species is one of the major obstacles to developing an effective vaccine. Progress is also hindered by the complexity of the virus-host interaction and a general lack of understanding regarding this interaction.

Despite these uncertainties, the first phase I trial of an HIV vaccine was conducted in the United States in 1987. Since then, more than 30 candidate vaccine have been tested in more than 70 phase I/II clinical trial both in the U.S. and in developing countries. Phase III trials of VaxGen's AIDSVAX conducted in Thailand and the U.S, have been disappointing. (see the VaxGen website for more information, http://www.vaxgen.com).

The HIV vaccine development program has followed three major overlapping paradigms. The first was directed at inducing neutralizing antibodies. The second aimed at stimulating CD8+ T lymphocyte cell responses. The newest strategies aim to optimize both the humoral and cellular immune response. In light of the success seen in trials with monkeys tested with SIV vaccines, one of the new strategies focuses on recombinant DNA and RNA viruses.

Scientists at the Dale and Betty Bumpers Vaccine Research Center (VRC), part of the National Institute of Allergy and Infectious Diseases, have introduced a new vaccine in November 2002 that incorporates HIV genetic material from the three most common HIV clades. This trial vaccine is a DNA vaccine, similar to vaccines previously found safe in clinical trials. The first phase of the trial, which is being conducted at the NIH in Bethesda, MD, will enroll 50 participants to test the vaccine's safety. Expanded tests are planned for several domestic sites as well as sites in Haiti and South Africa. For more information, including ways to volunteer, interested persons can call toll-free 1-866-833-5543 or TTY 1-866-411-1010 or they can email vrcforlife@mail.nih.gov.

Reports from the WHO-UNAIDS Vaccine Initiative address the challenge of distributing an effective vaccine worldwide if one is developed. Depending on the efficacy of the vaccine, especially if it is only 30 percent effective, the incidence of AIDS could rise as a result of false expectations. Finding candidates for vaccine trials brings its own set of problems. Informed consents for participants in developing countries need to be tested to assure that participants understand all aspects of the trials particularly that experimental vaccines do not mean they are protected from HIV infection. Participants in vaccine trials can also have false-positive test results for HIV antibodies. (Andrew J McMichael & Tomas Hanke, "HIV vaccines 1983–2003," *Nature Medicine*; 9(7) July 2003; NIAID News Press Release, Nov 02, "New Vaccine Holds Promise of Global Effectiveness," http://ww.niadid.nih.gov/newsroom/releases/newhivvacc.htm; International AIDS Vaccine Initiative, http://www.iavi.org).

AIDS wasting syndrome *see* Wasting syndrome

AIDS/HIV

AIDS/HIV is a term used to describe the disease caused by HIV infection that occurs both before and after the development of AIDS. Federal programs designed to help individuals with AIDS include provisions for individuals who have been infected with HIV but have not yet developed AIDS.

AIN *see* Anal intraepithelial neoplasia

Alaska natives

The U.S. Department of Health & Human Services helps to meet the health care needs of Alaska natives with HIV/AIDS through direct health services contracted by tribes and urban Indian health programs. Information on these programs can be found on the Internet at http://www.his.gov/MedicalPrograms/AIDS/.

Alkaline phosphatase

Alkaline phosphatase is an enzyme normally found in certain cells within the liver, bone, kidney, intestine, and placenta. When cells of these organs are destroyed, more of this enzyme leaks into the blood circulation, and alkaline phosphatase levels are elevated. In hepatitis and other diseases causing liver damage, alkaline phosphatase levels are used to assess liver health.

Allopathic medicine

Allopathic medicine is a term describing the use of conventional Western medical principles. Allopathic medicine is traditionally used to describe a system in which illness or disease is treated by producing a second condition that is antagonistic toward or incompatible with the first disorder. An example is an antibiotic used to treat an infection.

Alpha defensins

Alpha defensins or Human Neutrophil Proteins have three subtypes, alpha defensins 1–3. Defensins are cysteine-rich, carbohydrate-free molecules produced by neutrophils and macrophages (types of white blood cells). Defensins are able to chemically influence monocytes, and they possess cytotoxic (capable of destroying other cells) and antimicrobial activities.

Studies suggest that the binding of defensins to certain other macroglobulin protein receptors on macrophage cells can downregulate the inflammatory response to various pathogens. In 2002, scientists discovered that the one to two percent of people infected with HIV who have not yet developed AIDS have high levels of alpha defensin proteins. Termed non-progressors, these people, who have been studied since the early years of the epidemic, remain HIV positive but have not yet developed AIDS.

Alpha interferon (Interferon alpha, IFN-α)

Alpha interferon is one of three major classes of interferon chemicals secreted by the immune system in response to infection. In persons who are HIV positive, elevated interferon levels are regarded as an indication of disease progression. Synthetic alpha interferon compounds are used in the treatment of hepatitis in an effort to make the immune system work more effectively.

Alpha lipoic acid (ALA)

The dietary supplement alpha lipoic acid was recently investigated in NCCAM clinical trials for its value in HIV-infected persons unresponsive to HAART therapy. Because anti-retroviral drugs do not fully restore the immune system and patients often fail multi-drug treatment, there is a need for alternative and complementary medicine that can restore an immune system ravaged by HIV/AIDS. The use of ALA is based on the premise of a widespread deficiency of glutathione, which is vital to lymphocyte function, in patients with HIV/AIDS. Participants are still being recruited for this study, which is being held in San Jose, CA. For more information contact Brenda Cayme at 408-393-3207 or search the trial, Immune restoration by lipoic acid in AIDS, at http://clinicaltrials.gov

Alternative medicine

Alternative medicine, which is also known as complementary medicine, includes treatments that are not considered standard procedure in most Western countries, such as homeopathy, Traditional Chinese medicine (TCM), acupuncture and herbal medicine. Alternative medicine focuses on lifestyle changes, energy medicine, herbal medicines, and homeopathic preparations, as well as aromatherapy, bright light therapy, and spiritual healing.

The National Center for Complementary and Alternative Medicine (NCCAM), a branch of the National Institutes of Health, researches the use of alternative medicine in clinical trials. Currently, NCCAM is conducting nine clinical trials involving the use of complementary medicine in HIV at various locations throughout the country. For more information, see www.nccam.nih.gov/.

Alvac-HIV

Alvac-HIV is a genetically engineered HIV vaccine composed of a live, weakened canarypox virus into which parts of genes for non-infectious components of HIV have been inserted. When ALVAC infects a human cell, the inserted HIV genes direct the cell to make HIV proteins. These proteins are packaged into non-infectious HIV-like particles that bud from the cell membrane. These particles fool the immune system into mounting an immune response to HIV, primarily producing antibodies designed to fight HIV during a subsequent exposure to the virus. ALVAC can infect but not grow in human cells, which is an important safety feature.

Amebiasis

Amebiasis is an inflammation of the intestines caused by infestation with the ameba *Entamoeba histolytica*. Frequent, loose stools flecked with blood and mucus are typically seen in amebiasis. Amebiasis can occur as an opportunistic infection in patients with HIV infection.

Ameliorative therapy

Ameliorative therapies are treatments used to relieve symptoms; also known as palliative treatments, ameliorative therapies do not cure diseases but they make conditions better or more tolerable.

American Indians

The U.S. Department of Health & Human Services helps to meet the health care needs of American Indians with HIV/AIDS through direct health services contracted by tribes and urban Indian health programs. Information on these programs can be found on the Internet at http://www.his.gov/MedicalPrograms/AIDS/.

American Social Health Association (ASHA)

ASHA was founded in 1914 by a group of public health reformers committed to attacking what they perceived as an undesirable social condition (the incidence of STDs) that they believed could be improved through medical and educational means. Since this time ASHA has introduced school sex education programs, mounted educational campaigns to change behavior, testified before Congress, and lobbied to reduce high medical costs associated with disease control. ASHA also awards research grants and sponsors fellowships for postdoctoral studies in infectious disease control. ASHA was responsible for the passage of the Venereal Disease Control Act in 1938, and continues to study trends in STD rates while it engages in preventive efforts. ASHA sponsors resource centers and hotlines for many STDs, including herpes, syphilis and HIV. For more information see http://www.ashastd.org/.

Amino acids

Amino acids are the building blocks that make up proteins. There are 22 amino acids found in animals and humans, and each amino acid has its own three-letter DNA code or codon. For example, the nucleotide string C-T-C represents the amino acid leucine. Because the nucleotides may be in a variety of different orders or positions, each amino acid may have more than one codon. DNA is transcribed into messenger RNA. Transfer RNA brings the appropriate amino acids together to produce a protein.

Amniocentesis

Amniocentesis is a procedure in which a needle is used to withdraw amniotic fluid from the amniotic sac that surrounds the fetus in the uterus. During pregnancy, amniotic fluid is sometimes tested for signs of fetal maturity and infection and for the presence of certain genetic markers.

Amniotic fluid

Amniotic fluid is fluid contained within the amnion, or innermost membrane of the uterus that envelopes the fetus during pregnancy. Amniotic fluid can be infected with organisms associated with certain STDs if the mother has an infection during pregnancy.

Amphotericin B

Amphotericin B is an antibiotic drug used to treat disseminated fungal infections, such as cryptococcidiosis. Amphotericin B can have severe side effects including fever, chills, nausea, kidney toxicity, and bone marrow suppression. Toxicity may be reduced by administering the drug in a lipid-soluble form.

Amsler grid

The Amsler grid is a diagram of squares used to assess vision. Defects in the central visual field, including those caused by CMV retinitis, which is associated with cytomegalovirus infection, may be detected as breaks or unevenness in the lines of the grid.

Amyl nitrite

Amyl nitrite (popper) is a drug used as a vasodilator since 1859. In the 1980s, it became widely used as a sexual stimulant, especially in the gay population. At the beginning of the AIDS epidemic, some researchers suspected amyl nitrite as a cause. With the discovery of the HIV virus, this idea was disproved.

Anal cancer *see* Anal intraepithelial neoplasia (AIN)

Anal intercourse

Anal intercourse involves penile insertion into the partner's anus. Anal intercourse is a strong risk factor for the transmission of STDs, particularly the HIV virus. Condoms provide some protection, but the surgeon general reports that anal intercourse is still a dangerous practice, and condoms are more likely to break because of the greater amount of friction. In anal intercourse, the anus is subject to small tears, which facilitates the entry of infectious organisms directly into the bloodstream.

Anal intraepithelial neoplasia (AIN)

Anal intraepithelial neoplasia is an early form of anal cancer caused by certain strains of the human papilloma virus (HPV), particularly types 16 and 18. High grade AIN has been reported in 0.5 to 5.4 percent of HIV negative homosexual men and four to 15.2 percent of HIV positive men. The risk of AIN is reported to be 2.9 times higher in HIV positive men who have a CD4 count lower than 500 cells/mm^3

compared to men with CD4 counts higher than 500 cells/mm^3.

Kiviat, N.B., et al. "Association of anal dysplasia and human papillomavirus with immunosuppression and HIV infection among homosexual men." *AIDS* 7:43–49, 1993.

Anal lesions *see* Condylomata acuminata and Granuloma inguinale

Anal sex

Anal sex refers to insertion of the penis into the anus of both men and women. Anal sex carries a high risk of STD, particularly HIV, transmission because the anal area is likely to have small tears, facilitating entry of virus present in semen directly into the blood circulation. *See also* **Anal intercourse.**

Anal warts *see* Condylomata acuminata, Genital warts, and Human papilloma virus (HPV)

Anergy

Anergy refers to the loss or weakening of the body's immunity to an irritating agent, or antigen. Patients who are immunologically suppressed may be unable to produce a reaction to an antigen. For example, such patients may not produce a reaction to an antigen such as tuberculosis on a tuberculin (Mantoux) skin test. The lack of a reaction indicates anergy.

Researchers have shown that CD4+ T cells can be turned off by a signal from HIV that leaves them unable to respond to further immune system stimulation.

Angiogenesis

Angiogenesis is the process of forming new blood vessels. Angiogenesis is essential for the growth of tumors, especially Kaposi's sarcoma. Angiostatic agents are drugs that interfere with the ability of tumors to form new blood vessels.

Antibiotics

Antibiotics are naturally derived or synthetic chemical agents produced by various species of microorganisms (bacteria, fungi, actinomycetes), which are used to suppress or destroy other microorganisms. Antibiotics generally target certain related strains of bacteria and fungi, although some antibiotics are broad-spectrum, meaning that they are effective against a variety of gram negative and gram-positive bacteria. *See also* **Bacteria**; **Drug resistance**; and **Gram stain**.

Antibody

Antibodies are immunoglobulin proteins produced by the immune system in response to invasion by foreign molecules known as antigens. Antibody production is directed by T lymphocytes and carried out by B lymphocytes. Antibodies are specifically designed to react with or destroy the specific antigens that caused their production. Antibodies are identified on the basis of the infectious agent they target. For instance, antibodies produced in response to hepatitis B vaccines or infection are known as hepatitis B antibodies.

Antibodies remain long after the initial exposure to antigens. Many infectious diseases can be diagnosed by the presence of antibodies to specific organisms. Neutralizing antibodies destroy or inactivate infectious agents usually by blocking receptors on the cells or the virus, while enhancing antibodies promote infection. Although it has not been proved, enhancing antibodies are suspected of enhancing the ability of HIV to produce disease. Theoretically, enhancing antibodies could attach to HIV virions and enable macrophages to engulf the viruses. However, instead of being destroyed, the engulfed virus may remain alive within the macrophage. Macrophages then are able to carry the virus to other parts of the body.

Vaccines, which contain inactivated antigens, elicit the production of protective antibodies. Protective antibodies are intended to ward off infection on subsequent exposures to the antigen. Because antibodies generally prevent a subsequent infection, they are said to confer immunity.

Antibody-positive

Many diagnostic tests for infectious agents are designed to detect the presence of specific antibodies. After exposure to infectious or toxic agents, the immune system responds by producing specific antibodies against these agents. These antibodies can be used as diagnostic disease markers. For instance, a positive antibody test for HIV indicates past exposure to HIV or HIV infection. People who test positive for HIV antibodies for HIV are said to be HIV seropositive or seropositive for HIV. *See also* **Seroconversion** and **Seropositive**.

Anticonvulsant

Anticonvulsants are medications, such as phenytoin (Dilantin) used to prevent or lessen convulsions or seizures. Some anticonvulsants also have analgesic and antidepressant effects and may be used as adjuvant therapies for some STDs.

Antigens

Antigens are substances such as pollen or viral particles that can elicit an immune response. Although most antigens are proteins, antigens may be carbohydrates or lipids. When the immune system encounters foreign antigens, it reacts by producing specific antibodies capable of reacting with the antigen. The presence of antigenic proteins or DNA associated with specific STD organisms can be used as a specific disease marker for the diagnosis of acute or active infection.

Antiretroviral drug resistance

Viruses can mutate into strains that are resistant to specific antiretroviral agents. For instance, certain strains of HIV have become resistant to the drug AZT. Treatment failure usually reflects resistance to one or more of the drugs used in the patient's treatment protocol.

Antiretroviral drugs

Antiretroviral drugs are agents, such as zidovudine (AZT), that fight against retroviruses, including HIV. Many antiretroviral drugs are able to suppress the activity or replication of retroviruses. Antiretroviral drugs may be used as a specific therapy, or as part of a protocol in which several drugs are administered simultaneously. Some antiretrovirals are directed at specific stages of the viral life cycle. For example, reverse transcriptase inhibitors interfere with the reverse transcriptase enzyme necessary for RNA replication, and protease inhibitors with the translation of viral DNA.

Patients with HIV infection starting on antiretroviral drug therapy usually begin with two nucleoside reverse transcriptase inhibitors along with a third agent, consisting of another nucleoside reverse transcriptase inhibitor, a non-nucleoside reverse transcriptase inhibitor, or a protease inhibitor. A combination of three drugs is usually necessary to reduce the viral load to below-detectable levels. This is necessary to prevent the development of a resistant viral strain. *See also* **Antiretroviral drug resistance; Genotype (Genotypic) assay; Highly active antiretroviral therapy (HHART); Lipodystrophy; Non-nucleoside reverse transcriptase inhibitors (NNRTIs); Nucleoside/nucleotide reverse transcriptase inhibitors (NRTIs); Phenotype assay; and Protease inhibitors.**

Antisense

Antisense is a complementary piece of genetic material (DNA or RNA) that binds to another piece of DNA or RNA by base-pairing, preventing that DNA/RNA fragment from being used to synthesize new proteins. HIV antisense therapy uses a sequence of oligonucleotides that bind to HIV messenger RNA and block viral replication.

Antiviral Agents

Antiviral agents are medications that interfere with the life cycle of a virus. Antiviral agents also suppress viral replication or activity. *See also* **Antiretroviral drugs.**

Apthous ulcer (canker sore)

Apthous ulcers are small, often painful, shallow lesions that develop on the mucous membranes lining the mouth, esophagus or rectum. Recurrent aphthous ulcers (RAU) reappear frequently and are often unresponsive to treatment.

Arm

In clinical trials, arm refers to a cohort or group of participants who receive the same treatment; if given the treatment, they represent the treatment arm, whereas if they are given the control or placebo, they represent the control arm.

Arsenic

Arsenic compounds were used in the early 1900s as a syphilis treatment, although their toxicity often interfered with their effectiveness. The use of arsenic therapy ended with the discovery of penicillin. In 1943 penicillin was found to be an effective treatment for syphilis, and it has since remained the treatment of choice. *See also* **Salvarsan.**

Aspergillosis

Aspergillosis is an uncommon life-threatening infection caused by fungus of the *Aspergillus* family. Aspergillosis may occur in immunosuppressed individuals, including AIDS patients. If infection reaches the brain, it may cause dementia.

Etiology

The etiologic agent includes fungi of the *Aspergillus* species.

Epidemiology

Aspergillosis is increasingly seen in patients with advanced HIV disease and is considered an AIDS-defining illness.

Symptoms

Symptoms include cough, chest pain, fever, chills, respiratory tract disease, central nervous system infection, and breathing difficulty. Aspergillosis typically infects the lungs and sinuses, but can spread through the blood to other organs including the brain, heart, and spleen. Aspergilli have a tendency to invade blood vessels and cause infection, chest pain, and blood-tinged respiratory secretions.

Patients with central nervous system involvement usually have symptoms similar to that of a mass lesion or stroke due to the invasion of blood vessels. Symptoms include seizures and focal abnormalities. CT or MRI imaging tests may show single or multiple lesions, with bony invasion that may have spread from the sinuses. Sinus imaging films may also be abnormal. Patients with fungal sinusitis usually have classical features of fever, facial pain and swelling, nasal discharge, and headache. Often there is a history of recent sinus infection treated with broad-spectrum antibiotics.

The prognosis in aspergillosis is related to the fact that this fungal infection tends to occur in patients with advanced AIDS who may have other complications of end-stage HIV infection. Typically, in AIDS patients, treatment response is poor and death may occur within 2–4 months after diagnosis.

Diagnosis

Diagnosing invasive pulmonary aspergillosis may be difficult, with diagnosis requiring a lung biopsy showing fungal involvement. A presumptive diagnosis of invasive aspergillosis may be made in patients who have pulmonary symptoms and new chest radiographic abnormalities and positive *Aspergillus* bronchial or sputum cultures.

Treatment

Treatment is usually with amphotericin B, using 1.0–1.5 mg/kg/day, followed by life-long maintenance therapy with either amphotericin B or itraconazole, using 400 mg daily.

Risk Factors

Risk factors include neutropenia (low level of segmented neutrophilic white blood cells), use of corticosteroids and broad-spectrum bacterial therapy, and previous pneumonia, especially *Pneumocystis jiroveci* pneumonia. There is also evidence that aspergillosis may be a direct effect of advanced HIV disease and may occur in the absence of other predisposing factors. Patients typically have extremely low CD4+ lymphocytes counts and a history of other AIDS-defining opportunistic infections.

Assembly and budding

Assembly and budding are processes in the HIV viral cycle by which new HIV is formed in infected host cells. Viral core proteins, enzymes, and RNA gather just inside the cell's membrane, while the viral envelope proteins aggregate within the membrane. An immature viral particle is formed and then pinches off from the cell, acquiring an envelope and the cellular and HIV proteins from the cell membrane. The immature viral particle then undergoes processing by an HIV enzyme called protease to become an infectious virus. An understanding of the HIV life cycle helps researchers know what drugs, such as protease inhibitors, can effectively reduce HIV production in people who are infected with the virus. *See also* **Retrovirus replication.**

Asymptomatic

Individuals who do not feel or show outward signs of infection despite the presence of a disease-causing agent (for instance, antibodies to an infectious organism such as HIV or hepatitis) are said to be asymptomatic, meaning they are free of outward symptoms. For instance, individuals infected with HIV typically remain asymptomatic for five or more years after their diagnosis after a short initial period characterized by symptoms of acute infection.

Atovaquone (Mepron, formerly known as 566C80)

Atovaquone is an antimicrobial drug used as a treatment for *Pneumocystis jiroveci* pneumonia for individuals who cannot tolerate or fail on TMP-SMX or who are pregnant.

Autoinoculation

Autoinoculation refers to the spread of infection by an individual from one part of the body to another, usually by means of the hands.

Autologous

Autologous specimens are those derived from one's self, such as blood that is withdrawn and later re-introduced into the body. Autologous blood donors typically have units of blood drawn in the weeks prior to surgery so that it is available if a transfusion is needed.

Avascular necrosis (AVN)

AVN, which is also referred to as osteonecrosis, is a disease resulting from temporary or permanent loss of blood supply to the bone. AVN is a possible late complication in AIDS that may be associated with highly active antiretroviral therapy (HAART), particularly protease inhibitors, although this has not been confirmed. The most common site to be affected is the femoral head.

Many patients with AVN have other risk factors, including alcohol abuse, tobacco smoking; hyperlipidemia (elevated blood lipids); corticosteroid use; the use of lipid-lowering agents; hypercoagulability (increased clotting ability of the blood); and possibly the use of megestrol acetate (Megace). In its early stages, AVN may not cause symptoms, or it may cause only mild symptoms such as loss of range of motion, or mild pain. People infected with HIV who have risk factors for AVN even in the absence of symptoms should be tested with an MRI scan or a CT scan to assess damage. Routine imaging tests or radiographs are not recommended for diagnosing early AVN.

Azidothymidine *see* Zidovudine

Azole Drug

Azoles represent a class of drugs used to fight fungal infections. There are two subclasses of azoles: the imidazoles, such as clotrimazole and ketoconazole, and the triazoles, such as fluconazole and itraconazole.

AZT *see* Zidovudine

AZTEC

AZTEC is a controlled-release form of the anti-retroviral agent zidovudine (AZT).

B lymphocytes

B lymphocytes are white blood cells involved in antibody production during the immune response. B lymphocytes originate and mature within the bone marrow. During infections, B lymphocytes are transformed into plasma cells that produce large quantities of antibody directed at specific pathogens. In persons living with AIDS, the functional ability of both B and T lymphocytes is damaged, with the T lymphocytes being the principal target of HIV.

Bacillary angiomatosis (BA)

Bacillary angiomatosis is a skin condition first described in 1983 in HIV-infected patients with fever and subcutaneous nodules.

Etiology

The etiologic agents include *Bartonella henselae* and *Bartonella quintana*. *B. henselae* is also the most common cause of cat-scratch disease in persons who are immunocompromised.

Epidemiology

BA has only been seen in persons with HIV disease.

Symptoms

The clinical appearance is of very reddened subcutaneous nodules that may occasionally resemble Kaposi's sarcoma. Lymphadenopathy may be associated with these skin findings. In some instances *B. Henselae* infection may become disseminated, causing endocarditis, osteomyelitis, and hepatic lesions.

Diagnosis

Diagnosis is based on the characteristic appearance, but biopsy may be done to rule out other causes. Tissue studies show vascular proliferation and mixed inflammatory cells. With Warthin-Starry staining techniques, the organism can be seen.

Treatment

Treatment is with a macrolide antibiotic, either erythromycin orally, 250–500 mg every six hours, or doxycycline orally, using 100 mg every 12 hours for one to two months for skin disease and longer for other sites of infection.

Risk Factors

Risk factors include HIV disease. Exposure to cats, especially kittens, is associated with a higher risk of contracting BA and cat-scratch disease.

Bacteremia

Bacteremia is a transient blood infection caused by various infectious agents, including *Neisseria gonorrhoeae*. When present, bacteremia is considered a serious STD complication.

Bacteria

Bacteria are single-celled organisms that represent the simplest form of life. Neither plant nor animal, bacteria have many protective functions, such as helping with digestion and maintaining healthy tissue. However, some bacteria are toxic (pathogenic) to human beings and cause diseases, such as pneumonia and infection. Specific bacteria are responsible for many of the sexually transmitted diseases, such as syphilis and bacterial vaginosis.

Bacterial resistance

Bacterial resistance occurs when certain strains of a particular infectious agent become resistant to specific antibiotics. In becoming resistant, these organisms are able to thrive in the presence of the antibiotic, rendering the therapy ineffective. Since the advent of antibiotics, many organisms have developed specific antibiotic resistance. In dealing with STDs, bacterial resistance is often used to describe strains of *Neisseria gonorrhoeae* that are resistant

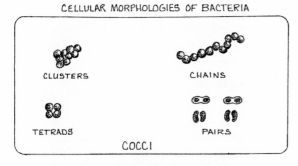

CELLULAR MORPHOLOGIES OF BACTERIA

CLUSTERS   CHAINS

TETRADS   PAIRS

COCCI

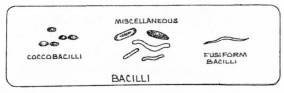

MISCELLANEOUS

COCCOBACILLI   FUSIFORM BACILLI

BACILLI

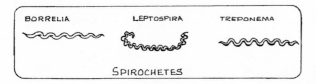

BORRELIA   LEPTOSPIRA   TREPONEMA

SPIROCHETES

Cellular morphologies of bacteria (Marvin G. Miller).

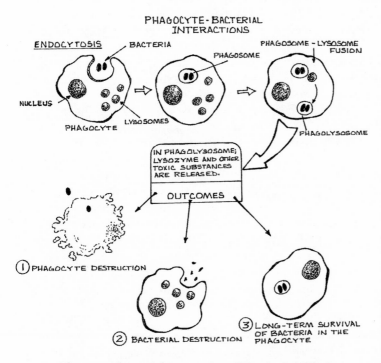

PHAGOCYTE-BACTERIAL INTERACTIONS

ENDOCYTOSIS   BACTERIA   PHAGOSOME-LYSOSOME FUSION

PHAGOSOME

NUCLEUS

LYSOSOMES

PHAGOCYTE   PHAGOLYSOSOME

IN PHAGOLYSOSOME; LYSOZYME AND OTHER TOXIC SUBSTANCES ARE RELEASED.

OUTCOMES

① PHAGOCYTE DESTRUCTION

② BACTERIAL DESTRUCTION

③ LONG-TERM SURVIVAL OF BACTERIA IN THE PHAGOCYTE

Phagocyte-bacterial interactions (Marvin G. Miller).

to penicillin. *See also* **Antiretroviral drug resistance.**

Bacterial vaginosis (BV)

Bacterial vaginosis is the leading cause of vaginal complaints in the United States, and it is often confused with yeast infections. However, vaginosis is not related to infection or inflammation. The vagina normally contains a number of different strains of bacteria, all with their own functions. In vaginosis, the vagina becomes less acidic, allowing certain bacterial strains to grow too quickly. This results in bacterial overgrowth, an imbalance of bacterial flora, and an alteration of the normal acidic pH (acid-base balance).

Etiology

Originally termed "nonspecific vaginitis," BV was first described in 1955 by Houston gynecologists who named the related organism *Haemophilus vaginalis*. The name was later changed to *Corynebacterium vaginale*. However, the responsible organism most often seen in BV has since been found to be unique and not a member of either of these species. This organism has since been named *Gardnerella vaginalis*. However, other bacteria can also cause BV, including *Mobiluncus* species, gram negative rods such as *Escherichia coli*, and *Mycobacterium hominis*. In BV concentrations of these organisms are 100 to 1,000 times higher than that seen in women without BV.

Epidemiology

Bacterial vaginosis is reported to occur in 35 percent of women visiting STD clinics, 15 percent of pregnant women, and 5–15 percent of women visiting gynecological clinics. Because bacterial vaginosis may not cause symptoms, it is hard to say how prevalent it is. BV is caused by a loss of the protective acid-producing bacteria known as lactobaccili, which produce a natural disinfectant, hydrogen peroxide. Normally, hydrogen peroxide combines with chlorine molecules found in the cervical mucus to prevent an overrun of certain less friendly bacteria.

The level of hydrogen peroxide produced by lactobacilli directly affects susceptibility to infection with BV. Without sufficient hydrogen peroxide, certain bacteria such as *Gardnerella vaginalis*, *Mycoplasma hominis* and *Mobuluncus curtisii*, organisms that are normally found in small amounts in the vagina, are able to freely proliferate, causing overgrowth. Because gardnerella are anaerobic (bacteria that thrive in the absence of oxygen), they tend to cause more problems. In BV, *Gardenerella* and other bacteria produce proteins that cause a fishy odor, and they change the normal acid pH of 3.5 to 4.5 to a high pH, usually above 5.0, which is more alkaline.

Symptoms

Half of all women with BV report having no symptoms. Signs of BV vary considerably among women. Typical symptoms include an unpleasant, fishy smelling vaginal odor and excessive vaginal discharge that can vary from gray to white with a consistency that may be thin or watery to creamy. This discharge may stain undergarments. The odor is particularly bad after sexual intercourse as semen mixes with vaginal secretions and some-

times before menstruations. Patients may complain of vaginal itching or burning but BV does not cause vaginal pain or pain during intercourse.

Diagnosis

Diagnosis is made by examination of the vaginal secretions using a wet prep microscopic examination. In BV, clue cells are seen microscopically. Clue cells, which are squamous epithelial cells covered with bacteria, are unique to BV and represent the best single criterion for BV diagnosis. Clue cells have a stippled or granular appearance, with borders that are obscure or finely speckled because of the adherence of bacteria. Vaginal pH can also be tested with commercial kits such as FemExam. The normal vaginal pH is around 3.5–4.4, whereas in BV, the pH is generally higher than 4.5. Cervical fluid has a higher pH than vaginal fluid and should not be used for testing pH.

Vaginal secretions may also be tested with a whiff test. This test is positive in BV and negative in yeast infections. Physical examination may show a layer of white or gray-white discharge that sticks to the walls of the vagina, whereas yeast is generally curdier and does not form a consistent layer. Gram stained smears of vaginal secretions show a shift in that lactobacilli (gram positive rods) are no longer predominant. Douching, recent intercourse, menstruation, and other infections can alter the appearance of the discharge in BV. Absence of an even white vaginal discharge should not rule out BV if other signs and symptoms of BV infection are present.

A recently introduced nucleic acid amplification test using specific oligonucleotide probes has been found capable of detecting high concentrations of *G. vaginalis* and simultaneously detects *Candida* species and *Trichomonas vaginalis*.

Treatment

Although BV is not an infection, it requires treatment because it can lead to other health problems. For instance, women with BV are more likely to have abnormal Pap smears with atypical cells. BV may also cause infection in the fallopian tubes and ovaries (pelvic inflammatory disease), and this may lead to fertility problems. BV also increases a woman's chances of contracting the HIV virus during pregnancy.

Patients are typically treated with the antibiotic metronidazole (Flagyl) using 500 mg orally twice a day for seven days or clindamycin 300 mg taken orally twice a day for seven days. Metronidazole may also be used in a 0.75 percent gel (Metro-Gel) using five grams intravaginally twice a day for five days. A two percent Clindamycin cream can also be used, using five grams intravaginally at bedtime for seven days. Single two-gram doses of metronidazole were once used but patients tended to experience recurrences of BV one month after treatment. Overall, most patients respond well to treatment, although BV can later recur. There are no over-the-counter treatments available for BV.

In clinical trials, purified Lactobacillus suppositories showed improvement in half of the test patients, but recurrences occurred in 29 percent of subjects. Antimicrobial agents such as tetracycline and erythromycin, which are effective in chlamydial or gonorrheal cervicitis, have limited activity against anaerobic bacteria such as *Gardnerella* and are considered poor treatment choices.

Risk Factors

Most experts agree that sexual intercourse with a number of different partners is the most likely risk factor. Although *Gardnerella vaginosis* is not transmitted during sex, male partners of women with BV have been shown to carry similar bacteria. In some instances semen contains chemicals that destroy protective lactobacilli. In these instances condoms may offer protection, but overall, condoms do not protect against the development of BV. It is also believed that anything introduced into the vagina, such as a dildo or toy, can inhibit lactobacilli, increasing the risk of BV. The use of intrauterine devices (IUDs) is also associated with a 20 percent rate of BV, compared to a six percent rate in women using other forms of birth control. Routine douching is also related to a higher incidence of BV, since douching kills off the protective lactobacilli.

Several studies have shown that treatment of male partners does not improve the clinical outcome of BV or reduce recurrence. The CDC guidelines do not recommend treatment of male partners.

Pregnancy

Untreated, bacterial vaginosis can lead to fertility problems or premature delivery in pregnancy. Pregnant women are also at special risk for developing BV because of the increased production of anaerobic bacteria in the vagina during pregnancy. This causes a greater likelihood of *Gardnerella* infecting the cervix and the membranes surrounding the amniotic sac cushioning the fetus. This may result in infection of the amniotic fluid, causing a condition of chorioamnionitis, aminiotic fluid infection, and premature labor. Treatment during pregnancy is generally administered orally, using 300 mg Clindamycin twice a day for seven days, or 250 mg metronidazole taken orally three times a day for seven days.

A series of studies in the United States, Scandinavia, and Australia that included women from different ethnic and socioeconomic groups has consistently demonstrated an increased risk for pre-term delivery and low birth weight among women with BV.

Complications

Other complications of BV include postpartum endometritis (abdominal wound infections following Cesarean section); vaginal cuff cellulitis (vaginal bacteria contaminating the operative field during hysterectomy); post-abortion pelvic inflammatory disease (PID); and PID not related to pregnancy. There is also growing evidence suggesting that the presence of BV or absence of lactobacilli may increase a woman's risk of developing HIV during heterosexual intercourse. Another study showed that women with BV were more likely to seroconvert to HIV (develop antibodies to the HIV virus) than women without clinical signs of BV.

Centers for Disease Control and Prevention. *Sexually Transmitted Diseases Treatment Guidelines 2002.* Atlanta: U.S. Dept. of Health and Human Services, 2002.

Stewart, Elizabeth G., and Paula Spencer. *The V Book: A Doctor's Guide to Complete Vulvovaginal Health,* New York: Bantam Books, 2002.

Baculovirus

The baculovirus is a virus found in insects, which is used in the production of some experimental HIV vaccines.

Balanoposthitis

Balanoposthitis is a condition characterized by inflammation of the glans and foreskin of the penis that may occur in STD infections, particularly chancroid.

Bath houses

In the early years of the HIV pandemic, before the nature of the infection had been determined, bath houses used as meeting places for homosexual men facilitated the spread of HIV infection.

Beta 2 microglobulin test

Beta 2 microglobulin is a protein tightly bound to the surface of many nucleated cells, particularly immune system cells. Elevated levels of this protein occur in a variety of diseases. Beta 2 microglobulin is not specific to HIV infection, but there is a correlation between this marker and the progression of HIV disease.

Bethesda System

The Bethesda System is a formal classification system used to grade Pap smears. The Bethesda System was first proposed by a 1988 National Cancer Institute Workshop on the Classification of Cervical and Vaginal Cytology in an attempt both to standardize diagnoses and to improve the reproducibility of reporting by pathologists for mild, moderate, and severe cell dysplasia. The Bethesda System, which has been widely adopted, replaces the older terms of atypia-mild-moderate-severe dysplasia.

In the Bethesda System, the term atypical squamous cells of uncertain significance (ASCUS) is used for cells observed to be abnormal but neither clearly reactive nor clearly dysplastic. Moderate and severe dysplasias are regrouped into high-grade squamous intraepithelial lesions (HGSIL) with mild dysplasia and the changes suggestive of HPV (koilocytosis) grouped as low-grade squamous intraepithelial lesions (LGSIL). The Bethesda System also evaluates the adequacy of the specimen as satisfactory, satisfactory for evaluation but limited, and unsatisfactory.

Infections reported in this system include: *Trichomonas vaginalis*; fungal organisms morphologically consistent with *Candida* species; predominance of coccobacilli consistent with shift in vaginal flora; bacteria morphologically consistent with *Actinomyces* species; cellular changes associated with herpes simplex virus; and squamous cell changes encompassing the human papilloma virus (HPV). *See also* **Human papilloma virus** and **Pap smear.**

Blood borne diseases

Blood borne diseases are diseases, such as hepatitis B, hepatitis C, and HIV/AIDS, that are primarily transmitted by blood to blood contact, including the use of contaminated medical instruments and equipment, and transfusions of blood products.

Blood tests

Blood tests are useful in diagnosing infections and in monitoring response to therapy. Infectious agents contain proteins that can be detected in blood tests, and they induce the production of antibodies that serve as markers for infection.

The first diagnostic STD test, the Wasserman test, was used to detect *Treponema pallidum*, the spirochete responsible for syphilis. At one time, blood tests for syphilis were performed as a state requirement for marriage. Today, blood tests for infectious diseases such as HIV and hepatitis are included in most prenatal profiles.

Blood transfusions

The blood supply in the United States is tested with the most sensitive techniques available for hepatitis A, hepatitis B, hepatitis C, HIV-1, HIV-2, HTLV-1, and syphilis. However, patients who are recently infected may not have seroconverted (produced antibodies) at the time of their blood donation. Consequently, their blood tests may be falsely negative. Although blood donors may be infected and able to transmit disease via blood products, infected individuals typically do not develop antibodies for three months. The newer NAT tests used to test blood donors for HIV and hepatitis in many parts of the United States are more sensitive and able to detect bacterial or viral particles soon after infection.

To reduce the incidence of using blood donors who may have been recently infected but have not yet seroconverted or do not yet test positive with available NAT tests, donors are screened by interview, with questions specifically relating to lifestyle factors, including sexual habits and injection drug use. The intention is to identify donors who may be at risk for HIV.

Despite the introduction of highly specific testing methods and the efforts of blood banks to identify donors who may be at risk, since 1999 there have been at least two documented instances in which patients contracted HIV from blood donors. In August 2000, a Texas heart patient became the first American infected with AIDS virus from donated blood since the rigorous testing methods of blood donors implemented in 1997. In July 2002, two people contracted HIV from blood transfusions provided by a regional Florida blood bank. Although the testing process now in use by blood banks is highly sophisticated, it is still considered experimental and fails to pick up people recently infected with HIV and other STDs.

Researchers at the University of California in San Francisco have studied the risk of transfusion-transmitted viral infection. The primary study, which involved 764 patients receiving autologous or allogenic red blood cell transfusions, showed no incidences of HIV or HTLV-1 transmission, but three patients showed serocoversion to Hepatitis B core antibodies, and two patients showed confirmed seroconversion for the Hepatitis C virus. Only one of two Hepatitis C conversions occurred before blood products were routinely screened for Hepatitis C by enzyme immunoassay. The study concluded that transfusion-associated seroconversions to hepatitis B and C markers were observed in the early 1990s despite testing donors for markers of both viruses. *See also* **Factor VIII.**

Transfusion Notes, *Medical Laboratory Observer*, May 2002 and September 2002.
Murphy, E.L. and M.P. Busch, et al. "A prospective study of the risk of transfusion-acquired viral infections," *Transfusion Medicine*, Sept. 1998; 8(3): 173–178.

Body cavity lymphoma (BCL)

Body cavity lymphoma represents a type of cancer known to develop in patients with HIV/AIDS. The DNA of human herpesvirus-8 (HHV-8), which causes Kaposi's sarcoma, has been found in BCL tissue. BCL is a unique B-cell neoplasm with a strong propensity for body cavity involvement. These lymphomas remain isolated and rarely disseminate into other tissues. BCL also has a poor prognosis.

Body piercing

Body piercing refers to the insertion of a needle into skin or mucous membranes in order to produce a permanent opening into which a ring or other form of jewelry is commonly attached. Body piercing in most states is an unlicensed and unregulated industry, and in most communities facilities for piercing are not subject to health inspections. The American Academy of Dermatology is opposed to the use of piercing of body parts, with the exception of earlobes. Genital piercing, in particular, poses risks for several different infections, including hepatitis B, hepatitis C, tetanus, and HIV. Both the United States and Canadian Red Cross organizations prohibit blood donations for one year after body piercing or tattoo because of the risk of transmitting blood borne diseases. Other risks include bleeding, scarring, and metal sensitivity.

Bone marrow

Bone marrow is the heart of the immune system. Bone marrow, a spongy, pulpy tissue, is found at the center of bone. The bone marrow functions to produce and store immune system cells (leukocytes or white blood cells), red blood cells, platelets, and stem cells, and it directs these cells to the blood circulation and other immune system organs as needed. Primordial bone marrow stem cells produced within the bone marrow differentiate and mature into various tissue cells depending on the body's needs.

The sternum, ileac crest of the hipbone, the ribs and the skull are all rich in bone marrow, which can be extracted or aspirated to study abnormal cell function. When the bone marrow is suppressed by immunosuppressant medications or infection, it is unable to produce adequate concentrations of immune system cells. In AIDS, immune system cells known as CD 4+ T lymphocytes are destroyed by the HIV virus.

Bone marrow suppression *see* Immunosuppression

Branched DNA assay (bDNA test)

The bDNA test, developed by Bayer, measures the amount of HIV and other viruses in blood plasma. Test results are calibrated in numbers of virus particle equivalents per milliliter of plasma. The bDNA is similar in results but not in technique to the polymerase chain reaction (PCR) test. The bDNA test is used to evaluate the effectiveness of drug treatment regimens and to gauge HIV disease progression. Newer versions, or generations, of these assays are undergoing development and will be able to detect smaller numbers of copies of HIV in blood samples. *See also* **Viral burden**.

Bug chasers

The term "Bug chasers" was introduced in 2003 to describe people who seek out others who are infected with HIV so that they can be exposed to the virus and, in turn, become infected. Members of this group primarily meet through Internet discussion groups where those infected with HIV are known as "Gift givers." In an article in *Rolling Stone*, Gregory Freeman describes interviewing members of this subculture and explains that a Yahoo! spokeswoman confirmed that the company shuts down such sites when it receives notice that subscribers are promoting HIV infection or other types of harm, but the company does not actively seek out these groups.

Condoms and safe sex are ridiculed on bug-chasing Web sites, and it is not unusual for people posting to write that the fear of HIV takes the fun out of sex. Others see it as a form of suicide, while still others mistakenly think that HIV infection has been cured or is easy to live with now that antiretroviral therapies are available. One person interviewed, who now has AIDS and regrets his decision, had no idea that antiretroviral drugs can have side effects that prevent their use or that drug failure can occur. Although many AIDS activists do not like to admit that this problem exists, the CDC reported an alarming increase in cases of syphilis among men who have sex with men between 2000 and 2001 and in late 2002, indicating that sex prevention advice is being ignored, particularly in several U.S. cities.

Freeman, Gregory A. "In Search of Death." *Rolling Stone*, February 6, 2003.

Burkitt's lymphoma

Burkitt's lymphoma is a common childhood tumor first associated with infection by Denis Burkitt, a medical missionary to East Africa in the 1950s. Burkitt's lymphoma also occurs in AIDS infection and in patients who are immunosuppressed. The Epstein-Barr virus (EBV) has been implicated as a causal factor in Burkitt's lymphoma. After initial infection with EBV, the virus is shed lifelong and provides a readily available source of infection.

Burkitt's lymphomas typically appear early in the course of AIDS, prior to profound immunosuppression, whereas immunoblastic lymphomas typically occur in late-stage AIDS when cellular immunity is compromised. EBV-positive AIDS-related lymphomas often are refractory to conventional chemotherapy, with rare complete remissions and an absence of durable clinical responses.

Calymmatobacterium granulomatosis

Calymmatobacterium granulomatosis is a type of bacterium responsible for the development of donovanosis (granuloma inguinale), a sexually transmitted disease more common to tropical regions. *See also* **Donovanosis** and **Granuloma inguinale**.

Canarypox

Canarypox is a virus that infects birds and is used as a live vector in the manufacture of HIV vaccines. The canarypox virus can carry a large amount of foreign genes, but it cannot grow in human cells.

Cancers related to STDs

Certain infectious organisms responsible for causing STDs are also known to cause specific cancers. Several specific strains of the human papillomavirus (HPV) are known to cause cellular changes that may progress to squamous intraepithelial lesions. These lesions may progress to cervical cancer, anal cancer or penile cancer, depending on the site of infection. The HTLV-I virus, the first human retrovirus to be discovered, causes adult T-cell leukemia/lymphoma.

Studies have also linked the human herpesvirus-8 (HHV-8) to Kaposi's sarcoma, body cavity cell lymphoma, and primary effusion lymphoma. About one in six individuals infected with HIV also has cancer. The most common cancers in HIV-positive patients are not cancers that are commonly found in the normal population.

Kaposi's sarcoma was the first cancer to be recognized as being associated with AIDS. To its list of AIDS related cancers, the CDC has added intermediate and high-grade non–Hodgkin's lymphoma, primary central nervous system lymphoma, and cervical cancer. The designation of cervical cancer is controversial because the relationship is more likely to be co-infection with HPV, rather than immunosuppression.

A suppressed immune system contributes to cancer development, whereas a healthy immune system works to prevent cancer. Normally, CD8+ lymphocytes and other cytotoxic cells destroy other cells showing cancerous changes.

Several other tumors have not yet been recognized by the CDC as AIDS-defining, but are clearly seen more often in AIDS patients. These include anal cancer, Hodgkin's disease, benign and malignant smooth muscle tumors in children, skin cancers, testicular cancer and cancers of the oral mucosa, head and neck, and possibly lung cancer. *See also* **Human papilloma virus** and **Kaposi's sarcoma.**

Klencke, Barbara, and Paul Volberding. "AIDS-relating Malignancies." Chapter 76 in *Sexually Transmitted Diseases*. 3rd Edition. Edited by King K. Holmes, et al. New York: McGraw-Hill, 1999.

Candidiasis

Genital candidiasis is a disease caused by infection with the yeast *Candida albicans.* The earliest reports of vulvovaginal candidiasis appear in the writings of Hippocrates and Galen, and the first clinical description of this disorder dates from 1792. Candidiasis is not usually sexually transmitted although it can be. Candidiasis is a very common cause of vaginitis and is primarily caused by yeast overgrowth related to antibiotic therapy. Candidiasis is more common in women who are pregnant or menstruating, and in diabetics. Occasionally, candidiasis is caused by the use of immunosuppressants, such as corticosteroids and chemotherapeutic agents. Candidiasis often occurs in patients who are immunosuppressed, including patients with HIV.

Etiology

Approximately 90 percent of all instances of candidiasis are caused by *Candida albicans* and most other instances are caused by *Candida glabrata*, a related strain that does not respond as well to

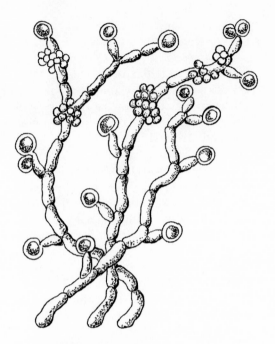

Candida albicans (Marvin G. Miller).

therapy. There is speculation that the incidence of *C. glabrata* is rising, in part due to indiscriminate use of over-the-counter anti-fungal creams, which allow *C. glabrata* to proliferate.

Epidemiology

In the United States, candidiasis is currently the second most common cause of vaginal infections, next to bacterial vaginosis. Women are affected more often than men, and an estimated 70 to 75 percent of women are reported to have candidiasis at least once in their lifetimes. Incidence of candidiasis occurs primarily in people 20 to 40 years old. Some studies show transmission through sexual intercourse, but most instances of candidiasis are not sexually transmitted. Penile colonization with candida has been demonstrated in 20 percent of male partners of women with candidiasis.

Symptoms

Women with genital candidiasis usually develop itching or irritation of the vagina and vulva, and they may have a vaginal discharge. The irritation may be severe even when the discharge is light. The vulva may also become reddish and swollen, and the skin may be raw and cracked. The vaginal wall is usually covered with a white cheese-like material, although it may look normal. Vaginal candidiasis is also known as monilia.

Men often have no symptoms, but the end of the penis (the glans) and the foreskin (in uncircumcised men) may be sore and irritated especially after sexual intercourse. Occasionally, men may notice a slight discharge from the penis. The end of the penis may be coated with a white cheese-like material.

Treatment

In women, candidiasis can be treated by washing the vagina with soap and water, drying it with a clean towel, and then applying an antifungal cream containing clotrimazole, miconazole, butoconazole, or ticonazole and terconazole. Alternatively, ketoconazole, fluconazole, or itraconazole can be taken orally. In men, the penis should be washed and dried before any antifungal cream (containing nystatin) is applied.

Precautions

Women who take oral contraceptives must stop using them for several months during treatment for candidiasis because they can worsen candidiasis. Vaginal *Candida* colonization rates in HIV-infected women are higher than among women who do not have HIV, although studies show that HIV-infected women have similar demographic characteristics and high-risk behaviors. The colonization rates in HIV appear to correlate with the severity of immunodeficiency. Therapy for women with HIV is the same as for those who are not HIV positive. Prophylactic therapy with fluconazole is not recommended for women with HIV.

Pregnancy

Management of candidiasis is more difficult during pregnancy, with clinical responses being blunted and recurrences more likely. Only topical azole therapies are recommended during pregnancy. Most topical antifungal agents are effective, especially when prescribed for longer periods, such as 1–2 weeks. Single application of high dose topical clotrimazole has also been shown to be effective. Oral nystatin may be used, but it is desirable to use topical treatment if possible.

Risk Factors

Risk factors include antibiotic therapy, tight restrictive clothing, diets high in sugar, diabetes, immunosuppression, unprotected sex, oral sex, and pregnancy. Women at risk for vaginal candidiasis, such as women with impaired immune function or who are taking antibiotics for extended periods, may need an antifungal drug as preventive therapy. Broad-spectrum antibiotics such as tetracycline, ampicillins, and oral cephalosporins are mainly responsible for candidiasis.

Recurrent Vulvovaginal Candidiasis

Recurrent vulvovaginal candidiasis (RVVC), which affects less than five percent of women, is usually defined as four or more episodes of symptomatic VVC each year. Most women with RVVC have no apparent predisposing or underlying conditions. *Candida glabrata* and other non-albicans *Candida* species are found in 10 to 20 percent of patients with RVVC.

Conventional anti-mycotic treatments are not as effective in RVVC. Each episode of RVVC caused by *C. albicans* responds well to short duration oral or topical azole therapy. However, to maintain clinical control, specialists recommend a longer duration of initial therapy, such as 7–14 days of topical therapy or a 150 mg dose of fluconazole repeated three days later, to achieve mycologic remission before initiating a maintenance antifungal regimen.

Maintenance antifungals are selected on the basis of pharmacologic characteristics of individual agents and route of administration. Recommended regimens include clotrimazole, using 500 mg dose vaginal suppositories once weekly, ketoconazole, using a 100 mg dose once daily; fluconazole, using a 100–150 mg dose once weekly; and itraconazole, using a 400 mg dose once monthly or a 100 mg dose once daily. Maintenance regimens should be continued for six months. Patients using ketoconazole should be monitored with liver function tests, since they may develop hepatotoxicity. Although maintenance regimens are effective in reducing RVVC, 30 to 40 percent of women will have recurrent disease once maintenance therapy is discontinued.

Severe Vulvovaginal Candidiasis

Severe vulvovaginitis with extensive vulvar erythema, edema, excoriation, and fissure formation, has lower clinical response rates in patients treated with short courses of topical or oral therapy. Either 7–14 days of topical azole or 150 mg fluconazole in two sequential doses, with the second dose 72 hours after the initial dose, is recommended.

Non-albicans Vulvovaginal Candidiasis

The optimal treatment of vulvovaginal candidiasis not caused by *Candida albicans* is unknown. Longer duration of therapy (7–14 days) with a non-fluconazole azole drug is recommended as first-line therapy. If recurrence occurs, 600 mg boric acid in a gelatin capsule administered vaginally once daily for two weeks is recommended. Additional options include topical four percent flucytosine, although a referral to a specialist is recommended. If non-albicans VVC continues to recur, a maintenance regimen of 100,000 units of nys-

tatin delivered daily via vaginal suppositories has been successful. *See also* **Oral Candidiasis (Thrush)** and **Yeast infections.**

Centers for Disease Control and Prevention. *Sexually Transmitted Diseases Treatment Guidelines 2002.* Atlanta: U.S. Dept. of Health and Human Services, 2002.

Canker sore *see* Aphthous ulcer

CARE Act *see* Ryan White Comprehensive AIDS Resources Emergency Act

CCR5

CCR5 is a cell surface molecule, which is needed along with the primary receptor, the CD4 molecule, in order for HIV to fuse with the membranes of the immune system cells. Researchers have found that the strains of HIV most often transmitted from person to person required the CCR5 molecule and CD4 molecule in order for HIV to enter the cell. In addition to its role in fusion, CCR5 is a receptor for certain immune-signaling molecules called chemokines that are known to suppress HIV infection of cells.

CDC *see* Centers for Disease Control and Prevention

CD4 cell count

The CD4 cell count measures the number of CD4+ T lymphocytes per cubic millimeter (mm3) of blood. The CD4 count is a good predictor of immunity. As the CD4 cell count declines, the risk of developing opportunistic infections increases. The normal adult range for CD4 cell counts is 500 to 1500 per cubic millimeter of blood.

The normal CD4 count for infants is much higher and declines to adult values by age six. CD4 counts should be performed at least every six to 12 months in patients with counts greater than 500/mm³. If the count is lower than 500/mm³, testing every three months is advised. Children with HIV children should be checked every three months regardless of the CD4 count. According to CDC criteria, a CD4 count of 200 or less is used to define AIDS.

U.S. Department of Health & Human Services, HIV/AIDS Bureau, 2003.

CD4+ T lymphocytes (CD 4+ cells)

Lymphocytes are white blood cells with a prominent nucleus and moderate cytoplasm. There are two primary classes of lymphocytes: T cells which guard the body against infectious and toxic agents, and B cells, which are directly involved in antibody production. The immune system also produces two different T lymphocyte subtypes with different surface proteins known as cluster designation or CD markers: 1) CD4+ T cells, which are helper cells, and 2) CD8+ T cells, which are suppressor cells. T helper cells fight infectious organisms, whereas T suppressor cells destroy cells that are infected, potentially cancerous, or which could cause autoimmune disorders. CD4 cells are targeted and destroyed by the HIV virus. Normally, people have 500–1500 CD4+ T lymphocytes/mm³. Untreated HIV infection causes an annual decline of 50–100 CD4+ cells/mm³.

Destruction of CD4+ lymphocytes is the major cause of the immunodeficiency observed in AIDS, and decreasing CD4+ lymphocyte levels appear to be the best indicator for developing opportunistic infection. Although CD4 counts fall, the total T cell level remains fairly constant through the course of HIV disease, due to a concomitant increase in the CD8+ T cells. The ratio of CD4+ to CD8+ cells is an important measure of disease progression.

CD8+ T lymphocytes

CD8+ lymphocytes are a subset of T lymphocytes that have CD8 or cluster designation 8 molecule on their surface. CD8+ cells are known as suppressor cells or cytotoxic lymphocytes (CTLs) because they function to destroy cells that are infected or damaged. Normally, the immune system maintains a balanced ratio of CD4+ and CD8+ lymphocytes. High levels of HIV-specific CD8+ T lymphocytes are seen throughout HIV disease. However, in advanced-stage disease CD8+ cells are no longer able to recognize the virus.

Cells

Cells are the basic building blocks of all living organisms. Different tissues in the body, including blood, contain specific types of cells. The human body is composed of about a trillion cells, although there are about 200 basic types of cells. Each cell contains a complete copy of the body's DNA genome in the form of chromosomes. Cells reproduce by dividing, and each new cell has DNA identical to the parent cell.

Centers for Disease Control and Prevention (CDC)

The CDC is recognized as the lead federal agency for protecting the health and safety of Americans at home and abroad, providing credible information to enhance health decisions, and promoting health through strong partnerships. The CDC, located in Atlanta, Georgia, is an agency of the U.S. Department of Health and Human Services. CDC serves as the national focus for developing and applying disease prevention and control, environmental health, and health promotion and education activities designed to improve the health of the people of the United States. Through its prevention services, surveillance data and treatment guidelines the CDC is able to report on the incidence of diseases as well as their risk factors and offer safe and efficacious treatment guidelines.

Centers for Medicare and Medicaid Services (CMS)

CMS is a federal agency within the U.S. Department of Health and Human Services. CMS runs the Medicare and Medicaid programs, two national health care programs that benefit about 75 million Americans. Along with the Health Resources and Services Administration, CMS runs the State Children's Health Insurance Program (SCHIP), a program that provides medical coverage for uninsured children in the United States. CMS also regulates all laboratory testing (except research) performed on human subjects in the United States. CMS was formerly known as the Health Care Financing Administration (HCFA).

Central nervous system (CNS) damage in HIV

Although monocytes and macrophages with CD4+ surface markers can be infected by HIV, they appear to be relatively resistant to cell destruction. However, these infected cells travel through the body and carry HIV to various organs, especially the lungs and the brain. Persons living with HIV often experience abnormalities in the central nervous system. Investigators have hypothesized that an accumulation of HIV in brain and nerve cells or the inappropriate release of cytokine chemicals or toxic byproducts of these cells may be to blame for the neurological manifestations of HIV disease.

Glossary of HIV/AIDS-Related Terms. 4th edition. Rockville, MD: HIV/AIDS Treatment Information Service, 2002.

Cervical cancer and precancer *see* Human papilloma virus, Pap smear

Cervicitis

Cervicitis is inflammation of the cervix generally caused by an infection. *See also* **Mucopurulent cervicitis.**

Cervix

The cervix is the mouth of the womb or lower terminus of the uterus that juts into the lower vagina. The cervix contains a narrow canal connecting the upper and lower parts of a woman's reproductive tract. The cervix is covered with squamous epithelial cells, and it is lined by mucus producing cells called columnar epithelial cells. These outer and inner layers of tissue meet at the squamocolumnar junction.

Chancroid (*Haemophilus ducreyi*)

Chancroid is a sexually transmitted disease characterized by painful ulcers and painful regional lymphadenopathy. Chancroid is also known as soft chancre (ulcus molle) and was first differentiated from syphilis (hard chancre) in France in the 1850s.

Etiology

Chancroid is caused by *Haemophilus ducreyi*, a small anaerobic gram-negative bacterium, shaped as a rod, which is transmitted by direct contact through the skin, presumably through minor abrasions. The organism is rounded at the ends and has an indentation at the sides and may be found both within and on the outside of neutrophils (type of white blood cell). *Haemophilus ducreyi* requires hemin (X factor), which is found in blood, for its growth. It has not been described in men having sex with men. Chancroid is usually transmitted through intercourse, but it may occur through fingers (autoinocculation), affecting the conjunctiva and other bodily sites.

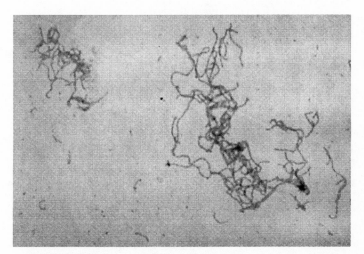

Haemophilis ducreyi in a patient with chancroid (Public Health Imaging Library, CDC).

Epidemiology

Most cases occur as a result of localized outbreaks clustered in certain states and generally involve traditional core STD populations, including prostitutes and their clients. In some areas of the United States, chancroid is endemic, and it is known to occur in discrete epidemics. About 10 percent of persons who have chancroid acquired in the United States are co-infected with syphilis or herpes simplex virus. Outside of the United States, this percentage is higher. Surveillance data in the United States indicates that about 10 times as many males are affected as females. Chancroid primarily occurs in younger adults, although it may occur at any age. The World Health Organization reports that the annual incidence of chancroid worldwide is about seven million.

The annual incidence in the United States decreased between 1950 and 1978. However, a dramatic rise in chancroid occurred in the 1980s, with approximately 5,000 new cases being reported annually. By 1995, the number had dropped to 1,000 new cases annually, with outbreaks confined to endemic clusters in New York City, New Orleans, and Jackson, Mississippi.

Diagnosis

A definitive diagnosis of chancroid requires identification of *H. ducreyi* using specimens from the base of the ulcer collected on cotton or calcium alginate swabs. For culture growth, the organism requires special culture media that is not widely available from commercial sources. Even when this media is available, sensitivity of detection is less than 80 percent. The organisms may also be seen on a gram stain taken from the lesion. On gram stain, *H. ducreyi* is seen as a "school of fish" with small, pleomorphic (able to change forms) gram-negative rods.

Currently, there are no FDA approved polymerase chain reaction tests for *H. ducreyi* available in the United States, although some commercial laboratories have developed methodologies. Diagnosis is usually made by excluding syphilis and herpes simplex virus, disorders that may also cause genital ulcers. Patients with chancroid also show evidence of lymphadenopathy (swollen painful lymph gland enlargement). The combination of a painful ulcer and tender lymphadenopathy in the groin, symptoms occurring in one third of patients, suggests a diagnosis of chancroid.

Symptoms

Symptoms generally develop 4–7 days after the initial infection. A papule or pustule erupts that typically erodes to form a painful ulcer with ragged margins. The ulcer may be very deep, and most patients develop multiple ulcers. Unlike the chancre of syphilis, the chancroid ulcer edge is soft and the ulcer changes shape when the edges are squeezed. Ulcers are usually 1–2 centimeters in diameter but can be larger.

The shape can be round, oval or irregular. The base of the ulcer is often yellowish-gray and exudes a foul smelling discharge. Several ulcers may merge to form larger ulcers.

Swollen lymph nodes in the inguinal or groin region typically appear 1–2 weeks after the primary lesion appears and affect 30 to 60 percent of patients. The typical enlarged gland associated with chancroid is unilateral, spherical, and painful. The lymph nodes may be firm and can rupture or ulcerate. The genital ulcer is usually present when the lymphadenopathy appears, unlike lymphogranuloma venereum, in which the primary lesion is usually transient and has already healed by the time most patients are examined.

In women, the most common sites of infection are the labia majora and minora, but ulcers can be found in the perianal area, in the vagina, on the clitoris or on the cervix. In women with intravaginal or cervical lesions, the chief complaint may be difficult or painful sexual intercourse or difficult or painful urination. Women may also note pain on defecation or a vaginal discharge. In men, the ulcers are usually found on the external or internal surface of the prepuce or foreskin. The glans, the meatus, and the shaft of the penis can also be involved.

Treatment

Prior to the introduction of antibiotic therapy, circumcision and saline soaks were standard forms of therapy. In 1938, patients were treated with sulfonamide antibiotics, which proved effective. Today, treatment for genital ulcers caused by chancroid includes azithromycin, using one gram orally in a single dose; ceftriaxone using 250 mg intramuscularly in a single dose; ciproflxacin using 500 mg given orally twice a day for three days; or erythromycin base using 500 mg orally three times daily for seven days. Ciprofloxacin should not be used in pregnant or lactating women. Men who are uncircumcised

and persons with HIV infection do not respond as well to treatment as those who are circumcised or who are HIV negative. All patients should be re-examined 3–7 days after initiation of therapy and advised to abstain from sexual intercourse until the infection is healed completely. Sex partners should also be examined and treated if they have symptoms or have had sex with the patient within the 10 days preceding onset of the patient's symptoms.

If treatment is successful, symptoms from the ulcers usually improve within three days and their appearance improves within seven days. If no clinical improvement is evident, the clinician must consider whether the diagnosis is correct, the patient is co-infected with another STD, the patient is infected with HIV, in which case resistance to infection is decreased, the treatment was not used as instructed, or the *H. ducreyi* strain causing the infection is resistant to the prescribed antibiotic. The time for complete healing depends on the size of the ulcer, with large ulcers requiring up to two weeks for complete healing. Also, healing is slower for some uncircumcised men who have ulcers under the foreskin. Swollen and inflamed lymph nodes may take longer to heal and may require needle aspiration or incision and drainage even when the ulcers have healed.

Pregnancy

The safety of azithromycin for pregnant and lactating women has not been established. Ciprofloxacin is contraindicated during pregnancy and lactation. Pregnant patients should be treated with ceftriaxone or erythromycin. No adverse effects of chancroid on pregnancy outcome have been reported.

Complications

Scarring can occur at the site of an extensive infection that is complicated by enlarged lymph nodes, and fistulous tracts may form. Phimosis (tightening and constriction of the foreskin of the penis caused by inflammation, making it impossible to bare the glans) and balanoposthitis (inflammation of the glans and foreskin of the penis) may occur, and lymph nodes can rupture. Large ulcers may require a longer time to heal and lymphadenopathy that fluctuates in severity may require a longer time to heal than the ulcers do.

Patients who also have HIV infections should be monitored closely, because as a group these patients are more likely to experience treatment failure and to have slower-healing ulcers. HIV infected patients may require longer courses of therapy than patients who are HIV negative. The use of azithromycin and ceftriaxone in HIV infected patients has not been well studied. Therefore the recommended protocols for these medications should only be used if follow-up visits are certain. Some specialists suggest using the erythromycin seven-day regimen for HIV infected patients.

Risk Factors

Risk factors include lower socioeconomic status, prostitution, unprotected sex and open lesions or abrasions. Trauma or abrasion is necessary for the organisms to penetrate the skin. Chancroid has been established as an important risk factor for heterosexual spread of HIV, and genital ulcers have been shown to be portals of entry for HIV.

Centers for Disease Control and Prevention. *Sexually Transmitted Diseases Treatment Guidelines 2002.* Atlanta: U.S. Dept. of Health and Human Services, 2002.

Ronald, Allan, and William Albritton. "Chancroid and Haemophilus ducreyi." Chapter 38 in *Sexually Transmitted Diseases.* 3rd Edition. Edited by King K. Holmes, et al. New York: McGraw-Hill, 1999.

Chemokines *see* Cytokines

Chemotherapy

Chemotherapy is a general term referring to the use of medications to treat disease. The term is more commonly used to describe medications primarily used to treat cancer. Chemotherapeutic agents are generally cytotoxic drugs that attack and destroy cancerous cells. This type of therapy commonly has adverse side effects that may include the temporary loss of the body's natural immunity to infections, loss of hair, digestive upset, and general feeling of malaise or illness.

Child Sexual Abuse

Children who are sexually abused are at risk for STDs, and multiple episodes of abuse increase the risk of infection. Vaginal or rectal penetration is also more likely to lead to detectable STD infection than fondling. Sexual assault is a violent crime that affects children of all ages, including infants. The U.S. Department of Justice reports that the majority of children who are sexually abused will have no physical complaints related either to trauma or STD infection. Most sexually abused children do not indicate that they have genital pain or problems. In children, the isolation of a sexually transmitted organism may be the first indication that abuse has occurred.

Although the presence of a sexually transmissible agent in a child over the age of one month is suggestive of sexual abuse, exceptions do exist. Rectal and genital chlamydia infections in young children may be due to a persistent perinatally acquired infection, which may last for up to three years. Between 80 and 90 percent of sexually abused children are female, and the average age is seven to eight years. Between 75 and 85 percent of sexually abused children were abused by a male assailant, an adult or minor known to the child, most likely a family member such as the father, stepfather, mother's boyfriend, or uncle. Over 50 percent of male victims of sexual abuse have experienced anal penetration. Vaginal penetration has been reported to occur in approximately one-half and anal penetration in one-third of female victims of sexual abuse.

Sexually Transmitted Diseases and Child Sexual Abuse. Washington, D.C.: U.S. Department of Justice, 1996.

Chimpanzees

Researchers at the University of Alabama were the first to determine in 1999 that the human immunodeficiency virus (HIV) is identical to the simian immunodeficiency virus (SIV) found in chimpanzees (SIVcz).

Chlamydia

According to the Centers for Disease Control and Prevention (CDC), infection with *Chlamydia trachomatis* (*C. trachomatis*) is the most prevalent sexually transmitted disease in the United States, with an estimated four million new cases developing each year. About 50 percent of men and 75 percent of women infected with chlamydia do not have symptoms and are often diagnosed during routine screening.

The name "trachoma" is derived from a Greek word meaning "rough," and refers to the pebble-like appearance of cells of a tissue infected by *C. trachomatis*. A Sicilian physician, Pedanius Dioscorides in A.D. 60, first used the term. In the next century, the scientist Galen conducted an in-depth study of *C. trachomatis*. During the crusades,

LIFE CYCLE OF CHLAMYDIAE

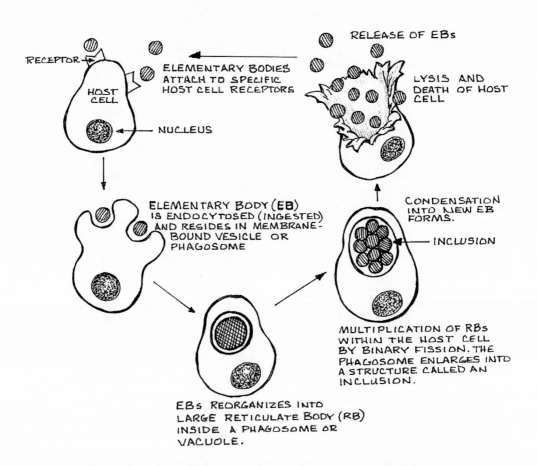

Life cycle of *Chlamydia trachomatis* (Marvin G. Miller).

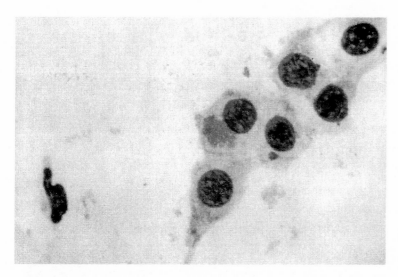

Chlamydia trachomatis in a urethral scraping (Dr. Wiesner and Dr. Kauffman, CDC).

a host cell in which it can replicate its genetic material. Condoms, used consistently and correctly, are very effective in preventing transmission of Chlamydia.

Symptoms and Complications

Chlamydia can infect the urinary-genital area, the anal area and occasionally the eyes, throat and lungs. Its primary target is the mucous membranes of the cervix (opening to the uterus) in women and the urethra (urine canal) in men. The highest rates of infection are seen in female teens because the cervical tissue of young females is very thin, making it more vulnerable to infection.

People infected with chlamydia may show no signs of infection. Alternately, they may show signs of infection anywhere from several weeks to many months after their initial exposure to the organism. About 30 percent of men and up to 75 percent of women will show no disease symptoms until complications arise.

• INFECTIONS IN WOMEN — When symptoms do occur, they are usually mild and may be confused with gonorrhea, a disease with similar symptoms. Women with chlamydia may experience frequent urination, burning during urination, low back pain, pain during intercourse, bleeding between menstrual periods, genital irritation, and a yellowish-green vaginal discharge. Left untreated, infection can spread to the uterus, fallopian tubes, and ovaries, causing a condition of pelvic inflammatory disorder (PID). It is estimated that approximately a third of all women who contract chlamydia go on to develop PID.

PID is most likely to occur in individu-

chlamydial infection spread from the Middle East to Europe. A fresh wave of infections called "Egyptian ophthalmia" occurred after Napoleon's Egyptian campaign.

Epidemiology

First recognized as an STD in 1970, chlamydia is transmitted through oral, genital or anal sex with an infected partner. Chlamydia may also be transmitted by autoinoculation, including finger to eye contact, or during childbirth. Chlamydia cannot be contracted by kissing, and it is not transmitted via towels, toilet seats or clothing. In 2001, more than 783,000 chlamydial infections were reported to the Centers for Disease Control. Seventy-five percent of all reported cases occurred in persons under age 25. Infection with *C. trachomatis* is responsible for a number of conditions, including trachoma; inclusion conjunctivitis; cervicitis; urethritis; epididymitis; proctitis; infantile pneumonia; and lymphgranuloma venereum.

Etiology

The etiologic agent is a tiny bacterium known as *Chlamydia trachomatis*. Like most bacteria, chlamydia responds well to antibiotic therapy, but like a virus, it needs als who have recurring chlamydia infections. Scarring as a consequence of PID can lead to infertility or to ectopic pregnancies (when a fertilized egg implants in the fallopian tubes instead of the lining of the uterus). Ectopic pregnancies can lead to pain, significant bleeding and death. Up to 10 percent of women with advanced cases of chlamydia may develop infertility.

• INFECTIONS IN MALES— In men, Chlamydia primarily causes urethral infections. Chlamydia is responsible for about 50 percent of the urethral infections in men that are not caused by gonorrhea. Symptoms include a clear, thin discharge from the penis, burning with urination, swelling in the scrotal area, itchiness or irritation in the urethral area, and redness at the tip of the penis. Symptoms in both men and women generally resolve about three weeks after the initial exposure.

However, left untreated, chlamydia can cause serious complications. In men, chlamydia infections can ultimately spread to the prostate gland and epididymis (convoluted tubule lying on the testicle, through which sperm pass from the testicle to the vas deferens gland), causing prostitis and epididymitis. This can result in scarring and infertility.

• OTHER ORGANS SUSCEPTIBLE TO INFECTION—Chlamydial eye infections cause conjunctivitis, an eye disorder characterized by inflammation and swelling of the inner rim of the eye with symptoms of redness, itching and pain. Conjunctivitis in newborns may develop during vaginal childbirth.

Anal infections are characterized by symptoms that include pain, fluid discharge and bleeding. Chlamydia may also cause proctitis, a condition characterized by an inflamed rectum.

Chlamydial throat infections contracted during oral sex may produce no symptoms or they may cause symptoms of a sore throat.

Diagnosis

Chlamydia can easily be tested using cervical specimens collected by a health-care provider with a culture swab. In men, a swab of fluid discharge from the penis can be cultured. When these specimens are cultured, they are allowed to grow on nutrient agar from which they can be identified. However, these tests can take up to three days for results.

More commonly, the swabs are tested by immunoassays that involve a polymerase chain reaction (PCR testing) to amplify DNA. In PCR, which is a form of nucleic acid amplification (NAT) testing, genetic material consistent with chlamydia is identified in a positive test. Urine specimens may also be tested for chlamydia using this detection method. NAT tests are recommended as the assays of choice in genitourinary disease except in cases of sexual abuse in children.

The CDC recommends testing all women who have symptoms of cervical inflammation or who have a compatible STD syndrome. They also recommend testing individuals who have had sexual contact with infected patients, victims of sexual assault or abuse, and all sexually active women younger than 25 years. The CDC also suggests testing all women older than 25 years who have had unprotected sex or who had more than one sex partner during the previous 90 days, or who have previously had an STD. Individuals at risk for infection should be tested once each year and during pregnancy.

The optimal timing of screening in pregnancy is uncertain. CDC guidelines recommend testing at the first prenatal visit. Screening early in pregnancy provides increased opportunities to improve pregnancy outcomes, including low birth weight and premature delivery. The CDC also reports that screening and treatment in the third trimester might be more effective at preventing transmission of chlamydial infection to the infant during birth by reducing the risk for reinfection. CDC guidelines updated in May 2002 recommend pregnant women less than 25 years of age and those at increased risk for chlamydia infection should be tested again for chlamydia and gonorrhea during the third trimester. Screening in early pregnancy and again in the third trimester helps reduce postnatal complications and helps protect the newborn from infection.

Treatment

Chlamydia can be treated with a number of different antibiotics, including one dose of azithromycin, or a seven-day course of doxycycline, amoxicillin, or erthyromycin. The results of clinical trials suggest that azithromycin and doxycline are equally efficacious, although if compliancy is questionable, a single dose treatment with azithromycin is more cost effective. Ofloaxacin is similar in efficacy to doxycycline and azithromycin, but it is more expensive and does not offer any advantages. Penicillin is not an effective treatment for chlamydia. Levofloxacin has not been evaluated in clinical trials but because of its similarity to ofloxacin, levofloxacin may be substituted in doses of 500 mg daily for seven days. Other quinolone drugs either are not reliably effective against chlamydial infection or have not been adequately evaluated.

When PID, prostate infection or epididymis infections are present, the prescribed course of antibiotics is longer. Although antibiotics successfully kill chlamydia bacteria, any damage done by the bacteria cannot be reversed. To minimize further transmission of infection, patients undergoing treatment for chlamydia should refrain from sexual intercourse for seven days after a single-dose therapy or until the completion of seven-day therapeutic regimens. A test of cure (a negative test confirming that treatment was effective) can be performed three weeks after the completion of therapy. If tests are performed earlier, false positives may occur due to the presence of dead organisms. The CDC recommends screening women 3–4

months after treatment is complete to reduce the incidence of PID.

Pregnant women are usually prescribed erythromycin or amoxicillin because other antibiotics, such as doxyclycline and ofloxacin, may be harmful to a developing fetus. With treatment, the newborn should not be at risk for developing a chlamydia infection. To help prevent chlamydial eye infections, hospital nursery employees routinely treat the eyes of newborns with prophylactic silver nitrate or antibiotic ointment shortly after birth. Patients with a co-existing HIV infection should use the same therapy for chlamydia as patients who are HIV negative.

• VACCINES—Researchers at the National Institute of Allergy and Infectious Disease (NIAID) are currently working on methods to prevent infection, such as topical antibiotic preparations and vaccines.

Recurrence

A high prevalence of C. trachomatis infections is found in women who have had chlamydial infection in the preceding several months. Most post-treatment infections result from reinfection, often because sexual partners were not treated or because the patient resumed sex among a network of persons with a high prevalence of infection. Repeat infection causes an increased risk of PID and other complications when compared to patients with an initial infection. For this reason, patients are advised to have repeat testing 3–4 months after finishing treatment.

Pregnancy

Chlamydia can readily be transmitted from mother to baby as the baby passes through the vaginal canal during childbirth. Approximately 50 percent of babies born to mothers with chlamydia acquire eye infections, and another 10 percent develop lung infections. Neonatal infections can result in blindness, lung disease, and fatal pneumonia. For this reason, screening for chlamydia is included in most prenatal screening programs. However, if testing is not performed until years after the initial infection, the fallopian tubes may already be scarred. In pregnant women, there is some evidence that chlamydia infections can lead to premature delivery. All pregnant women should have a screening test for chlamydia in early pregnancy and women younger than 25 years or who are at high risk should be tested again in the third trimester.

Clinical experience and preliminary data suggest that azithromycin is a safe and effective chlamydia treatment in pregnancy. Erythromycin is also safe and effective, but patients may not comply with the full treatment dose because of the drug's side effects. The CDC recommends that pregnant patients be treated with erythromycin base, 500 mg orally taken four times daily for seven days, or amoxicillin 500 mg orally three times daily for seven days.

Alternative regimens include 250 mg erythromycin taken four times daily for 14 days, erythromycin ethylsuccinate using 800 mg orally four times daily for seven days or 400 mg four times daily for 14 days; or azithromycin, using one gram orally as a single dose. The compound erythromycin estolate should not be used in pregnancy because it may cause liver problems.

• NEONATAL INFECTIONS—*C. Trachomatis* infection of neonates results from exposure to the mother's infected cervix during delivery. The prevalence of infection among pregnant women does not vary by race, ethnicity, or socioeconomic status. Babies who are born to infected mothers can develop chlamydial infections in their eyes and respiratory tracts. Chlamydia is a leading cause of early infant pneumonia and conjunctivitis (inflammation of the conjunctiva, the inner rim of the eye) in newborns.

Preventive ocular treatment with silver nitrate solution or antibiotic ointments does not prevent perinatal transmission of chlamydia from mother to infant. However, ocular prophylaxis with those agents does prevent eye infection. Initial perinatal infection with chlamydia involves the mucous membranes of the eyes, oropharynx and throat, urogenital tract and rectum. Infection is most often recognized by conjunctivitis that develops 5–12 days after birth. Chlamydia is the most frequent identifiable infectious cause of ophthalmia neonatorum, a condition of neonatal eye infection.

Chlamydia is also a common cause of subacute, afebrile (absence of fever) pneumonia with onset from 1–3 months of age. Infections with mild or no symptoms can also occur in the respiratory tract, genital tract, and rectum of neonates. Treatment for neonates consists of erythromycin base or ethylsuccinate 50 mg/kg/day administered orally into four doses daily for 14 days. Treatment is effective in approximately 80 percent of patients. Therefore, a second course of therapy and follow-up of infants is recommended. Neonates with conjunctivitis should also be evaluated for pneumonia.

Characteristic signs of chlamydial pneumonia in infants include a repetitive staccato cough with rapid breathing and hyperinflation, and bilateral diffuse infiltrates on a chest scan. Wheezing is rare and infants are typically afebrile. Diagnosis is made by NAT testing performed on nasopharyngeal swabs or tracheal aspirates.

Precautions

Until a physician determines that there are no signs of infection on a follow-up visit, individuals with chlamydia should refrain from all sexual contact. All of the individual's partners should be checked and treated for chlamydia even if they have no signs of infection. This will prevent the individual from developing a recurring case of chlamydia. In some states, all cases of chlamydia must be reported to the state health department by the facility that performs the testing.

Complications

Possible complications include pelvic inflammatory disease, ectopic pregnancy (pregnancy in which the fetus grows outside the womb) and infertility in women. In men, possible complications include epididymis and infertility. The autoimmune thyroid disorder, Reiter's syndrome, is known to occur in some people with chlamydia, even after the infection has been treated with antibiotics. In addition, compared to women who do not have chlamydia, women infected with chlamydia may also have a higher risk of acquiring HIV infection from an infected partner.

Risk Factors

The CDC reports that risk factors include young age, lower socioeconomic status, non-married status, multiple sexual partners, a new sex partner, history of gonorrhea, and lack of barrier contraceptive devices. Persons who engage in sexual behaviors that can place them at risk for STDs should use latex or polyurethane condoms every time they have sex. A condom put on the penis before starting sex and worn until the penis is withdrawn can help protect both the male and female partner from chlamydia infection.

Individuals diagnosed with chlamydia should notify all recent sex partners so that they can see a health care provider and receive treatment. Sex partners of infected individuals should receive treatment even if they show no signs of infection. Infected individuals should not have sex until both partners have completed drug treatment. *See also* **Conjunctivitis; Epididymitis; Eyes; Lymphogranuloma venereum; Mucopurulent cervicitis; Ophthalmia neonatorum; Trachoma;** and **Urethritis.**

CDC. *Sexually Transmitted Diseases Treatment Guidelines 2002.* Appendix E, "Chlamydia trachomatis Screening Recommendations." Atlanta: U.S. Dept. of Health and Human Services, 2002.

National Institute of Allergy and Infectious Disease, 2002.

NIAID/Centers for Disease Control and Prevention. *Sexually Transmitted Disease Surveillance 2001 Supplement: Chlamydia Prevalence Monitoring Project.* Atlanta, GA: U.S. Dept. of Health and Human Services, 2001.

Chlamydia Prevalence Monitoring Project

The Centers for Disease Control and Prevention's (CDC) Chlamydia Prevalence Monitoring Project is a collaborative effort among the Regional Infertility Prevention Projects, STD project areas, state epidemiologists and public health laboratory directors, the U.S. Department of Labor and the Indian Health Service. The purpose of this project is to monitor the prevalence of genital chlamydia trachomatis infections among women screened for this infection in the United States through publicly funded programs. The data from this effort is included in the CDC's annual STD Surveillance Report.

In 2001, the median state-specific chlamydia test positivity among 15 to 24 year old women who were screened at selected family planning clinics in all states, the District of Columbia, Puerto Rico, and the Virgin Islands was 5.6 percent. At selected prenatal clinics in this same population, median chlamydia test positivity was 7.4 percent. Among women entering juvenile or adult corrections facilities in 22 states, the median chlamydia test positivity was 14.8 percent.

Chlamydia Trachomatis (C. Trachomatis)

Chlamydia trachomatis is the infectious agent responsible for several different types of chlamydial infections. *See also* **Chlamydia.**

Choraphor

Choraphor is a patent herbal preparation used for the external treatment of herpes infections. Choraphor contains the herb St. John's Wort (Hypericum), ammoniated acid and copper sulphate in a solution of deionized water. Clinical studies have found Hypericum extract effective in reducing the frequency and severity of recurrent episodes of cold sores (herpes labalis) and genital herpes.

Choraphor is not a preventative medication. Rather it is an antiviral topical application that helps to heal herpes lesions, blisters or sores and reduces further recurrences. According to the manufacturer, it has been demonstrated to end outbreaks successfully in many cases.

Because the herpes virus remains dormant within the nervous system, it is impossible to fully eradicate. However, Choraphor is reported to attack the virus as it surfaces, reducing the viral load and accelerating recovery time. Patient testimonials and product information can be found at the manufacturer's web site, http://www.choraphor.com.

Chromosome

Chromosomes are strands of DNA that contain the genetic code for many different genes. Chromosomes occur in identical pairs. During reproduction, one chromosome from each parent combines. Each human cell contains a full complement of 23 chromosome pairs. 22 chromosomes hold the genetic code for approximately 30,000 different genes, and a pair of sex chromosomes designated X or Y determines the gender of an offspring.

Chronic idiopathic demyelinating polyneuropathy (CIPD)

CIPD is a syndrome characterized by a chronic, spontaneous loss or destruction of myelin, the protective sheath that surrounds nerve fibers. Patients with CIPD show progressive, usually symmetric weakness in the upper and lower extremities. Patients with clinical progression of symptoms after four to six weeks are by definition said to have CIPD. Treatment typically consists of IV immune globulins administered for four to five days or plasmapheresis using five to six exchanges over two weeks. *See also* **Acquired immune deficiency syndrome (AIDS)**.

City-county health departments

City and county health departments keep track of STD statistics for their area, contact the partners of individuals infected with STDs, and provide information regarding resources available for persons with HIV infection administered under the Ryan White Care Act.

Clade

The HIV-1 virus can be further categorized into three subgroups: major (M), outlier (O), and N. Group M of HIV-1 can be further divided into subtypes or clades named A–J. Clades are related HIV isolates classified according to their degree of genetic similarity (such as the percentage of identity within their envelope genes). The clade B of subgroup M of HIV-1 is responsible for nearly all HIV infections in North America and Western Europe. The clades or subtypes A and C are found predominantly in Africa. Subtype E occurs in Thailand. Other M clades are found primarily in Africa and Asia.

Clap *see* Gonorrhea

Clinical trials

Various branches of the National Institutes of Health, including the National Institute of Allergies and Infectious Diseases and the Centers for Disease Control and Prevention's Division of STDs and HIV, conduct clinical trials to evaluate newly developed STD treatments. Participants in clinical trials are given the opportunity to try out new medications before they are available to the general public, and receive diagnostic tests free of charge. In some trials, participants are also paid a fee to cover their time and travel expenses.

Based on the results of an initial decrease in viral load, drugs under investigation for HIV may be given accelerated approval in which phases of the trials are combined or drugs approved before the completion of studies. *See also* **Phase I trials, Phase II trials, Phase III trials**, and **Phase IV trials**, and also the Clinical Trials list in the resource section at the end of this book.

Clue cells

Clue cells can be seen in vaginal or cervical exudates screened by wet prep tests and sometimes during a microscopic examination of the urine. Clue cells are square-shaped superficial epithelial cells from the vaginal wall that are studded with bacteria particularly along the cell edges. Clue cells are diagnostic for bacterial vaginosis. *See also* **Bacterial vaginosis (BV)**.

Coccidiomycosis

Coccidiomycosis is an infectious fungal disease caused by the inhalation of spores of *Coccidioides immitis*, which are carried on windblown dust particles. It is considered an AIDS-defining opportunistic infection in persons with HIV infection.

Etiology

The etiologic agent is *Coccidioides immitis*, a dimorphic fungus found in the soil in the desert around the Southwestern United States and Northern Mexico, as well as in focal areas of Central and South America. Infection follows inhalation of arthrospores, which form endospores and spherules within the lung. Mature spherules release new endospores, which perpetuate infections.

Epidemiology

Coccidiomycosis, which is also known as desert fever, San Joaquin Valley fever, or Valley fever, is endemic in hot, dry regions of the Southwestern United States and Central and South America. Infection tends to occur in situations where soil is disturbed, such as construction sites, and usually causes a self-limited respiratory illness. People with HIV infection develop more severe, disseminated disease. Both new primary infection and reactivation occur in persons with HIV infection.

Symptoms

Most patients, especially if their CD4+ lymphocyte cell count is less than 250,000, develop pneumonia, presenting with fever, weight loss, night sweats, cough and dyspnea (shortness of breath), with symptoms lasting from several weeks to several months before the disease is diagnosed. Disseminated or systemic disease occurs in at least 30 percent of cases and results in generalized lymphadenopathy, skin nodules or ulcers, peritonitis, liver abnormalities, and bone and joint involvement. A type of meningitis with symptoms of lethargy, fever, headache, nausea, vomiting, and confusion occurs in about 10 percent of patients. In meningitis, the

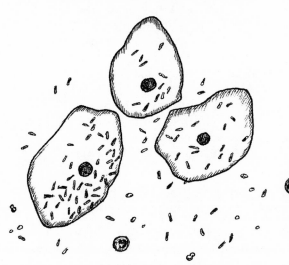

Clue cell (**Marvin G. Miller**).

cerebrospinal fluid typically contains a predominance of lymphocytes and more than 50 cells/ml of fluid.

Diagnosis

Coccidiomycosis is diagnosed by culturing the organism from clinical specimens such as sputum or by demonstrating the typical spherule during tissue examination. Blood cultures are positive in a minority of patients. Tests for antibodies to *Coccidiodes* are usually positive but can be negative in up to 25 percent of patients with disseminated infection.

Treatment

Amphotericin B, using 0.5–1.0 mg/kg/day, is the mainstay of therapy and should be used initially in patients with diffuse pulmonary or disseminated disease. Fluconazole, using 400–800 mg/day administered orally, may be used alternatively for patients with mild disease. Complete eradication is unlikely and chronic suppressive therapy with either fluconazole, using 200–400 mg/day, or itraconazole, using 200 mg every 12 hours, is needed. Successful treatment with itraconazole or fluconazole has been reported in approximately 80 percent of patients who develop meningitis.

Prevention

Preventive therapy is not recommended. However, persons with HIV traveling to areas where Coccidiomycosis is endemic are advised not to disturb the soil and to avoid windy, dusty areas.

Co-existing STDs

Co-existing STDs is a term referring to more than one STD entity occurring in one person. Having one STD is a risk factor for acquiring other STDs. The presence of co-existing STDs must be considered when selecting an optimal treatment.

Colposcopy

Colposcopy is a procedure employing a lighted magnifying instrument known as a colposcope to examine the lower genital tract and, if indicated, to aid in obtaining cervical biopsy specimens. Colposcopy is commonly performed as a follow-up procedure in women with HPV who show evidence of abnormal cell morphology on Pap smears. *See also* **Human papilloma virus** and **Pap smear.**

Community Programs for Clinical Research on AIDS (CPCRA)

The CPCRA, founded in 1989 by the National Institute of Allergy and Infectious Diseases, and called the Terry Beirn Community Programs for Clinical Research on AIDS since 1992, is a network of research units composed of community-based health care providers who offer their patients the opportunity to participate in research at locations where they receive their health care. The 15 CPCRA units comprise a variety of clinical settings, including private physicians' practices, university, and veterans' hospital clinics; drug treatment centers; and freestanding community clinics.

Patients attending these clinics are eligible for participation in CPCRA studies. The CPCRA is targeted to serve populations under-represented in previous clinical trials efforts. The research focus and scientific agenda of the CPCRA is identifying and improving treatment options in the day-to-day clinical care of people with HIV. More information can be found on their internet address, http://www.cpcra.org/.

Complementary DNA (cDNA)

Complementary DNA refers to a double helical DNA copy of an RNA molecule. Complementary DNA is formed during viral replication.

Condoms

Condoms are thin rubber or latex tubes that fit over a man's erect penis. When the man ejaculates he ejaculates into the condom, which prevents sperm from entering the vagina. The word condom is derived from the Latin *condos*, meaning receptacle.

The oldest illustration of a condom was found in Egypt, and dates back more than 3,000 years. The oldest condoms discovered were found in the foundations of Dudley Castle near Birmingham, England, and were apparently washed and re-used. Made of fish and animal intestines, these condoms date back to 1640, soon after the first syphilis epidemic threatened Europe.

Condoms made of sheep intestines are still available today, although they are now used once and disposed of. Sheepskin condoms are not effective against the HIV virus. Rubber condoms were first mass-produced after 1844, when Charles Goodyear patented the vulcanization of rubber. Latex, the sap from a rubber tree, is the raw material used for condoms. In 1995 plastic condoms went on the market in the United States.

The CDC reports that correct and consistent use of the male latex condom can reduce the risk of STD transmission. Lubricated condoms offer more protection from breakage and leakage of semen. However, no protective method is 100 percent effective, and condom use cannot guarantee absolute protection against any STD. The CDC also notes that condoms lubricated with spermicides are no more effective than other lubricated condoms in protecting against the transmission of HIV and other STDs.

Male Condoms

When used consistently and correctly, male latex condoms are effective in preventing the sexual transmission of HIV infection, and can reduce the risk for other STDs. However, because condoms do not cover all exposed areas, they are likely to be more effective in preventing infections transmitted by fluids from mucosal surfaces, for instance gonorrhea and HIV infections, than in preventing those transmitted by skin-to-skin contact, such as herpes simplex virus (HSV); human papilloma virus (HPV); and syphilis.

Condoms are regulated by the Food and Drug Administration (FDA) as medical devices and are subject to tests for product safety and effectiveness. Each latex condom manufactured in the United States is tested electronically for holes before packaging. In the United States, rates of condom breakage during sexual intercourse and withdrawal are low (approximately two broken condoms for every 100 used). Condom failure usually results from inconsistent or incorrect use rather than breakage.

Male condoms made of materials other than latex are available in the United States. Although they have had higher breakage and slippage rates, they are equally effective as latex condoms used as a barrier for pregnancy. Non-latex condoms (those made of polyurethane or other synthetic material) can be used for persons with latex allergy.

The proper use of male condoms includes: using a new condom with each act of sexual intercourse (e.g. oral, vaginal and anal); handling the condom carefully to avoid damaging it with fingernails, teeth or other objects that could result in a tear; putting the condom on after the penis is erect and before any genital contact with the partner, ensuring that no air is trapped in the tip of the condom; and using only water-based lubricants (such as K-Y Jelly, Astroglide, AwualLube, and glycerin) with latex condoms. Oil-based lubricants, such as petroleum-based jelly, mineral oil, massage oils, hand lotions, baby oil and body lotions, can weaken latex and should not be used. Ensure adequate lubrication during intercourse, using lubricants if needed, and remove condoms from their wrappers gently, never using teeth, scissors or sharp nails. Hold the condom firmly against the base of the penis during withdrawal, and withdraw while the penis is still erect to prevent slippage.

Condoms have an expiration date, stamped on the box or wrapper, and the expiration date should be checked before use. The expiration date is not the same as the manufacturing date. Condoms lubricated with the spermicide N-9 are not recommended because they cost more and have a shorter shelf life than other lubricated condoms. In addition, condoms with N-9 have been associated with an increased risk of bacterial urinary tract infections in women. Extreme temperatures can cause latex to become brittle and break easily. For this reason, condoms should not be stored in glove compartments or other places subject to extreme temperatures.

Female Condoms

Laboratory studies indicate that the female condom (Reality), which consists of a lubricated polyurethane sheath with a ring on each end that is inserted into the vagina, is an effective mechanical barrier to viruses, including HIV. With the exception of one investigation of recurrent trichomoniasis, no clinical studies have been completed to evaluate the efficacy of female condoms in providing protection from STDs, including HIV. If used consistently and correctly, the female condom may substantially reduce the risk for STDs. When a male condom cannot be used properly, sex partners should consider using a female condom. *See also* **Dental dams; Diaphragms; Spermicides;** and **Sponges.**

Centers for Disease Control and Prevention. *Sexually Transmitted Diseases Treatment Guidelines 2002.* Atlanta: U.S. Dept. of Health and Human Services, 2002.
"Male Latex Condoms and Sexually Transmitted Diseases." CDC Fact Sheet for Public Health Personnel, July 2001.

Condylomata acuminata

Condylomata acuminata is a condition characterized by genital warts, which typically appear around the vagina, penis or rectum.

Etiology

Condylomata acuminata is caused by the human papilloma virus (HPV), generally types 16 and 18.

Epidemiology

There is limited epidemiological data on the incidence of condylomata acuminata. Reports from France, which are similar to those of other developed countries, suggest that about 107 of every 100,000 people develop condylomata acuminata annually.

Symptoms

Condylomata acuminata has a cauliflower-like appearance and often occurs on moist skin. In homosexual men, condylomata acuminata generally causes warts in the perianal area or in the anal canal. These warts rarely extend into the rectum. Perianal condylomata acuminata appear as raised pink-brown papules, usually in clusters, and occasionally as large cauliflower-like masses.

Condylomata acuminata may appear on the lips, tongue, or palate as a rare manifestation of infection. Most of these patients also have other genital or perianal warts and most give a history of oral sex.

Diagnosis

Diagnosis is made by physical examination with detection of the characteristic warts sufficient for diagnosis.

Treatment

No treatment is completely satisfactory. External genital warts may be removed by laser, cryotherapy (chemical freezing), or surgery using local anesthetics. Chemical treatments, such as podophyllum resin or purified toxin or trichloroacetic acid, can be applied directly to the warts. However, chemical treatments, which seldom work, require many applications over weeks to months and may burn the skin. Excisional treatments include curettage, electrosurgery, scissors excision or laser vaporization. Injectable treatments include interferon or 5-fluorouracil/epinephrine gel implant.

Patient-applied treatment includes podofilox (Condylox) solution and gel, and imiquimod (Aldera) cream. Podofilix 0.5% solution has the advantage of not needing to be washed off after application. Applied with a cotton swab, it is used twice daily for three days. Imiquod 5% cream, which stimulates immune system chemicals, is applied with fingers three times weekly for up to 16 weeks. The treatment area is washed with mild soap and water 6–10 hours after application of cream.

Precautions

Patients with compromised immune function due to malignancy or HIV infection are more likely to have frequent recurrences of extensive lesions which may be resistant to treatment. Treatment with topical podophyllin can cause burns when used for warts present in the anal canal.

Risk Factors

Unprotected sex, anal sex, smoking, multiple sex partners and the presence of another STD. *See also* **Genital warts** and **Human papilloma virus.**

Condylomata lata

Condylomata lata are moist papules or lesions similar to warts that frequently occur in secondary syphilis. *See also* **Syphilis.**

Conjunctivitis

Conjunctivitis refers to inflammation of the conjunctiva, the clear membrane covering the white of the eye and the inside of the eyelid. The conjunctiva produces a fluid that lubricates the cornea and eyelid. Conjunctivitis can be caused by infection with a number of different organisms that cause STDs. The three most common causes are *Chlamydia trachomatis*, herpes simplex virus, and *Neisseria gonorrhoeae*. Other sources of infection include *Treponema pallidum*, which causes syphilis, and cytomegalovirus.

Conjunctivitis can be endemic such as is seen in trachoma. Conjunctivitis can also be transmitted during sexual intercourse, autoinoculation or during childbirth. Most states require that nursery staff administer prophylactic optical treatment to neonates following childbirth to help protect against conjunctivitis related to childbirth. *See also* **Chlamydia; Cytomegalovirus; Eyes; Gonorrhea; Herpes simplex virus; Syphilis;** and **Trachoma.**

Contact tracing

In contact tracing, a policy initiated in the 1930s, health care workers contact the sexual partners of individuals with reportable STDs and encourage them to report for treatment. Contact tracing, which is a form of STD control, also includes contacting treated individuals and having them come in to be re-examined to ensure that they have been cured. By identifying a patient's sexual contacts, these individuals could be apprised of the possibility of infection, and be tested and treated, if needed. *See also* **Partner notification programs.**

Core protein

Core protein refers to the protein capsule surrounding a virus's RNA or DNA. Distinct antibodies can be formed against the core protein of the hepatitis or HIV virus as well as the viral envelope. In some early infections, such as hepatitis, only antibodies to core protein may be present. In HIV, p55, the precursor molecule to the core, is broken down into the smaller protein molecules of p24, p17, p7, and p6. HIV's core protein is primarily composed of p24.

Counseling

Counseling is an important part of STD treatment. STD counselors provide information on what to expect from medical treatment. In addition, counselors explain any complications to watch for, and explain if and why past and future partners should be notified. Counselors also explain risk factors and preventive strategies, and help the patient cope with emotional issues related to having an STD.

Crabs *see* Pubic lice (*Pediculus pubis*)

Cryptococcosis

Cryptococcosis is an opportunistic infection that occurs in five to 10 percent of patients with HIV infection in North America, where it is the most common invasive fungal disease.

Etiology

The etiologic agent is *Cryptococcus neoformans,* a fungus found worldwide as a soil organism. About five percent of patients who have HIV infection in the Western world develop a disseminated form of cryptococcosis, affecting multiple organs and bodily systems. It is thought that transmission occurs via inhalation of the spores and unencapsulated form of the fungus, which leads to colonization of the airways and subsequent respiratory infection. Without an intact immune system response, the organism is free to proliferate and disseminate throughout the body.

Cryptococcus neoformans can cause infection in humans and animals, but human infection is thought to proceed from environmental sources rather than from animals suffering from cryptococcosis.

Pigeons and pet birds are often healthy carriers, excreting these yeasts with their excrements. Cryptococcal infection may arise from inhalation of contaminated dust.

Epidemiology

Cryptococcosis is more prevalent in Sub-Saharan Africa than it is the United States, where it primarily occurs in patients with AIDS or who are otherwise immunosuppressed. Most cases of infection occur in patients with CD4+ lymphocytes counts less than 50,000 per cubic millimeter.

Symptoms

Cryptococcosis usually presents as a subacute meningitis or meningoencephalitis with symptoms of fever, malaise, and headache. Symptoms are usually present for 2–4 weeks before diagnosis. Classic symptoms of meningitis such as neck stiffness and light sensitivity occur in about one-third of patients. Some patients show signs of encephalitis such as lethargy, altered mental faculties, personality changes, and memory loss. About one-half of patients have evidence of pulmonary involvement with cough and shortness of breath, as well as abnormal chest radiographic films. Skin involvement is also common, and several types of skin lesions may occur. The most common form is a lesion resembling molluscum contagiosum.

Clinical deterioration in Cryptococcus infection may be due to cerebral edema. Cryptococcal meningitis requires lifelong suppressive therapy.

Diagnosis

Latex antigen agglutination tests performed on cerebrospinal fluid or serum are used as a preliminary screening test for Crypotococcus infection. A high titer of cryptococcal antigen is almost always detectable in cerebrospinal fluid. False complexes can occur as a consequence of prozones and immune complexes containing antigens bound to antibody.

Serum antibody detection tests are also available and are valuable in early disease and in localized infection in which antigen production is low. Screening tests can be confirmed using culture technique or DNA probe assays. DNA probe analysis reveals that recurrent *C. neoformans* infection results from reactivation of the original infecting strain rather than reinfection.

Treatment

Untreated, Cryptococcus meningitis is fatal. For Cryptococcus meningitis, Amphotericin B using 0.7mg/kg daily along with flucytosine, using 25 mg/kg every six hours is used for the first two weeks, followed by lifelong therapy with fluconazole.

Risk Factors

Risk factors include a CD4 count less than 200,000 cells/cubic millimeter of blood and contact with pet birds. Patients infected with HIV are advised to avoid contact with pigeons and pet birds.

Cryptosporidium

Cryptosporidium is a type of coccidian protozoa that causes an opportunistic infection of cryptosporidiosis in persons with HIV infection. *Cryptosporidium* was rarely seen before 1982.

Etiology

Cryptosporidium parvum, the species most likely to infect humans, is a small protozoan that may inhabit the gastrointestinal, respiratory, and biliary tracts of a variety of animals, including humans. Widely seen among the animal population, *Cryptosporidium* was first reported in 1976 in a young immunocompetent child. Numerous waterborne and swimming pool outbreaks have since occurred, culminating in 1993 in the largest waterborne outbreak in U.S. history. The outbreak involved more than 400,000 people in Milwaukee. Infection usually occurs from three to 14 days after exposure. *Cryptosporidium* may be spread from domestic pets and from person-to-person contact. Since large numbers of *Cryptosporidium* cysts can be present in feces and the infectious dose is very small, fecal-oral contamination through sexual contact may also contribute to transmission.

Epidemiology

Outside of outbreaks, cryptosporidiosis affects about 2.1 percent of individuals with symptoms of diarrhea. Infection rates are highest in developing countries.

Symptoms

Symptoms of cryptosporidiosis depend on the immune status of the person infected. In healthy individuals, infection results in a flu-like, non-inflammatory gastrointestinal illness with symptoms of malaise, anorexia, vomiting, abdominal pain and cramps, and occasional fever. Diarrhea lasts on average 6–14 days, although it may last much longer. In persons who are immunocompromised, including AIDS patients, infection may cause severe prolonged diarrhea, respiratory infection, and liver involvement. Cryptosporidiosis may also involve the gallbladder, the biliary tract, the bronchi, and the lungs.

Diagnosis

Diagnosis is made by an examination of stool specimens for the presence of oocysts. Examination of at least two fecal smears may be necessary for diagnosis. Enzyme linked immunosorbent (ELISA) assay methods are also available for the detection of fecal cryptosporidial antigens. Blood tests are also available to detect IgM and IgG antibodies to *Cryptosporidium*.

Treatment

In severe diarrhea, intravenous fluids may be necessary to treat dehydration. There is no effective pharmaceutical therapy, although modest benefits have been observed with the use of paromomycin. Anti-diarrheal agents such as loperamide or paregoric may be helpful in controlling symptoms but have no effect on the causative organism. It is important to differentiate cryptosporidiosis from cyclosporidiosis because treatment with cotrimoxazole is effective in the latter infection.

Prevention

CDC guidelines for prevention include avoidance of fecal exposure during sexual contact, careful hygiene, including hand washing when handling pets, avoiding new pets under six months old, and drinking bottled water in regions that may not have a safe water supply. *See also* **Cyclospora cayetanensis.**

Cultural differences

Epidemiology studies show that different populations are more likely to develop STDs. Studies show that the primary reason for these differences is the availability of health care resources, with minority groups typically being underserved or less likely to seek healthcare services. Drug abuse, especially intravenous drug use, also differs among different ethnic groups and accounts for a higher rate of STDs in certain groups. STDs rates are also higher in prison inmates, a population primarily composed of minority groups.

Cultural influences

Cultural influences, particularly attitudes toward casual sex, frequent sex partners, and condom use influence STD development. Studies show that alcohol and drugs used before sex only contribute slightly to risky sex behavior in women. Prior use of condoms had a higher association with women's demands that their partners used condoms, although the risk increased when women had sex with new partners.

Intravenous drug use and partners who are intravenous drug users are high risk factors for STD transmission primarily because of the many STDs transmitted through needle sharing. Intravenous drug use is also associated with a higher incidence of risky sexual behavior.

Other factors reported to increase risky behavior and STD development include unsupervised time for teenagers and peer pressure. A study of U.S. teens conducted by the RAND Corporation and reported in *Pediatrics* found that 80 percent of teens who spent at least 30 hours unsupervised each week said they were sexually active, a behavior reported by only 68 percent of teens who spent less than five weekly hours unsupervised. In addition, 91 percent of teens who reported having sex indicated that the sexual encounter had occurred at a home, either theirs or someone else's. Boys who spent more than five hours per week after school without an adult present were twice as likely as other boys to have gonorrhea or chlamydia.

Culture and sensitivity (C&S)

In the culture and sensitivity (C&S) test, a biological specimen, such as blood, urine, or exudate from a lesion, is inoculated onto a plate of culture media, usually a type of agar containing growth nutrients. The culture plates are incubated at 37°C and observed for 48 hours for evidence of bacterial or fungal growth. Bacterial and fungal colonies are further tested and identified.

The isolated colonies are tested with a number of different antibiotics in the sensitivity portion of the test. Organisms that grow in the presence of specific antibiotics show resistance. Growth that is prohibited by antibiotics can be measured and the rate of susceptibility quantified. This enables the physician to see which antibiotics are most effective for treating the specific infection.

Cutaneous lymphoma

Cutaneous T-cell lymphomas and occasionally B-cell lymphomas can present in the early stages of HIV infection. The skin may be involved secondary to systemic disease. Cutaneous lymphoma may occur as more benign skin tumors or as a form of Non-Hodgkin's lymphoma (NHL), which is an AIDS-defining illness. Cutaneous lymphoma of NHL origin occurs in two forms: an aggressive form with plaques, tumors, and ulcerating lesions or nodules that responds poorly to therapy and is associated with a CD8+ infiltrate in immunocompromised patients; and a more typical cutaneous patch/plaque type of disease.

Cutaneous lymphoma is diagnosed by skin biopsy, and patients should be evaluated for signs of systemic lymphoma. Treatment depends on the extent of the lesions and the immunocompetence of the patients. Chemotherapy is often used, but it can seriously impair an immune system that is already suppressed.

CXCR4 (fusin)

CXCR4 or fusin is a cell molecule that acts as a cofactor or co-receptor for the entry of HIV into immune system cells. Early in the AIDS epidemic, CD4 molecules were found to be the primary receptor for HIV on immune system cells. Recent data suggest that a second molecule, CXCR4, is also required for fusion and entry of certain strains of HIV into host cells. New studies indicate a multistage interplay between HIV and two receptors on white blood cells. After binding to the receptor CD4, the virus fuses with a second receptor, CXCR4, which normally binds to cytokines. This double clasp may then signal the receptors to move the virus into the cells. Drugs intended to block the CXCR4 receptor are under development.

Cyclospora cayetanensis

The protozoan Cyclospora causes symptoms similar to those of *Cryptosporidium* in persons with AIDS. It is important to distinguish between the two infections because cyclosporidiosis responds to treatment with cotrimoxazole whereas cryptosporidiosis does not.

Cytokines

Cytokines are immune system chemicals such as interferon and various growth factors that are released during the immune response. Studies of the relationship between HIV and cytokines have shown that complex exchanges occur when HIV and white blood cells meet. Research shows that HIV-1 needs access to cytokines receptors on the cell surface to infect the cell. Several cytokines known as RANTES, MIP-1A, and MIP-1B, interfere with HIV replication by occupying and blocking these receptors. Findings suggest that one mechanism these molecules use to suppress HIV infectivity is to block the process of fusion used by the virus to enter and infect host cells.

Cytomegalovirus (CMV)

The cytomegaloviruses include a number of different CMV viruses that are commonly found in humans.

Etiology

The CMV virus belongs to the beta herpesvirus family and is also known as human herpes virus-5 or HHV-5. Although it is widespread, CMV is a significant human pathogen. Following a primary infection with CMV, excretion of virus can persist for weeks, months, or years before becoming latent. Periods without symptoms can alternate with periods of viral shedding that persist for years after the primary infections. Although most maternal CMV infections are mild and do not cause symptoms, fetal CMV can have serious consequences.

Infection requires close or intimate contact, including sexual contact and childbirth. The instance of infection in infants is higher in areas where breastfeeding is a common practice. Children attending day care centers also have a higher incidence of CMV infection, presumably from contact with saliva on hands and toys.

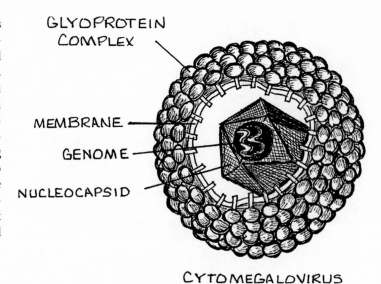

CYTOMEGALOVIRUS

Cytomegalovirus (CMV) (Marvin G. Miller).

Epidemiology

Infection with CMV is endemic and does not have a seasonal variation. Studies show the presence of CMV in every population studied worldwide. The presence of antibodies to CMV increases with age, and the prevalence of infection is higher in developing countries and among lower socioeconomic groups. Higher rates of CMV are seen in people with multiple sex partners and histories of STDs.

Studies of women of childbearing age in the United States show a prevalence ranging from less than 50 to 85 percent. Transmission occurs by person-to-person contact, and sources of contact include urine, mouth and throat secretions, cervical and vaginal secretions, semen, milk, tears, blood, transfusions of blood products, and transplanted organs. Blood products that have white blood cells removed (leukoreduced) shortly after blood collection do not pose risk for CMV transmission. Of the women who develop CMV during pregnancy, 30 to 40 percent transmit the virus to their fetuses.

Symptoms

Symptoms include fever, increased production of atypical lymphocytes, enlarged spleen, rash, and enlarged lymph nodes. Gastrointestinal symptoms may also oc-

cur, including colitis, fever, abdominal pain, and bloody or watery diarrhea. Rarely, gastrointestinal CMV infection can lead to the development of intestinal ulcer.

Diagnosis

Diagnosis is made by microscopic examination of exudates, with diagnosis confirmed by the demonstration of intranuclear inclusion bodies within infected cells. CMV can also be cultured from urine. Blood can also be tested with nucleic acid amplification testing using a polymerase chain reaction (PCR), which identifies viral DNA. However, infection diagnosed by PCR does not differentiate past exposure from active disease since antibodies to CMV persist after previous exposure.

Treatment

There is no safe, effective treatment for congenital CMV infection. The most encouraging results have been obtained with Ganciclovir, although toxic side effects, including immune suppression, may occur.

Neonatal Complications

The symptoms of intrauterine CMV infection are different and far more serious than usually seen in CMV infection. Vasculitis (inflammation of blood vessels), bruising, abnormal bleeding, and clotting problems are likely to develop and growth may be retarded. Microcephaly (a head circumference of less than the fifth percentile) may occur and brain function may be impaired. Deafness is the most common handicap caused by congenital CMV infection.

Multiple organs are often involved, although the most common occurrence is enlarged liver. Jaundice may occur if the liver is affected. Death occurring during the first year of life is usually caused by progressive liver disease or failure to thrive. Deaths from CMV infection occurring after the first year usually occur in severely neurologically handicapped children and are related to malnutrition, aspiration pneumonia, and severe infection. Long-term complications include hearing loss, mental retardation, microcephaly, optic atrophy, language delay, and learning disabilities.

Perinatal (occurring around or shortly after birth) infections are generally not as severe as congenital infections and may not cause symptoms.

Risk Factors

The risk of acquiring CMV during pregnancy poses the most serious consequences. Sexual transmission can be prevented by barrier methods, including condoms and spermicides. Another risk factor in pregnancy is exposure to children who are actively shedding the CMV virus. Immunocompromised patients are also at increased risk for developing CMV.

CMV in Persons with HIV/AIDS

CMV is one of the most common opportunistic organisms and the one most likely to cause visual loss in persons with HIV/AIDS. CMV infects many tissues, including the lungs, gastrointestinal tract, and brain, but its most common target is the eye, where it causes CMV retinitis.

CMV retinitis accounts for up to 85 percent of all CMV infections in AIDS patients. The optimal method for evaluating the progression of CMV retinitis and its response to treatment is with fundus photographs. Typically, CMV retinitis occurs late in the course of AIDS, when CD4 counts have declined to 50 or less. Treatment usually consists of ganciclovir and foscarnet administered intravenously or directly into the vitreous. *See also* **Acquired immune deficiency syndrome; Conjunctivitis; Herpesviruses; Human herpesviruses;** and **Mononeuritis multiplex (MM).**

Dane particle

The Dane particle is the original name for the hepatitis B virus, the etiologic agent of hepatitis B. The Dane particle refers to HBV virion or DNA.

DdC *see* Zalcitabine

DdI *see* Didanosine

Defensins *see* Alpha defensins

Dendritic cells (dendrites)

Dendrites, primarily macrophages, are immune system cells that may begin the HIV disease process by carrying the virus from the site of the infection to the lymph nodes, where other immune system cells become infected. Dendrites travel through the body and bind to foreign antigens, such as HIV, especially in external tissues, such as the skin and the membranes of the gut, lungs, and reproductive tract. They then ferry the foreign substance to the lymph nodes to stimulate T cells and initiate an immune response. In laboratory experiments, the dendrites that carry HIV also bind to CD4+ T cells, thereby allowing HIV to infect these cells, which are the primary target of HIV infection.

Dental dams

In oral sex with women, dental dams may be used. A dental dam is a six-inch square piece of thin latex that is available in dental and medical supply stores. Home-made dams can be made by cutting a rolled condom to the center and spreading it open. The dam should cover the entire vulva and should be held at both edges. It is important not to turn the dam inside out during oral sex. Both men and women can use dental dams for oral-anal sex to help prevent STDs.

To use a dental dam, rinse the powdery talc from the dental dam, pat dry or allow to air dry; place water-based lubricant on the side that faces either the female genitals (vulva) or the anus; place the barrier on the genitals or anus. Do not move the barrier back and forth between the vagina and anus, since this can cause infection. Throw the dental dam away after using. Dental dams should not be re-used.

Alternately, plastic wrap can be used, although there are no studies showing that it is effective against HIV transmission. However, it has been proved to block the herpes virus, which is a smaller molecule than the HIV virus. Also, plastic wrap should not be microwavable, since this type of wrap is porous.

"How to use a dental dam." Gay Men's Health Crisis, Fact Sheet, NYC, 1996. www.gmnc.org.

Dentistry

Although HIV transmission is possible in health care settings, the CDC reports that it is extremely rare. In 1990, the CDC reported on an HIV-infected dentist in Florida, Dr. David Acer, who apparently infected some of his patients while doing dental work. Studies of viral DNA sequence linked the dentist to six of his patients who were infected. The CDC has not determined exactly how transmission took place, but it is suspected that Acer used dental equipment that he had previously used on himself, since dentists primarily use disposable cleaning tips and other disposable equipment to reduce the risk of transmission. There have been no other confirmed reports of patients infected with AIDS during dental procedures.

Deoxyribonucleic acid (DNA)

DNA, which is the principal constituent of chromosomes, is the genetic material containing the life code or genome for all living organisms. DNA is found in genes within the nucleus of each cell. DNA carries the genetic information that enables cells to reproduce. The DNA genome consists of a very long string of four molecules called nucleotides. Each nucleotide contains a specific arrangement of the nucleosides adenine, cytosine, guanine, and thymine. The order in which the nucleotides are arranged determines the proteins for which the genes code. In most organisms DNA is first transcribed into ribonucleic acid (RNA), which is then converted into the specific proteins.

The spiral structure formed by two strands of DNA (primary and complementary) forms a double helix. The nucleotide strands of the helix are mirror images of one another. When a cell divides in reproduction the strands unwind, each serving as a template or model for the construction of a new complementary strand.

d4T *see* Stavudine

Diaphragms

Diaphragms used as vaginal contraceptives offer protection against cervical chlamydia, gonorrhea, and trichomoniasis. However, the effectiveness of diaphragms as prevention for HIV has not been evaluated, and the use of diaphragms is not recommended as protective against viral and other STDs. Diaphragm use has been associated with an increased risk of bacterial urinary tract infection in women.

Didanosine (ddl)

Didanosine (Videx) is a nucleoside reverse transcriptase inhibitor (NRTI) used as an antiretroviral agent in the treatment of HIV.

Direct access testing

Direct access testing (DAT) is the ability to order one's own laboratory tests without a doctor's prescription. As of 2001, 34 states allow DAT, but 18 states still prohibit the practice.

DNA mutations

DNA mutations are changes in the amino acids that make up DNA that result in a new inheritable characteristic. During the course of HIV disease, mutated HIV strains may emerge in an infected individual. These mutated strains, which are still HIV viruses, may differ widely in their ability to infect and kill different cell types, as well as in their rate of replication, and response to anti-retroviral agents. Single mutations in HIV can result in resistance to one or more antiretroviral drugs. Thymidine analog mutations (TAMS) in HIV initially occurred in patients on zidovudine (AZT) therapy.

DNA sequences *see* Nucleotide sequences

Donovanosis (*Granuloma inguinale*)

Donovanosis is a chronic ulcerative disease that generally affects the skin and sub-

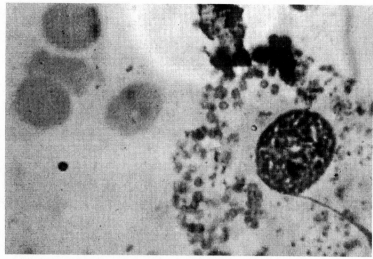

Donovan bodies in skin scrapings in *Granuloma inguinale* (Susan Lindsley, CDC).

cutaneous tissue (tissue directly below the surface skin) of the genital, inguinal, and anal regions. Donovanosis is caused by the bacteria *Calymmatobacterium granulomatosis*, an organism that multiplies within tissue cells. Granuloma inguinale is rare in temperate climates, such as the Northern United States, but it is common in some tropical and subtropical areas. *See also* **Granuloma inguinale**.

Douches

Douches are solutions of warm water, often containing chemicals, which are used to irrigate and cleanse the vagina. The practice of douching dates back to ancient Egyptian times. According to a 1988 federal survey, 37 percent of American women douche regularly, and women of lower socioeconomic backgrounds were found more likely to douche. However, douching can destroy the normal bacterial flora of the vagina, allowing pathogenic organisms to proliferate, thus promoting infection.

Douching cannot prevent STDs. On the contrary, women who douche are more likely to develop STDs because they generally have a significantly greater number of lifetime sexual partners, including partners with high numbers of sexual contacts.

The short-term relief provided by douching for irritating symptoms can make matters worse by promoting bacterial growth. Douching allows vaginal bacteria to travel through to the cervix and uterus, increasing the likelihood of pelvic inflammatory disease. Women who douche are reported to have a 73 percent greater risk of PID compared to women who do not douche.

The high pressure caused by douching can also disrupt the mucus plug that normally protects the opening of the womb. Studies also show an increased likelihood of ectopic pregnancy in women who douche.

Stewart, Elizabeth G. *The V Book: A Doctor's Guide to Complete Vulvovaginal Health.* New York: Bantam Books, 2002.

Drug pilot programs

Drug pilot programs distribute drug therapies to specific populations and later evaluate the results of this intervention. Examples are programs that deliver free anti-retroviral drugs to patients with HIV/AIDS. Obstacles to these programs include the cost of the medications for the sponsoring agency, stigma for recipients, lack of infrastructure and lack of trained personnel to monitor the programs.

Drug resistance

Bacteria and viruses can mutate into strains with resistance to specific antibiotics. For instance, some strains of *Neisseria gonorrhoeae* are resistant to penicillin and fluoroquinolone antibiotics. In the case of penicillin resistance, the mutated strains traditionally were found to produce penicillinase, an enzyme which breaks down penicillin. Penicillin resistance may also be caused by chromosomally mediated resistance to penicillin. Development of bacterial resistance has been linked to many different factors, including excess prescribing of antibiotics, easy access to antibiotics, and self-medicating by high-risk groups such as commercial sex workers.

To determine susceptibility or resistance, laboratories must perform a sensitivity test in which they culture the infectious agent and then subject the isolated colonies to therapeutic concentrations of various antibiotics. Uncontrolled growth in the presence of an antibiotic shows resistance.

When antibiotic therapy is prescribed without the benefit of a culture and sensitivity, ineffective treatment may be prescribed. This is why patients are sometimes told to come back for follow-up appointments or to return if symptoms persist to make sure their condition has been properly treated.

Surveillance studies conducted by the CDC showed that overall, 20.9 percent of *N. gonorrhoaea* isolates were resistant to penicillin, tetracycline, or both. Resistance to ciprofloxacin was first identified in 1991. From 1991 to 1998, fewer than nine ciprofloxacin-resistant isolates were identified each year in the United States. However, by 2001, 38 resistant isolates were identified in the United States, and in Honolulu, 20.3 percent of gonorrhea isolates showed resistance to ciprofloxacin. The rate of resistant strains also showed a significant increase in California. As a result, in early 2002, the California STD Program recommended that fluorquinolones no longer be used for gonorrhea treatment in California.

Resistance to anti-retroviral therapy has also been established in HIV infection, allowing the virus to replicate rapidly even in the presence of therapy. *See also* **Antibiotics** and **Culture and sensitivity**.

Early Intervention Services (EIS)

Early intervention services include activities designed to identify individuals who are HIV positive and get them into care as quickly as possible. As funded through Titles I and II of the CARE Act, EIS includes outreach, counseling and testing, information and referral services. Under Title III of the CARE Act it also includes comprehensive primary medical care for individuals living with HIV/AIDS.

Ebers Papyrus

The Ebers Papyrus is a compendium of medical practices written in 1550 B.C. The first written prescription for a contraceptive (barrier method) can be found in the Ebers Papyrus.

Ehrlich, Paul (1854–1915)

The renowned German immunologist Paul Ehrlich discovered the syphilis remedy Salvarsan (606) in 1919. Salvarsan was the first compound to target specifically an infectious agent. Salvarsan, an arsenic derivative or arsphenamine, replaced the more toxic mercury compounds, which had previously been used as a treatment for syphilis. Arsenic was proved to kill effectively *Treponema pallidum*, the bacteria responsible for syphilis.

ELISA test *see* Enzyme-linked immunosorbent assay

Emergence of AIDS *see* AIDS history

Emergency response workers

As a provision of the Ryan White Act, police officers and other employees who are exposed to HIV in their line of duty, have a right to counseling and treatment if blood tests on the source person are positive; emergency response workers also have the right to receive blood testing and management after occupational exposures.

Employment issues

Individuals with STDs including HIV/AIDS are protected from job discrimination under the Americans with Disabilities Act.

Endemic

Endemic refers to diseases that are prevalent or more likely to be found in specific populations. For instance, trachoma is endemic in certain developing countries.

Enteritis

Enteritis is a sexually transmitted gastrointestinal syndrome that predominantly occurs among persons whose sexual practices include oral-fecal or oral-genital contact. Enteritis usually results in diarrhea and abdominal cramping without signs of proctitis or proctocolitis. In otherwise healthy persons, the parasite *Giardia lamblia* is most frequently implicated.

Among HIV-infected patients, some infections that usually are not sexually transmitted may occur via anogenital transmission, including cytomegalovirus, *Mycobacterium avium*-intracellulare, Shigella species, Salmonella species, Cryptosporidium, Microsporidium, and Isospora. Multiple stool examinations for ova and parasites or a direct antigen test on the stool may be required to direct *Giardia lamblia*. Stool cultures are required to identify other pathogens. Additionally, enteritis may occur as a primary symptom in HIV infection. *See also* **Cryptosporidium**; **Giardiasis**; **Mycobacterium avium**-complex; **Parasites**; and **Shigellosis**.

Envelope protein

The envelope protein is a protective fatty membrane that forms the outer shell of many viruses, including HIV, the AIDS virus. In HIV, the envelope is known as gp 120 because it is a glycoprotein with a molecular weight of 120,000 daltons. Glycoproteins are proteins with attached carbohydrate molecules. Many hormones and antibodies are also composed of glycoprotein molecules.

Enzyme-linked immunosorbent assay (ELISA)

The ELISA refers to a specific laboratory assay methodology used to detect antibodies to a specific antigen. The ELISA is a simple test, employing a tiny shard of an antigen, such as a virus. This antigen is capable of reacting with antibodies to this virus. Patients with hepatitis or HIV have antibodies in their serum that develop from about six weeks to six months after they are infected. The presence of antibodies to a specific virus demonstrates that the patient has been infected with this virus. Most primary assay methods for HIV or hepatitis use the ELISA methodology. Positive results are generally confirmed with a more specific test, such as the Western Blot assay, which shows evidence of specific viral proteins.

The original HIV ELISA tests developed by Robert Gallo and manufactured by Abbot had sensitivity and specificity problems, resulting in many false positive and false negative assays in the first years that they were in use. The early tests could not detect antibodies to the core viral proteins of HIV, which are the first antibodies to develop after HIV infection. Thus, many individuals in the early stages of HIV infection were falsely identified as negative.

The ELISA HIV test developed by the French, which was manufactured by Genetic Systems, received patent approval months after the American patent was approved, although the Institut Pasteur had applied for American patent rights months before the American team. Although studies by the Red Cross showed the Pasteur test did not have the same problems with false negatives, politics and concerns over patent royalties allowed Abbott, using Gallo's test, to have an exclusive contract for testing the American blood supply. This test has since gone through many modifications, and now is highly sensitive and specific for HIV antibodies.

Epidemic

An epidemic refers to a disease that occurs clearly in excess of normal expectation and spreads rapidly through a demographic segment of the human population, such as everyone in a given geographic area, military base, school, or similar population unit, or everyone of a certain age or sex or cultural group. Epidemic diseases can be spread from person to person or from a contaminated source such as food or water.

Epidemiology

Epidemiology is the branch of medical science that studies the incidence, distribution, and control of disease in a population.

Epididymitis

Epididymitis refers to an infection of the epididymis, the convoluted tubule lying on the testicle through which sperm pass from the testicle to the vas deferens gland.

Etiology

Among sexually active men younger than age 35, epididymitis is most often caused by *C. trachomatis* or *N. gonorrhoeae* infections. Epididymitis caused by sexually transmitted enteric organisms, such as *Escherichia coli*, also occurs among men who are the insertive partner during anal intercourse. Sexually transmitted epididymitis usually is accompanied by urethritis, which may cause no symptoms.

Epididymitis may also occur as a nonsexually transmitted urinary tract infection caused by Gram-negative enteric organisms. Non-sexually related epididymitis frequently occurs in men older than 35 years who have recently undergone urinary-tract instrumentation or surgery and men who have anatomical abnormalities of the urinary tract.

Symptoms

Symptoms of epididymitis include unilateral (one-sided) testicular pain and tenderness, hydrocele (accumulation of serous fluid in the scrotum), and palpable swelling of the epididymis. Testicular torsion, a surgical emergency, should be considered in all cases, but it occurs most often among adolescents and in men with no other signs of infection or inflammation. Emergency testing for torsion may be indicated when the onset of pain is sudden, pain is severe, or initial test results do not suggest urethritis or a urinary tract infection.

Diagnosis

Physical examination and history show unilateral testicular pain and tenderness. Swelling and enlargement of the epididymis usually are present. Testicular torsion, a surgical emergency, should be considered in all cases, but it occurs more frequently among adolescents and in men without evidence of inflammation or infection. In questionable diagnoses, a specialist should be consulted immediately.

A gram stain of urethral discharge shows more than five segmented white blood cells/oil immersion field. If the cause is gonorrhea, gram negative diplococci will be seen in the cytoplasm of these cells. The urine can also be examined for the presence of white blood cells, and patients should have blood tests for syphilis and HIV.

Treatment

For epididymitis most likely caused by gonococcal or chlamydial infection, the antibiotics ceftriaxone, 250 mg given in a single dose intramuscular (IM) injection, or doxycycline using 100 mg orally twice a day for 10 days, are prescribed. If swelling and treatment persist at the end of treatment, other causes, such as fungal epididymitis, tumor, and abscesses, should be investigated. For epididymitis most likely caused by enteric organisms, for patients allergic to cephalosporin antibiotics or tetracyclines, or for epididymitis in patients older than 35 years, the recommended treatment is ofloxacin 300 mg given orally twice a day for 10 days or levofloxacin 500 mg given orally once daily for 10 days.

Failure to improve within three days of the initiation of treatment requires a reevaluation of both the diagnosis and treatment. Swelling and tenderness that persist after completion of antibiotics should be evaluated comprehensively and other causes such as testicular cancer and TB should be investigated.

Partners of patients with gonococcal or chlamydial infections should be treated, and intercourse should be avoided until therapy is completed in the patient and any partners. Sex partners from within 60 days prior to onset of symptoms should be contacted so that they can receive treatment if indicated.

Precautions

Patients with HIV infection who have uncomplicated epididymitis should receive the same treatment as patients who are HIV negative. However, in patients with HIV, fungi and mycobacteria are more likely to be the source of infection. Although most patients can be treated on an outpatient basis, hospitalization should be considered when severe pain suggests other diagnoses, such as torsion, testicular infarction or abscess, or when patients have fevers or might be noncompliant with an antibiotic regimen.

Centers for Disease Control and Prevention. *Sexually Transmitted Diseases Treatment Guidelines 2002.* Atlanta: U.S. Dept. of Health and Human Services, 2002.

Epstein-Barr virus (EBV)

The Epstein-Barr virus is a human herpesvirus known to cause infectious mononucleosis. EBV is a beta human herpesvirus and is also known as human herpesvirus-4 or HHV-4.

EBV almost certainly also plays a role in some nasopharyngeal carcinomas, Burkitt's lymphoma, Hodgkin's lymphoma, lymphoproliferative disorders, the hyperproliferative disorder oral hairy leukoplakia, and in other lymphoproliferative disorders in individuals who are immunosuppressed. EBV has been found in most cases of body cavity lymphoma and primary effusion lymphoma, causing researchers to suspect that EBV assists human herpesvirus-8 (HHV-8) in the development of these diseases.

The most common test for EBV is the rapid slide test (Monospot), which is performed on blood specimens. This test shows the presence of heterophile antibody and is not specific for EBV, although in patients with symptoms of infectious mononucleosis, it offers a rapid diagnosis in conjunction with other supportive tests, such as the complete blood count (CBC). Researchers speculate that EBV, resulting from minor childhood colds or infectious mononucleosis in adolescents, can remain latent, persisting throughout one's lifetime.

The presence of EBV antibodies to early antigens (EA), viral capsid antigens (VCA), and nuclear antigens (EBNA) occurs in sequence, with EA appearing early in chronic EBV infection. In EBV infection, EBV antibodies occur in blood and in tissue specimens from patients with lymphoproliferative disease.

Erythema multiforme

Erythema multiforme is a type of hypersensitivity reaction or rash that occurs in response to medications, infections, or illness. Its origin is unknown, although 90 percent of cases are associated with herpes simplex or mycoplasma infections. This disorder occurs primarily in children and young adults. A severe form of this condition is called Stevens-Johnson Syndrome.

Esophagitis

Esophagitis is a condition caused by inflammation of the esophagus. Esophagitis is one of the gastrointestinal manifestations that may occur in patients with HIV infection. The most common causes of esophagitis include candida, cytomegalovirus, idiopathic ulcers, and herpes simplex virus. These disorders are most likely to occur in patients with CD4 counts of 100 cells per cubic millimeter or less.

Most patients with esophagitis experience pain while swallowing and retrosternal chest pain. Patients with esophagitis are tested for acid reflux and treated if acid reflux is seen. Otherwise, they are treated for candidiasis. If the symptoms do not improve after five days, upper endoscopy and biopsy are recommended.

Exposure Category

In describing HIV/AIDS cases, exposure category refers to the mode of transmission or how a person may have been exposed to HIV, such as intravenous drug use, transfusion of blood products, male-to-male sexual contact, and heterosexual contact.

Eyes

The eyes can be affected by a number of different STDs, including chlamydia, gonorrhea and syphilis, which frequently cause conditions of conjunctivitis or retinitis in infants, children and adults. Infants can be infected in utero and during passage through the cervical canal. Adults are generally infected by autoinoculation or finger to eye transmission. In children, child-to-child transmission of chlamydia commonly occurs in trachoma endemic areas. Several hundred million people are known to be afflicted with trachoma, and millions have been blinded. Poor hygiene and unsanitary conditions contribute to the spread of trachoma, which affects most children by two years of age in trachoma endemic areas.

Eye diseases also commonly occur in persons with HIV/AIDS who have developed other opportunistic infections. The most common cause is CMV. Symptoms include retinal changes that cause visual changes resembling cotton-wool spots, decreased visual function and color vision, and retinal hemorrhages. Some drugs such as rifabutin used in the treatment of Mycobacterium avium in AIDS patients may cause uveitis. Children infected with HIV may develop loss of retinal pigment and retinal lesions. *See also* **Acquired immune deficiency syndrome; Conjunctivitis; Cytomegalovirus; Gonorrhea; Herpes simplex virus; Syphilis** and **Trachoma.**

Factor VIII

Factor VIII (also known as anti-hemophilia factor or AHF) is a blood substance necessary for blood clotting. Individuals with hemophilia are deficient in Factor VIII and require frequent transfusions of this product to prevent episodes of uncontrolled bleeding.

Factor VIII is made in lots containing the blood of thousands of different blood donors. In 1984, after a number of patients with hemophilia became infected, it was discovered that one large lot of Factor VIII had been tested and found to be contaminated with the AIDS virus. Although heated products, known to destroy the virus were then available and the risks of using untreated AHF were known, untreated products were kept in use in some countries until mid–1985. Officials deemed that the cost of heat-treating or simply destroying the contaminated products outweighed any costs associated with future infections.

In mid–1998, in a trial held in Tokyo, it emerged that the Japanese government had known of the risks involved with using untreated blood products a year before it approved their use in 1984. When the government finally banned the use of untreated products in 1985, several hundred hemophiliacs had been infected with the HIV virus.

On May 6, 1985, U.S. public health officials expressed concern that untreated AHF continued to be used in the United States, although there was no shortage of the treated product at that time. In May 1997, the four principal American manufacturers of clotting factors, Alpha Therapeutics, Armour Pharmaceuticals, Cutter Laboratories, and Baxter Healthcare agreed to pay $100,000 to each of more than 6,000 HIV infected hemophiliacs or their survivors, who had charged the companies with negligence in a class-action lawsuit.

The companies were charged with having failed to provide heat-treated products in early 1984. According to records, the officials calculated the cost and decided it would be too expensive to destroy the contaminated lot or treat it, even though some individuals would be infected with HIV and there was no shortage of heated Factor VIII. The companies also agreed to reimburse the federal government nearly $12.2 million for payments made by federal health insurance programs. In February of 1985, Margaret Heckler, secretary of the U.S. Department of Health and Human Services, misled the public with her announcement that a positive test for HIV did not mean one would eventually develop AIDS.

On May 9, 1985, in France, Michael Garretta wrote the minister of social affairs of his intention to continue distributing Factor VIII that had not been heat-treated through July of 1985. In a highly politicized case in Paris, Garretta was convicted of selling contaminated products. Upon his release from jail, he was again convicted under an older law related to poisoning.

Jean-Pierre Allain, who had tried to warn Garretta of the dangers of contaminated blood, was also convicted despite acknowledgement by the prosecution that he had tried to convince Garretta. Others charged included Georgina Dufoix, the former minister for social affairs, Prime Minister Laurent Fabius, and Edmond Hervé, France's minister of health. In France, 1,000 of the country's 5,000 hemophiliacs had been infected with AIDS. In the United States, which also used untreated Factor VIII in 1985, by 2002 as many as 3,000 hemophiliacs had died of AIDS.

Female reproductive organs

The female reproductive organs include the vagina (a muscular passage that the connects the external genital organs), the cervix, the uterus, the ovaries, and the fallopian tubes.

The vagina is a fibromuscular tube that extends from the cervix to the vestibule of the Laboria minora. The vagina receives the penis and semen during sexual intercourse and also provides a passageway for menstrual blood flow. The cervix is the opening extending from the vagina to the uterus. The cervical canal is the narrow passage from the cervix to the uterus. The ovaries are glands that produce hormones. The ovaries contain follicles, in which eggs

develop. Mature follicles rupture and the developing egg is ejected from the ovary into the fallopian tubes during ovulation. The fallopian tubes begin as funnel-shaped passages extending from the ovaries. The uterus is a hollow cavity about the size of a pear that exists to house a developing fertilized egg. The thick wall of the uterus is composed of three layers. The inner layer is called the endometrium.

FemExam

The FemExam is a diagnostic test kit used to determine vaginal pH and detect proteins that are associated with bacterial vaginosis. Normally, the vagina has an acidic pH of 3.0 to 4.0. In vaginosis or trichomoniasis, the Ph is elevated usually to 6.0 or 7.0.

Fertility

Fertility refers to the ability to reproduce. Fertility can be compromised by a number of different STDs affecting both men and women. Some STDs such as chlamydia and gonorrhea, which can cause pelvic inflammatory disease in women, are particularly detrimental to reproductive health.

5-Fluorouracil (5-FU, Effudex)

5-Fluorouracil is a chemotherapeutic drug used topically as a cream to prevent or treat abnormal skin growths, neoplasias (especially cervical cancer) and warts.

Fluorquinolones *see* Quinolones

Folliculitis

Folliculitis refers to inflammation of the hair follicle. Fol-

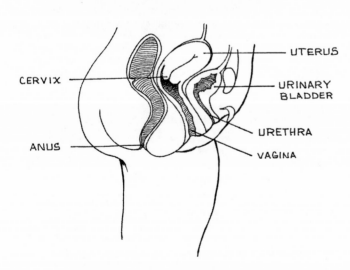

Female reproductive organs (Marvin G. Miller).

liculitis is seen in STD patients and in HIV-infected individuals. A hair follicle-based pustule is the primary lesion that occurs, although folliculitis can present as papules, sometimes with erosions and crusts. The usual causes include infection with *Staphylococcus aureus*, gram-negative bacteria, mites, and physical or chemical injuries, including razor burns.

A type of folliculitis causing an increased eosinophil count may be seen in HIV infected persons with CD4 counts less than 200 cells per cubic millimeter of blood. This disorder manifests as a chronic condition with itchy papules covering the face and upper trunk. Treatment consists of topical steroids and oral itraconazole therapy.

Food and Drug Administration

The Food and Drug Administration is a federal agency within the U.S. Department of Health and Human Services responsible for ensuring the safety of the U.S. food supply and also the safety and effectiveness of drugs, biologics, vaccines, and medical devices used in the diagnosis and treatment of disease. The FDA rigorously oversees the testing of all medications before they are approved for use in specific conditions. The FDA also works with the blood banking industry and the American Red Cross to safeguard the nation's blood supply.

Fusion inhibitors

Fusion inhibitors belong to a class of antiretroviral agents that binds to the gp41 envelope protein of HIV and blocks the structural changes necessary for the virus to fuse with the host CD4 cell. When the virus cannot penetrate the host cell membrane and infect the cell, HIV replication within that host cell is prevented.

Fusion mechanism

Fusion is an integral step in the process whereby HIV enters host cells. Researchers have found that in addition to the primary receptor, the CD4 molecule, other cofactors such as CCR5 and CXCR4 are needed for HIV to fuse with the membranes of the host's immune system cells.

GAG *(gag)*

Gag is a gene of HIV that codes for the core protein p55, which is the precursor of HIV proteins p17, p24, p7 and p6. These proteins form HIV's capsid, the inner protein shell surrounding HIV's strand of RNA.

Gallo, Robert, MD

Former director of Tumor Cell Biology at the National Cancer Institute, Robert Gallo is one of the best-known AIDS researchers. While dismissing and criticizing the findings of the French scientists who first isolated the AIDS virus in early 1983, Gallo attempted to take credit for this discovery. Although Gallo won numerous awards for his widely-published findings, it was eventually determined that scientists at the Institut Pasteur, with whom Gallo had consulted, had been the first to isolate HIV.

In numerous publications, Gallo described an allegedly new strain of the Human T-cell Leukemia Virus (HTLV), a retrovirus known to cause leukemia, as the infectious agent responsible for AIDS. Calling this virus HTLV3, Gallo based his research on an isolate contaminated with LAV, the true AIDS virus, which was discovered months earlier by researchers at the Institut Pasteur of Paris. Because of early confusion, the AIDS virus was later re-named as Human Immunodeficiency Virus or HIV-1.

In 1992 Gallo was investigated and found guilty of intellectual recklessness of a high degree by the National Academy of

Sciences and of scientific misconduct by the NIH's Office of Research Integrity. After charges of misconduct against Gallo's top researcher Mikulas Popovic were overturned, the charges against Gallo were reversed because of a lack of evidence. Whether Gallo and his team had intentionally contaminated their isolate with the LAV virus could never be proved although gene sequencing showed Gallo's strain to be identical to the French isolate.

The original ELISA method for testing HIV, the HTLV3 test developed by Gallo and his team, was not as specific or sensitive as the AIDS test developed by the Institut Pasteur. Gallo's test resulted in numerous HIV negative people testing positive for HIV, whereas many HIV infected patients had negative test results. This had critical ramifications for the nation's blood supply, which relied on Gallo's test although the Red Cross had early reported that the Pasteur test was far superior. The French test was superior in that it detected the antibodies to Gp41 that show up in early infection, whereas the American test did not. Later modifications to the American test by Abbott also enabled it to detect this particular HIV antibody.

Gallo was later removed from his position at the National Cancer Institute and became the acting director of the Institute for Human Virology in Maryland. He is credited with discovering the retrovirus HTLV-1, which causes leukemia, and T-Cell Growth Factor. He is also known for publishing many scientific papers linking the retrovirus now known as HIV to HIV/AIDS disease.

Crewdson, John. *Science Fictions: A Scientific Mystery, A Massive Cover-Up and the Dark Legacy of Robert Gallo*. New York: Little, Brown, 2002.

Gardnerella vaginale

Gardnerella vaginale, which is named after the Texas physician who first reported it, is the strain of bacteria most commonly responsible for bacterial vaginosis (BV). *See also* **Bacterial vaginosis.**

Genes

Genes are the basic units of DNA that contain the genetic code for specific proteins; the genetic code contains instructions for the gene's transcription, which results in certain characteristics. Genes are contained by, and arranged along the length of, chromosomes. Alteration of either gene number or arrangement can result in mutation. The human genome contains approximately 30,000 genes that are contained in chromosomes. Certain viruses, such as HIV, change the genome of cells that they infect.

Genital ulcer disease

In the United States, most young, sexually active patients who have genital ulcers have genital herpes, syphilis, chlamydia, or chancroid. The relative frequency of each disease differs by geographic area and patient population, with certain of these diseases being more prevalent in different parts of the country. Patients with genital ulcers may also have more than one of these STDs. Most genital ulcers occur as a result of STDs, but not all genital ulcers are caused by sexually transmitted infections.

Diagnosis

Diagnosis cannot accurately be made from a medical history and physical examination. The CDC recommends that all patients with genital ulcers have serologic tests for syphilis and a diagnostic evaluation (either antigen test or culture) for herpes. In areas where chancroid is prevalent, patients should also be tested for *Haemophilus ducreyi*. Currently, there are no FDA-approved DNA amplification tests available for *H. ducreyi*, but polymerase chain reaction (PCR) nucleic acid amplification tests are available through commercial laboratories that have developed their own tests. Type-specific serology for the herpes virus HSV type 2 may also be helpful in identifying persons with genital herpes. Biopsy of ulcers may also be helpful in identifying the causative agent in ulcers that do not respond to initial therapy.

CDC recommendations include HIV testing for patients with syphilis or chancroid and a consideration of HIV testing for patients with ulcers caused by HSV.

Treatment

Health care providers must often initiate treatment before all test results are available because early treatment decreases the possibility of ongoing transmission. Also, successful treatment of herpes depends on prompt therapy. Physicians should treat the condition most likely to be responsible for genital ulcers in the individual patient. Even after complete diagnostic evaluation, at least 25 percent of patients with genital ulcers do not receive a laboratory-confirmed STD diagnosis. *See also* **Chancroid**; *Chlamydia trachomatis*; **Herpes simplex virus**; and **Syphilis**.

Genital warts

Genital warts are raised papules occurring on the skin that can be visualized without the aid of magnification.

Etiology

Genital warts are caused by the human papilloma virus (HPV). There are four distinct morphologic types of genital warts: condylomata acuminata, which have a cauliflower-like appearance; papular warts, which are flesh-colored, dome-shaped papules, usually 1–4 mm in diameter; keratotic warts, which have a thick, crust-like layer and may resemble common skin warts or seborrheic keratosis, and flat-topped papules which appear macular to slightly raised. Condylomas usually occur on moist, partially keratinized or hardened skin, and flat papular warts occur on either partially or fully keratinized epithelium. Most genital warts are caused by HPV type 6, and to a lesser extent type 11.

Epidemiology

Human papilloma virus (HPV) infects half to two-thirds of sexually active people at some time in their lives. About five million new cases are reported each year in the United States.

Symptoms

Genital warts usually appear one to six months after the initial infection. Most genital warts occur on the penis, scrotum, urethral meatus, and perianal area in men and on the vulva, perineum and perianal area in women. Occasionally they may develop on the cervix and vaginal walls in women and on the pubic area or upper thighs in both men and women. They begin as tiny soft, moist, pink or red swelling, which grow rapidly and may develop stalks. Multiple warts often grow in the same area, and their rough surfaces give them the appearance of small cauliflowers. The warts may grow very rapidly in pregnant women, in people with impaired immune systems, for instance people with HIV or who are on immunosuppressant medications, and in individuals with inflammatory skin conditions.

Occasionally, patients report itching, burning, pain or bleeding, although many people do not have symptoms. Women with external genital warts may report an abnormal vaginal discharge, which is likely related to a co-existing vaginal vaginosis such as bacterial vaginosis.

Genital warts may appear on the lips, tongue or palate as a rare manifestation of infection. Most of these patients also have other genital or perianal warts and most give a history of oral sex.

Diagnosis

Speculum exam for vaginal and cervical warts is recommended for women with external genital warts. Colposcopy is indicated for women with cervical warts, and anoscopy for men and women with recurrent perianal warts and a history of anal intercourse. Urethroscopy is recommended for men with warts at the distal urinary meatus or who show signs of blood in their urine or exhibit an abnormal urinary stream.

Treatment

No treatment is completely satisfactory. External genital warts may be removed by laser, cryotherapy (chemical freezing), or surgery using local anesthetics. Chemical treatments, such as podophyllum resin or purified toxin or trichloroacetic acid, can be applied directly to the warts. However, chemical treatments, which seldom work, require many applications over weeks to months and may burn the skin.

Warts in the urethra may be treated with anticancer drugs such as thitepa or fluoracil. Alternatively, the warts may be removed from the urethra by endoscopic surgery.

Precautions

Although condoms can reduce the risk of HPV transmission, condoms do not cover all exposed areas, and HPV may be transmitted by exposure to uncovered areas with warts. *See also* **Condylomata acuminata** and **Human papilloma virus.**

Genitourinary tract

The genitourinary tract, which is also called the genitourinary system, urogenital system, or urogenital tract, refers to the organs concerned with the production and excretion of urine and those concerned with reproduction.

Genotype (genotypic) assay

The genotype assay, which is also known as the genotypic antiretroviral resistance assay, or GART, is a blood test used to determine if HIV has become resistant to the antiviral drugs that a patient is using. The test analyzes a sample of the virus from the patient's blood to identify any mutations in the virus that are associated with resistance to specific drugs. Mutations at certain positions in the HIV genes are linked to drug resistance. For example, a muta-

tion at position 30 of the protease gene results in resistance to the protease inhibitor nelfinavir. Genotypic assays are typically less expensive than phenotypic assays, but still cost approximately $300 to $600, and results can take as long as one week.

A major detriment to the genotype assay is that it will miss unknown or new gene mutations. Also, although the effects of some mutations are clear-cut, this is not always true. A mutation that does not cause resistance on its own could cause resistance when combined with other mutations. Resistance to one drug also sometimes results in increased sensitivity to another drug. For example, resistance to lamivudine reduces resistance to zidovudine.

Germinal centers

Germinal centers include a series of follicles or cavities found near the periphery of lymph nodes. Germinal centers are the sites of antibody production and are populated mostly by B lymphocytes, but include a few T lymphocytes and macrophages. In HIV infection, as the disease progresses, the germinal centers gradually decay.

Giardiasis

Giardia is a condition caused by infection with the parasite *Giardia lamblia*. Giardia may be sexually transmitted, especially in men who have sex with men and through oral-anal contact. Giardiasis is typically an infection of the small intestine, although it is often found in association with amebiasis.

Symptoms of giardiasis include diarrhea, abdominal cramps, bloating, and nausea. Multiple stool examinations are often necessary to detect Giardia. Metronidazole using 250 to 500 mg three times daily for seven days is the recommended treatment, although it has a 10 to 20 percent failure rate. Other therapies include paromomycin and furazolidone. *See also* *Enteritis* and *Parasites*.

Global Fund to Fight AIDS, Tuberculosis and Malaria

The U.S. Department of Health and Human Services was established in January 2002, in Geneva, Switzerland. Secretary Tommy Thompson heads the fund. The fund coordinates research and humanitarian efforts toward fighting AIDS, tuberculosis, and malaria worldwide. Countries worldwide support the fund. As of April 1, 2003, the U.S. had pledged $1.65 billion to the fund, and is expected to remain its single largest donor.

A recent Government Accounting Office (GAO) study (GAO-03-601) found that the fund has made noteworthy progress in establishing essential governance and other supporting structures and is responding to challenges that have impeded its ability to quickly disburse grants. However, the report found that the fund's ability to approve and finance additional grants is threatened by a lack of sufficient resources. Pledges made through the end of 2003 are insufficient to cover more than a small number of additional grants and without significant new pledges, the fund will be unable to support all of the already approved grants beyond their initial two-year agreement.

According to the United Nations, about $10 billion will be needed in 2005, increasing to $15 billion in 2007, to fight AIDS alone; malaria and tuberculosis will require billions more. With infection rates remaining as high as 38 percent in the developing world, and 10 million children orphaned by AIDS, supporting the Global Fund is essential. The complete GAO report can be found at http://www.gao.gov/cgi-bin/getrpt/GAO-03-601.

Clinton, William J. "Turning the Tide on the AIDS Pandemic." *New England Journal of Medicine*, May 3, 2003, 348:1800–1802.

Glycoprotein (gp)

Glycoproteins are conjugated proteins consisting of a protein molecule linked to a carbohydrate molecule.

Gonococcal infections

Gonococcal infections refer to infections caused by *Neisseria gonorrhoeae* and are commonly called gonorrhea.

Gonococcal Isolate Surveillance Project (GISP)

GISP is a branch of the CDC established in 1986 that studies isolates of gonorrhea from patients to determine the rates of drug resistance to quinolones and other antimicrobials. GISP studies conducted in approximately 26 states help in establishing a rational basis for gonococcal therapies, including the CDC treatment guidelines.

In 2000, GISP found that 0.4 percent of gonorrheal strains found in the United States showed minimum inhibitory concentrations greater than 1.0 mcg/ml to ciprofloxacin. In Honolulu, such isolates represented 14.3 percent of all samples. The GISP samples about three percent of all men in the United States with gonococcal infections and is a mainstay of surveillance.

Gonorrhea (Clap, GC)

Gonorrhea is the second most prevalent STD among reported communicable infections in the United States. Chlamydia is first.

Etiology

Gonorrhea is caused by the bacteria *Neisseria gonorrhoeae*, a gram-negative, oxidase positive diplococcus. Gonorrhea bacteria can grow in the warm, moist areas of the reproductive tract, including the cervix, uterus, and fallopian tubes in women, and in the urethra in women and men. *N. gonorrhoeae* can also grow in the mouth, throat, and anus.

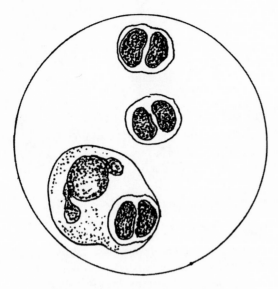

Neisseria gonorrhoeae (Marvin G. Miller).

Epidemiology

Gonorrhea remains one of the most prevalent bacterial sexually transmitted diseases in the United States, with an estimated 650,000 new cases reported annually. Gonorrhea is spread through sexual contact (vaginal, oral, or anal). This includes penis to vagina, penis to mouth, penis to anus, mouth to vagina, and mouth to anus contact. Ejaculation does not have to occur for gonorrhea to be transmitted or acquired. Gonorrhea can also be spread from mother to child during childbirth. Gonorrhea may also be spread to the eyes, causing conjunctivitis or ophthalmia neonatorum.

According to data from the Gonococcal Isolate Surveillance Project, GC rates increased steadily from 1964 to 1975 and then declined steadily until 1997. However, 1998 showed an eight percent increase in the rate of new cases compared to 1997, and rates for 1999 rose another 1.2 percent. GC rates are particularly high in the Southeastern United States, among minorities, and among adolescents from all ethnic and racial groups. The CDC recommends testing individuals who had sexual contact with infected patients, have a different compatible STD, are at risk for STDs, or who are victims of sexual abuse.

Symptoms

Up to 80 percent of gonorrhea cases in women affect the endocervix and are asymptomatic (cause no symptoms) until complications occur. Left untreated, gonorrhea can lead to pelvic inflammatory disease in 10 to 40 percent of affected women, with the potential risk of ectopic pregnancy, salpingitis, infertility, and chronic pelvic pain. Gonorrhea is asymptomatic in 85 percent of women and five percent of men.

In women, the first symptoms may appear seven to 21 days after infection. However, symptoms may not develop for weeks or months and may not be discovered until a woman's male partner shows signs of infection. Early symptoms of infection may be mild and can be mistaken for a bladder or vaginal infection. The initial symptoms and signs in women include a painful or burning sensation when urinating and a vaginal discharge that is thick in consistency and may be white, yellow, or occasionally bloody.

In men, symptoms usually appear two to five days after infection, but in some cases symptoms can take as long as 30 days to appear. Symptoms generally start with mild discomfort in the urethra, followed a few hours later by mild to severe pain during urination and a thick yellow discharge of pus from the penis. Men may also experience a frequent and urgent need to urinate, and the urge worsens as the disease spreads to upper parts of the urethra. The penile opening may also become red and swollen. In men, gonorrheal infection can cause acute urethritis. Left untreated, urethritis can develop into epidiymitis, prostatitis (causing low back pain), and urethral stricture. In both men and women, infected individuals can transmit gonorrhea to others even when they are free of symptoms.

Symptoms of rectal infection in both

men and women who engage in anal sex include rectal discharge, anal itching, soreness, bleeding, and sometimes painful bowel movements. The area around the anus may become red and raw, and the stool may be coated with mucus and pus. During a physical examination of the rectum, mucus and pus may be visible on the wall of the rectum.

Oral sex with an infected partner may cause gonorrhea of the throat (gonococcal pharyngitis). Infections in the throat may cause few symptoms, although they may cause a sore throat and discomfort during swallowing.

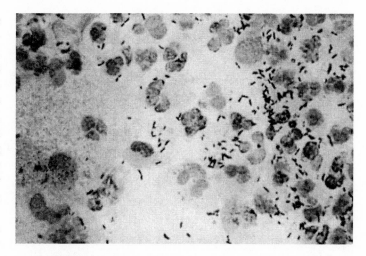

Neisseria gonorrhoeae gram stain — rectal smear (Joe Miller, CDC).

In the newborn, gonorrheal infection can cause severe conjunctivitis, which can result in blindness if untreated and, rarely, sepsis with associated meningitis, endocarditis, or arthritis. Infection in the newborn can also cause bacteremia, meningitis, arthritis and scalp infection. Between 30 and 50 percent of infants exposed to gonococci will develop ophthalmia in the absence of treatment.

Diagnosis

Neisseria gonorrhoeae can be cultured from genital discharge or secretions. GC should be tested for in patients with endocervicitis, urethritis (males), PID, urethral syndrome, bartholinitis, epididymitis, perihepatitis (Fitz-Hugh-Curtis syndrome in females), proctitis, disseminated gonococcal infections, and conjunctivitis.

A microscopic examination shows the presence of gram negative intracellular diplocci located within segmented neutrophilic leukocytes (white blood cells), and the gram stain remains a good presumptive test for gonorrhea. The gram stain test can be used as a point-of-care test for males with urethral discharge. Endocervical specimens collected on swabs

and urethral specimens collected on swabs can also be tested using a qualitative PCR based assay that detects *Neisseria gonorrhoeae* DNA. In asymptomatic males, the first urine specimen of the day, provided more than two hours have passed since prior urination, can be used for DNA testing.

Nucleic acid amplification testing (NAAT) methods are the most sensitive and specific diagnostic techniques because they measure the DNA of specific organisms. A key advantage is that the test may be performed on urine specimens in men and do not require a pelvic exam. A disadvantage is that the specimens can contain amplification inhibitors that cause false-negative results. Most test kits include controls that can identify inhibition if it occurs. FDA-approved testing methods include nucleic acid hybridization (nucleic acid probe) tests, nucleic acid genetic transformation tests, enzyme immunoassays (EIA), and direct fluorescence assays (DFA tests).

Treatment

2002 CDC treatment guidelines for uncomplicated infections of the cervix, urethra and rectum include: cefixime, using 400 mg in a single dose; or ceftriaxone, 125 mg administered intramuscularly (IM) in a single dose; or ciprofloxacin, 500 mg orally in a single dose; or ofloxacin, using 400 mg in a single dose; or levofloxacin, using 250 mg in a single dose. When a co-existing chlamydial infection has not been ruled out, CDC treatment recommendations include: azithromycin, using one gram orally in a single dose; or doxycycline, using 100 mg twice daily for seven days. Treatment recommendations are the same for patients who also have HIV. Other antimicrobials are active against *N. gonorrhoeae*, but none have substantial advantages over these regimens.

Although it does not provide the sustained therapeutic blood levels seen with ceftriaxone, an advantage of cefixime is that it can be administered orally. In clinical trials, cefixime has a cure rate of 97.4 percent for uncomplicated urogenital and anorectal infections. Ceftriaxone in a single 125 mg injection provides high bactericidal blood levels. In clinical trials, ceftriaxone has a 99.1 percent cure rate. In clinical trials, 500 mg ciprofloxacin has a cure rate of 99.8 percent.

• ALTERNATIVE REGIMENS—Alternative regimens for people who cannot tolerate or are resistant to cephalosporins and quinolones include spectinomycin, using two grams in a single, IM dose, which has a cure rate of 98.2 percent for uncomplicated infections. Single-dose cephalosporin regimens, other than ceftriaxone and cefixime, include ceftizoxime, using 500 mg administered IM. Single-dose quinolone regimens include gatifloxacin, using 400 mg orally; norfloxacin, using 800 mg orally; and lomefloxacin, using 400 mg orally. *See* the passage on quinolone resistance later in this entry.

• TREATMENT FOR GONOCOCCAL INFECTIONS OF THE PHARYNX—Gonococcal infections of the pharynx are more difficult to eradicate than urogenital and anorectal infections. CDC treatment guidelines include ceftriaxone, using 125 mg IM in a single dose, or ciprofloxacin, using 500 mg orally in a single dose. If a co-existing infection with chlamydia cannot be ruled out, recommended treatment includes azithromycin using one gram orally in a single dose, or doxycycline, using 100 mg orally for seven days.

Follow-Up

Patients with uncomplicated gonorrhea who are treated with recommended regimens need not return for a confirmation test to show that they are cured. However, patients with symptoms that persist after treatment should be evaluated by a culture for *N. gonorrhoeae*; if the organism is isolated, tests for antimicrobial susceptibility should be performed to see what antibiotics are effective. Infections identified after treatment usually result from reinfection by an infected partner rather than treatment failure. Persistent symptoms may also be caused by chlamydia infection.

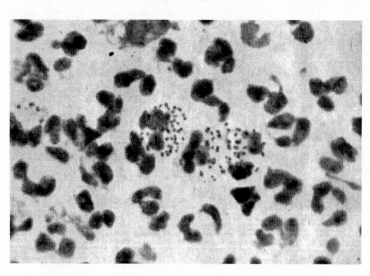

Gram stain of gonorrhea from urethral discharge (Navy Environmental Health Center Training and Health Communication Branch, CDC).

Gonococcal Conjunctivitis Treatment

In the only published study of gonococcal conjunctivitis in the United States, all 12 study participants responded to a single one-gram IM injection of ceftriaxone. CDC guidelines note that a single lavage of the infected eye with saline solution should also be considered.

Adverse Effects of Treatment

Some individuals may be allergic or develop adverse reactions to certain antibiotics. Persons who cannot tolerate cephalosporins or quinolones should be treated with spectinomycin. Because spectinomycin is only 52 percent effective against pharyngeal infections, patients with suspected pharyngeal infections should have a culture evaluated 3–5 days after treatment to verify eradication of infection.

Fluoroquinolones are not recommended for persons younger than 18 years because of potential damage to articular cartilage. However, no joint damage attributable to quinolone therapy has been observed in those treated with prolonged ciprofloxacin regimens.

Management of Sex Partners

Patients should be instructed to refer their sex partners for evaluation and treatment. All sex partners of patients with gonorrhea and chlamydia should be evaluated and treated if they had sex within 60 days of onset of symptoms in the infected partner. If a patient's last sexual partner was more than 60 days ago, that partner should still be treated. Patients should be instructed to avoid intercourse until the completion of therapy and until they and their sex partners no longer have symptoms.

Pregnancy

Pregnant women should not be treated with quinolones or tetracyclines. Infected women should be treated with a recommended or alternative cephalosporin. Women intolerant of cephalosporins should be administered a single, two-gram dose of spectinomycin IM. Co-existing chlamydial infections are treated with either erythromycin or amoxicillin.

Neonatal Gonorrhea

Gonococcal infection among infants usually results from exposure to infected cervical exudates at birth. It usually causes an acute illness that presents at two to five days after birth. The prevalence of infection depends on the prevalence of infection among pregnant women or whether pregnant women are screened for gonorrhea, and on whether newborns receive prophylactic treatment for ophthalmia shortly after birth. The most severe manifestations of gonorrheal infection in newborns are ophthalmia neonatorum

Gonococcal Ophthalmia (Navy Environmental Health Center Training and Health Communication Branch, CDC).

and sepsis, including arthritis and meningitis. Less severe manifestations include the nasal inflammatory condition rhinitis; vaginitis; urethritis; and inflammation at sites of fetal monitoring. Ophthalmia neonaturum can cause severe conjunctivitis and lead to corneal scarring, abscess, and permanent blindness. Blindness due to ophthalmia neonatorum declined dramatically with the institution of silver nitrate prophylactic programs for newborns.

Infants at increased risk of gonococcal ophthalmia include those who do not receive ophthalmia prophylaxis and those whose mothers have had no prenatal care or whose mothers have a history of STDs or substance abuse. Ophthalmia prophylactic treatment is required in many states and includes applications of one percent silver nitrate, 0.5 percent erythromycin, or one percent tetracycline administered as an ophthalmic ointment in a single application. In all cases of neonatal conjunctivitis, conjunctival exudates or secretions should be cultured for *N. gonorrhoeae.*

N. gonorrhoeae infection in newborns may also cause gonococcal scalp abscesses. Other rare complications include sepsis, arthritis, and meningitis. Localized gonococcal infection of the scalp can result from fetal monitoring using scalp electrodes. Detection of gonococcal infection in neonates with sepsis, arthritis, meningitis, or scalp abscesses requires cultures of blood, cerebrospinal fluid (CSF), and joint aspirate. Treatment includes ceftriaxone, using 25–50 mg/kg/day, administered IV or IM in a single daily dose for seven days, with a duration of 10–14 days if meningitis is documented; or cefotaxime, using 25 mg/kg IV or IM every 12 hours for seven days, with a duration of 10–14 days if meningitis is documented.

Because infants born to mothers with gonorrhea are at high risk for infection, prophylactic treatment with ceftriaxone using 25–50 mg/kg IV or IM, not to exceed 125 mg, using a single dose, is recommended.

Children

Sexual abuse is the most frequent cause of gonococcal infection in pre-adolescent children. Vaginitis is the most common manifestation of gonococcal infection in preadolescent girls. PID following infection is less common in children than in adults. Among sexually abused children, anorectal and pharyngeal infections with *N. gonorrhoeae* are common and frequently do not cause symptoms.

Because of the legal implications of a diagnosis of gonorrhea in a child, standard culture procedures for the isolation of *N. gonorrhoeae* should be used for children. Non-culture procedures such as NAAT testing can be used diagnostically but should not be used alone. Specimens from the vagina, urethra, pharynx, or rectum should be used. Isolates should be preserved to enable additional or repeated tests.

Recommended treatment for children weighing less than 45 kg who have uncomplicated gonococcal vulvovaginitis, cervicitis, urethritis, pharyngitis, or proctitis includes ceftriaxone, using 125 mg administered IM in a single dose, or spectinomycin, using 40 mg/kg with a maximum dose of two grams administered IM in a single dose. While cefixime is sometimes used because it can be administered orally, there are no published reports substantiating its safety or effectiveness when used for this purpose.

Recommended treatment for children weighing less than 45 kg who have bacteremia or arthritis includes ceftriaxone, using 50 mg/kg with a maximum dose of one gram, administered IM or IV in a single dose for seven days. Recommended treatment for children who weigh more than 45 kg and who have bacteremia or arthritis include ceftriaxone, using 50 mg/kg administered IM or IV in a single dose daily for seven days.

Complications

Untreated, gonorrhea may lead to disseminated gonococcal infection (DGI), which results from gonococcal bacteremia (transient blood infection). DGI often results in petechial (small bruising on the skin surface) or pustular (forming pustules) skin lesions; arthralgia, which is asymmetrical (not confined to one side of the body); tenosynovitis (inflammation of the tendon sheath); or septic arthritis. The infection is complicated occasionally by perihepatitis (infection of the covering of the liver causing pain similar to that of gallbladder disease), and rarely by endocarditis (inflammation of the lining of the heart), or meningitis. Some strains of *N. gonorrhoeae* that cause DGI may cause minimal genital inflammation.

Hospitalization is recommended for initial DGI therapy and recommended treatment consists of ceftriaxone administered IM or IV using one gram every 24 hours; or cefotaxime, with one gram administered IV every eight hours; or ceftizoxime, using one gram IV every eight hours; or ciprofloxacin, using 400 mg IV every 12 hours; or ofloxacin, using 400 mg IV every 12 hours; or levofloxacin, using 250 mg IV daily; or spectinomycin, using two grams IM every 12 hours. Protocols should be continued for 24–48 hours after improvement begins. At this time patients may be switched to one of the following protocols for one week: cefixime, using 400 mg orally twice daily; or ciprofloxacin, using 500 mg orally twice daily; or ofloxacin, using 400 mg orally twice daily; or levofloxacin, using 500 mg orally once daily.

Other complications include gonococcal meningitis and endocarditis. Therapy for meningitis should be continued for 10–14 days, and therapy for endocarditis should be continued for at least four weeks. The CDC recommends treatment with ceftriaxone, administering one to two grams IV every 12 hours.

Precautions

Epidemiologic studies provide strong evidence that gonococcal infections facili-tate HIV transmission. Although gonococcal infections in women often do not cause symptoms, the progression of infection can have serious consequences, including infertility. Antimicrobial resistance in *N. gonorrhoeae* remains an important challenge to controlling gonorrheal gonococcal strains that may be resistant to penicillins, tetracyclines, spectinomycin, and fluorquinolones.

Risk Factors

The U.S. Preventive Services Task Force recommends screening for asymptomatic women in several risk categories: young women (age <25 years) with more than two sex partners in the past year; women with repeated gonorrheal infection; and commercial sex workers. Approximately 79 percent of gonorrhea is found in persons aged 15 to 29 years of age. The highest rates of infection are found in 15 to 19-year-old women and 20 to 24-year-old men. In 1999, 77 percent of reported cases occurred in African-Americans.

Risk factors include multiple sex partners, drug use, unprotected sex, and commercial sex work. Used properly, male latex condoms provide a barrier, protecting against gonorrheal infection. Increases in gonorrhea prevalence have been noted since 1993 among men who have sex with men.

Antimicrobial Resistance

Some strains of *N. gonorrhoeae* have mutated into forms with antimicrobial resistance. During the 1980s, gonococcal resistance to penicillin and tetracycline became widespread. Consequently the CDC recommends cephalosporins as first-line treatment for GC. The emergence of numerous penicillin resistant strains caused the CDC to no longer recommend penicillin therapy for gonorrhea. Antimicrobial resistance occurs as plasmid-mediated resistance to penicillin and tetracycline, and chromosomally-mediated resistance to penicillins, tetracyclines, spectinomycin, and fluorquinolones.

Quinolone Resistance

Quinolone (also known as fluorquinolone) antibiotics include ciprofloxacin (Cipro); oflxacin (Floxin); levofloxacin (Levaquin); lomefloxacin (Maxaquin); norfloxacin (Noroxin); and enoxacin (Penetrex). Quinolone resistant strains of N. gonorrhoeae (QRNG) continue to spread, making treatment of gonorrhea with quinolones inadvisable in many areas, especially parts of Asia and the Pacific, including Hawaii. According to a 2000 WHO report, resistance to CDC-recommended doses of ciprofloxacin and ofloxacin exceeds 40 percent in some Asian countries. In the United States, QRNG is becoming increasingly common in areas of the West Coast, particularly California.

Therefore, the use of fluorquinolones in California as a treatment for gonorrhea is no longer recommended. Instead, the cephalosporins, such as ceftriaxone or cefixime, are used as a first-line therapy. However, as of March 2003, cefixime is no longer available in the United States through its primary manufacturer, Wyeth Pharmaceuticals. In the absence of cefixime, ceftriaxone is the only CDC-recommended gonorrhea treatment option for young children and pregnant women in the United States. *See also* **Ophthalmia neonatorum; Pelvic inflammatory disease; Quinolones;** and **Urethritis.**

Centers for Disease Control and Prevention. *Sexually Transmitted Diseases Treatment Guidelines 2002.* Atlanta: U.S. Dept. of Health and Human Services, 2002.

Goosby, Eric, MD

A San Francisco physician, Dr. Eric Goosby has been involved in HIV/AIDS since the beginning of the epidemic. In 1986 he was appointed AIDS Activity Division Attending Physician, and in 1987 he was appointed associate medical director of San Francisco General Hospital's AIDS Clinic. During his tenure, he developed a new method for providing treatment to intravenous drug users with badly scarred veins. Dr. Goosby acted as principal investigator for numerous AIDS Clinical Trial Group (ACTG) studies.

In 1991, he was promoted to director of HIV Services at the U.S. Public Health Service/Health Resources and Services Administration. While there, he administered the Ryan White CARE Act and helped establish the 52 AIDS epicenters located throughout the United States and its territories. In 1994, he was appointed director of the Office of HIV/AIDS Policy in the U.S. Department of Health & Human Services, working with Congress on all AIDS-related issues. In 1995, Dr. Goosby created and chaired the DHHS Guideline Committee on Standards for the Use of Protease Inhibitors. In 2000, he served as deputy director of the National AIDS Policy Office, and was instrumental in creating the Minority AIDS Initiative. In 2002, Dr. Goosby returned to San Francisco to serve as chief executive officer and chief medical officer for the Pangaea Global AIDS Foundation.

Government resources

The Unites States Government has created a number of different agencies dedicated to the research, education, treatment, and prevention of STDs. These agencies work together to administer a number of different programs and services, including clinical trials, treatment and research centers, drug assistance programs, housing programs, general assistance, educational websites, hotlines, fact sheets, slide shows, and educational brochures. See the list of government resources in the resources section at the end of this book for more information.

Gp41 (gp41)

Gp41 is the transmembrane protein of the HIV virus that connects the viral envelope to the viral core or center. A glycoprotein, gp41 has a molecular weight of

41,000 daltons and is embedded in the outer envelope of HIV. GP41 plays a key role in HIV's infection of CD4+ T cells by facilitating the fusion of the viral and the cell membranes. *See also* **Retrovirus replication**.

Gp160 (gp160)

Glycoprotein 160 is a precursor of the HIV envelope proteins gp41 and gp120.

Gp120 (gp120)

Gp120 is the envelope protein of the HIV virus. Gp 120 protrudes from the surface of HIV and binds to CD4+ T cells. In a two-step process that allows HIV to breach the membrane of T cells, gp120-CD4 complex refolds to reveal a second structure that binds to CCR5, one of several chemokine co-receptors used by the virus to gain entry into host T cells. A glycoprotein, gp120 has a molecular weight of 120,000 daltons and is the largest of the HIV proteins. Both gp120 and gp41are products of a larger protein, gp160. Accurate tests for HIV must include methods to detect antibodies to both gp120 and gp41.

Gram stain

The gram stain is a laboratory procedure used to help in the identification of bacteria and yeast. A biological specimen collected from various sources, including secretions from the vagina, cervix, penis, or from lesions, is smeared onto a glass slide and allowed to dry. After heat fixation, the slide is stained with crystal violet and iodine, decolorized and counterstained with safranin. Depending on the composition of their cell walls, bacteria will appear as gram positive (purple) or

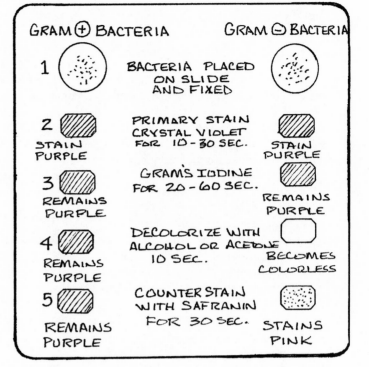

Gram stain test (Marvin G. Miller).

gram negative (red). The shape and size of bacteria seen on a gram smear help in their identification. Definitive identification is made when the organisms are cultured. A report of gram negative intracellular diplococci in genital secretions is diagnostic for gonorrhea.

Granuloma inguinale (Donovanosis)

Granuloma inguinale is a sexually transmitted disease caused by the bacterium *Calymmatobacterium granulomatosis*. Infection results in chronic inflammation of the genitals. Donovanosis is also known as serpiginous ulceration of the groin; lupoid form of groin ulceration; ulcerating granuloma of the pudenda; granuloma genitoinguinale; granuloma venereum; genitoinguinale; infective granuloma; granuloma inguinale tropicum; chronic venereal sores;

and ulcerating sclerosing granuloma. Donovanosis was first described in Calcutta in 1882.

Etiology

Granuloma inguinale is rare in temperate climates, such as the northern United States. It is common in some tropical and subtropical countries such as New Guinea, India, central Australia, and the Caribbean. This disease occurs more often in males than females and is more common in homosexual men. Donovanosis typically occurs in individuals between 20 and 40 years of age. The exact mode of transmission is uncertain, but the disease is most often seen in those who practice anal intercourse, although the disease is known to spread from the genital area to the anal region.

Symptoms

Symptoms begin about one to 12 weeks after the initial infection. The first symptom is a painless, pruritic (itchy) red nodule that slowly grows into a round, red lump that may ulcerate. The lesions are highly vascular with a beefy red appearance and bleed easily on contact. Sites of infection include the penis, scrotum, groin and thighs in men and the vulva, vagina and surrounding skin areas in women. In women, the lesions may resemble those of cervical cancer.

In both men and women, the anus, buttocks, and face may become infected. Over time, the raised bumps may cover the genitals. Healing is slow, and scar tissue forms. The lesions in donovanosis may become infected with other organisms. Untreated, the infection may spread systemically, affecting the bones, joints, or liver, causing severe weight loss, fever, and anemia. Lesions that are located in the anal canal may be associated with rectal bleeding. Infection may also occur in the lip, gum, cheek, palate, throat, and chest, although affected patients usually have co-existing genital lesions.

Four types of donovanosis have been described: 1) ulcergranulomatous, the most common type, which causes fleshy, exuberant, single or multiple, beefy-red ulcers that bleed readily when touched; 2) hypertrophic, which is characterized by an ulcer or growth with a raised, irregular edge, that may be completely dry and have a walnut-like appearance; 3) necrotic, usually a deep, foul-smelling ulcer that destroys the underlying tissue; and 4) sclerotic, characterized by extensive formation of fibrous (hardened) and scar tissue.

Diagnosis

Diagnosis is made by examination in which the characteristic bright red lumps are present. Specimens taken from the edge of the lumps can be examined microscopically for the presence of intracellular organisms known as Donovan bodies.

Treatment

Any of several antibiotics may be prescribed, including streptomycin, tetracycline, azithromycin, erythromcycin, doxycycline, and trimethoprim. The 2002 CDC guidelines recommend oral doxycycline using 100 mg daily for three weeks, or trimethoprim-sulfamethoxazole (Bactrim), using one double-strength (800mg/160mg) orally twice a day for at least three weeks. Alternative regimens include ciprofloxacin, using 750 mg orally twice a day for at least three weeks; or erythromycin base, using 500 mg orally four times daily for at least three weeks; or azithromycin, using one gram (1000mg) orally once per week for at least three weeks.

Therapy should be continued at least three weeks or until all lesions have completely healed. Some specialists recommend the addition of an aminoglycoside antibiotic (for instance, gentamicin using 1mg/kg intravenously every eight hours) to the above regimens if improvement is not evident within the first few days of therapy.

Patients should be followed clinically until signs and symptoms have resolved and they should have follow-up visits six months after treatment to ensure that the infection has been cured. Examination and treatment, if indicated, of all partners is recommended. Before the advent of antibiotics, antimony compounds were successfully used to treat this condition.

Persons who have had sexual contact with a patient with granuloma inguinale within the 60 days preceding the onset of symptoms should be examined and offered therapy. However, the value of therapy for people without clinical signs and symptoms has not been established.

Risk Factors

Risk factors include anal intercourse, poor personal hygiene, and tropical climate.

Pregnancy

Erythromycin is safely used as a treatment during pregnancy and for women who are breastfeeding. Consideration should be given to the addition of a parenteral aminoglycoside antibiotic such as gentamicin. Doxycycline and ciprofloxacin should not be used during pregnancy.

Complications

Carcinoma may occur either as a complication or sequel to donovanosis, occurring in 0.25 percent of 2,000 cases. The most frequent complication is pseudoelephantiasis, which is more common in women, occurring in up to five percent of all cases. Ulcerated lesions may allow transmission of other STDs, including HIV. Patients with both granuloma inguinale and HIV infection should receive the same regimen as patients who are HIV negative. Consideration should be given to the addition of an aminoglycoside antibiotic.

Centers for Disease Control and Prevention. *Sexually Transmitted Diseases Treatment Guidelines 2002.* Atlanta: U.S. Dept. of Health and Human Services, 2002.

Group B strep infections *see* Streptococcal vaginitis

Group M subtypes of HIV-1

HIV-1 is categorized into major (M), outlier (O), and N groups. Group M is further divided into subtypes or clades A to J. Subtypes are identified by gene sequence analysis of the envelope, pol, and gag viral genes. Subtype B of Group M is most common in North America and Western Europe. Subtypes A and C of Group M are found predominantly in Africa. Subtype E of group M occurs in Thailand, and other M clades are found primarily in Africa and Asia.

Haemophilus ducreyi

H. ducreyi is a small gram-negative bacterium rod responsible for chancroid. *See also* Chancroid.

HbsAG

HbsAG is an acronym for the hepatitis B surface antigen. The presence of this antigen can be used as a diagnostic tool for active hepatitis B, with a positive HbsAg test indicative of current hepatitis B infection.

Health Care Financing Administration (HCFA) *see* Centers for Medicare and Medicaid Services (CMS)

Health departments *see* City-County Health Departments

Health Disparities Initiative

One of the goals of the U.S. Department of Health & Human Services is the elimination of health service disparities among different socioeconomic groups. This initiative was designed to start with the millennium and meet its objectives by 2010 through the Healthy People 2010 project.

Health disparities include health-related differences that occur by gender, race or ethnicity, education, income, disability, geographic location, or sexual orientation. According to the CDC, race and ethnicity correlate with persistent, and often increasing, health disparities among U.S. populations in all these categories.

Race and ethnicity in the U.S. are risk markers that correlate closely with other more fundamental determinants of health status, such as poverty, access to quality health care, health care seeking behavior, illicit drug use, and living in communities with high prevalence of STDs. In describing the need for changes, the CDC guidelines state that acknowledging the disparity in STD rates by race or ethnicity is one of the first steps in empowering affected communities to organize and address these problems.

Studies show that African-Americans, Hispanics, American Indians and Alaska Natives, and Native Hawaiian and other Pacific Islanders have experienced poorer health status than the rest of the nation. In addition, CDC STD surveillance data show that the South, an area with an increased minority population, has consistently had higher rates of gonorrhea and both primary and secondary syphilis compared with other regions throughout the 1980s and 1990s. In 2001, six of the 10 states with the highest chlamydia rates were in the South.

The United States has a large and growing Hispanic population. In 2000, Hispanics represented 13 percent of the U.S. population (including residents of Puerto Rico), but accounted for 19 percent of the total number of new U.S. AIDS cases reported that year. A 2003 CDC study showed that Hispanic women have an alarming rate of cervical cancer, which is now known to be exclusively related to infection with the human papilloma virus (HPV).

African-Americans have the highest STD rates in the nation. Compared to whites, African-Americans are 27 times more likely to have gonorrhea and 16 times more likely to have syphilis. Genital lesions that occur in these diseases are directly related to a higher incidence of HIV infection in this population. Co-infection with both HIV and another STD increases the risk of transmitting HIV to another person.

The situation of health disparities requires attention, given that the minority groups listed above are expected to grow as a proportion of the total U.S. population. Current information about the biological and genetic characteristics of minority populations does not explain the health disparities experienced by these groups compared with the white, non–Hispanic population of the United States. These disparities are believed to be the result of genetic variations, environmental factors — particularly poverty — and specific health behaviors.

These disparities were clearly demonstrated in the U.S. Department of Health and Human Services study, *Report of the Secretary's Task Force on Black and Minority Health*, which revealed large and persistent gaps in health status among different racial and ethnic groups. In response, the U.S. Department of Health and Human Services created the Office of Minority Health in 1985. In 1990, Congress passed the *Disadvantaged Minority Health Act of 1990* to improve the health status of underserved populations, including racial and ethnic minorities.

Because disparities continue to affect the United States, in 1998, the CDC created its own Office of Minority Health in an effort to address this problem. In addition, an initiative entitled Healthy People 2010 was established to increase quality and years of healthy life, and to eliminate health disparities. *See also* **African-Americans; Healthy People 2010; and Hispanics.**

CDC STD Surveillance 2001. *Special Focus Profiles: STDs in Racial and Ethnic Minorities.* Centers for Disease Control and Prevention Division of the U.S. Dept. of Health and Human Services, Atlanta, 2001.

Health insurance

In the United States, health insurance can be obtained through group plans, employment or membership in labor unions, professional associations and various organizations, or it can be purchased as an individuals plan. For individuals over age 65 and for disabled persons, Medicare health coverage is also available.

For group plans obtained through employment, coverage can be continued if employment is severed, although the premiums generally become much higher. Through the Consolidated Omnibus Budget Reconciliation Act of 1985 (COBRA), health insurance coverage can be extended for up to 18 months. For individual plans, non-cancellable policies can be obtained. These are also called guaranteed renewable policies. These policies remain in effect indefinitely as long as the premium is paid. Insurance regulations vary in different states. All states have a State Insurance Program that will work with people when disputes over coverage occur.

There are three major types of consumer health insurance: Fee-For-Service or Traditional plans, health maintenance organizations (HMOs), and Preferred Provider Organizations (PPOs). The latter two plans, although generally less expensive, limit which physicians a patient can see. In general, with these plans the patient pays a co-pay for each visit to a physician and for each prescription medicine. In addition, a referral is needed to see any type of specialist. Traditional plans generally cost more, but patients usually only pay out-of-pocket expenses up to a certain annual amount or "cap." Traditional plans also have the option of major medical or basic plans. Higher premiums are paid for more comprehensive coverage.

Long-term care insurance coverage can also be purchased to help cover the costs associated with long-term care, including nursing home or hospice care. In addition, each state has a state insurance commission that works to investigate insurance problems and protect patient rights. Most hospitals also have business representatives or social workers who can assist patients in completing insurance claims. Social Security disability provisions are also available for people with disabling conditions such as AIDS who have qualified for Social Security disability. *See also* **Centers for Medicare and Medicaid Services** (CMS) and **Social Security Disability for** HIV/AIDS.

Health Insurance Portability Privacy Act (HIPPA)

HIPPA is a federal act intended to protect patient privacy while allowing patients access to their medical information. Guidelines effective in April 2003 also mandate that patients be informed of agencies that have access to their medical information. Patients can also authorize spouses and relatives to receive their medical information, and patients must provide signed authorization if they want health care information left on their answering machines. Disclosure of protected health information is to be disclosed only to those involved in the treatment, payment procedures and health care operations of individuals.

Health Care Providers Rights

Health care providers must follow guidelines that state medical information can be used to coordinate medical treatment or services, sharing information with technicians, doctors and other providers and with family members or others who are involved in a patient's medical care. Information may also be disclosed to insurance providers, such as the plan's third party administrator. Information disclosures may also be made to third party "business associates" that perform various activities, such as physical therapy, necessary to provide quality care.

Health care providers are also allowed to disclose protected health information to health departments and related agencies when required to do so by federal, state, or local law. Health care providers may also disclose protected health care information when necessary to prevent a serious threat to the safety and health of the patient or others who may be affected. Any disclosure, however, would only be to someone able to help prevent the threat.

Health information may be also disclosed if it is related to public health activities, such as: to report births and deaths; to report child abuse or neglect; to report adverse medical reactions; to notify people of recalls of products they may be using; to notify people who may have been inadvertently exposed to a disease; or who may be at risk for contracting or spreading a disease or condition.

Health information may also be disclosed to a health oversight agency for activities authorized by law, such as activities necessary for the government to monitor the health care system, government programs, and compliance with civil rights laws.

Health information may be disclosed in response to a court or administrative order, or in response to a subpoena, discovery request, or other lawful process by someone else involved in a lawsuit or dispute, but only after efforts have been made to inform the patient about the request. Health information may also be disclosed to law enforcement agencies in response to a court order; to identify or locate a suspect, fugitive, material witness or missing person; to help in criminal investigations resulting in death; and in emergency circumstances to report a crime, the location of the crime or victims, or the identity, description or location of the person who committed the crime.

Health information may also be disclosed to military officials for activities deemed necessary by appropriate authorities, to determine eligibility by the Department of Veterans Affairs, and to federal officials conducting national security and intelligence activities. Health information of inmates may be disclosed to physicians and others involved in one's medical care.

Under the law, health care providers must make disclosures to patients when required by the secretary of the Department of Health and Human Services to investigate compliance with HIPAA. Other uses and disclosures of protected health information can be made only with the patient's written permission. Patients also have a right to revoke this permission in the future.

Patients' Rights Under HIPPA

Patients have the right to inspect and copy protected health information contained in a "designated record set," which contains enrollment, medical and billing records, and any other records used to determine medical benefits. Health care information used for medical decisions must be requested in writing from health care providers or medical records departments of hospitals.

Under federal law, patients may not inspect the following records: psychotherapy notes; information compiled in reasonable anticipation of, or use in, a civil, criminal, or administrative action or proceeding; and protected health information that is subject to law that prohibits access.

Patients may also request that protected health care information not be disclosed for the purposes of treatment, payment, or healthcare operations. Patients may also request that any part of their protected health information not be disclosed to family members or friends who may be involved in their health care. Requests must state the specific information to be withheld and state to whom the restriction applies. Health care providers may not comply with this request if they feel the information is needed for the specified parties to provide emergency treatment.

Patients also have the right to amend their protected health information and they have the right to receive an accounting of certain disclosures of protected health information made to other parties. Patients can request that they only be communicated with at specific locations or by mail. Patients may make written complaints relating to compliance with HIPPA to their health care providers or to the secretary of Health and Human Services. Patients also have a right to ask for copies of the specific HIPPA compliance policies of their health care providers.

Health Resources and Services Administration (HRSA)

HRSA is the agency of the U.S. Department of Health & Human Services that administers various primary care programs, including the Ryan White CARE Act, for the medically underserved. HRSA is responsible for coordinating the AIDS Drug Assistance Program (ADAP), which provides FDA-approved medications to low-income individuals with HIV disease who have limited or no private insurance or Medicaid. HRSA also functions to maintain a reimbursement and accounting system for CARE funds, and to establish AIDS education and training centers throughout the country. For more information about HRSA and the Ryan White CARE Act, see http://hab.hrsa.gov/.

Healthy Life Choices Project

The Healthy Life Choices Project is a dietary and behavioral protocol being evaluated in National Center for Complementary and Alternative Medicine (NCCAM) clinical trials for its effect on diarrhea related to HIV infection. The study will de-termine whether changes in diet and behavior lessen the number of times HIV positive people experience soft or loose stools. Trials are being conducted at Columbia University's School of Nursing/ Center for Aids Research in New York City. For more information contact Ann Chung at 212-305-0216 or amc103@columbia. edu.

Healthy People 2010

The Healthy People 2010 Project is a federal initiative dedicated to the principle that every community and ethnic group deserves equal access to comprehensive health care systems. Healthy People 2010 includes a set of health objectives for the United States to achieve over the first decade of the new century. This initiative builds upon the national health objectives set forth in the following Surgeon General's Reports: the 1979 report, *Healthy People*; the 1980 report, *Promoting Health/ Preventing Disease: Objectives for the Nation*; and the 2000 report, *Healthy People 2000: National Health Promotion and Disease Prevention Objectives.*

Healthy People 2010 is designed to achieve two overarching goals: 1) to increase the quality and years of healthy life through disease prevention and equality of treatment services for everyone; and 2) to eliminate health disparities among different segments of the population that occur by gender, race or ethnicity, education or income, disability, geographic location, or sexual orientation.

Healthy People 2010 identified ten leading health indicators (LHIs) that are major public health concerns in the U.S. The LHIs were chosen as "determinants of health." As such, they are critical influences or conditions that precede a variety of health problems. The LHIs were chosen based on their ability to motivate action, the availability of data to measure their progress, and their relevance as broad public health issues. The indicators include: physical activity; overweight and obesity; tobacco use; substance abuse; responsible sexual behavior; mental health; injury and violence; environmental quality; immunization; and access to health care.

This project also has a well-defined objective intended to reduce the incidence of sexually transmitted diseases with responsible sexual behaviors. The following table describes these goals.

HELLP Syndrome

HELLP syndrome is a rare but potentially life-threatening syndrome that rarely occurs in the 3rd trimester of pregnancy and includes maternal hemolysis (breakdown or lysis of red blood cells, which can cause acute blood loss), elevated liver enzymes, and low platelets. This syndrome is caused by mitochondrial toxicity. Mitochondrial toxicity causes fatty acid oxidation of

Healthy People 2010 Sexually Transmitted Diseases Objective Status

Objective	Baseline Year	Baseline	1997	1998	1999	2000	2001	2010 Objective
1) Reduce the proportion of adolescents and young adults with *Chlamydia trachomatis* infections								
a) Females aged 15–24 yrs attending family planning clinics	1997	5.0%	5.0%	6.1%	5.6%	5.9%	5.8%	3.0%
b) Females aged 15–24 yrs attending STD clinics	1997	12.2%	12.2%	13.5%	13.7%	13.5%	13.3%	3.0%
c) Males aged 15–24 yrs attending STD clinics	1997	15.7%	15.7%	16.9%	17.0%	16.4%	17.0%	3.0%
2) Reduce gonorrhea (cases per 1000,000 population)	1997	123		122.4	131.9	132.3	129.0	128.5	19.0
3) Eliminate sustained domestic transmission of primary and secondary syphilis (cases per 100,000 population)	1997	3.2	3.2	2.6	2.4	2.1	2.2	0.2
4) Reduce the proportion of adults aged 20 to 29 yrs with genital herpes infection	1998–1994	17.0%	—	—	—	—	—	14.0%
5) Reduce the proportion of females aged 15 to 44 yrs who have ever required treatment for pelvic inflammatory disease (PID)	1995	8.0%	—	—	—	—	—	5.0%
6) Reduce the proportion of childless females with fertility problems who have had an STD or who have required treatment for PID	1995	27.0%	—	—	—	—	—	15.0%
7) Reduce congenital syphilis (cases per 100,000 live births)	1997	27.0	27.8	21.3	14.5	14.0	11.1	1.0

Adapted with permission of the Centers for Disease Control and Prevention. STD Surveillance 2001 Healthy People 2010. Appendix, Table 25-1.

mitochondria. The use of nucleoside analog reverse transcriptase inhibitor (NRTI) drugs in HIV infection may increase susceptibility to this syndrome. *See also* **Pregnancy** and the sections on pregnancy in **Acquired immune deficiency syndrome (AIDS)**.

Helper/suppressor ratio (of T cells)

T cells are a subgroup of white blood cells known as lymphocytes. Two major types of T cells exist: T helper (CD4+) cells, and T suppressor (CD8+) cells. The HIV virus destroys both of these T cell subtypes, but it primarily targets CD4+ T helper cells. The normal ratio of helper T cells to suppressor T cells is approximately 2:1. This ratio becomes inverted in persons with AIDS, but may also be temporarily abnormal in other conditions, including some autoimmune diseases.

Hemophilia

Hemophilia, including hemophilia A and hemophilia B, is the most common congenital blood clotting disorder known. Hemophilia affects one in 10,000 persons. Primarily affecting males, hemophilia is a condition caused by a deficiency of Factor VIII, a blood component necessary for proper blood clotting. This condition is caused by a defect on the X chromosome, with the result that hemizygous (having no corresponding gene on the Y chromosome) males are primarily affected. Hemophilia varies in severity, with severe disorders causing bleeding into joints or muscles and excessive postoperative bleeding. Patients with hemophilia are treated with transfusions of recombinant (human derived) Factor VIII concentrate or cryoprecipitate blood products.

In the early to mid–1980s, thousand of hemophiliacs developed AIDS as a result of transfusions of human-derived Factor VIII products that were contaminated with the HIV virus. Heat-treating destroys HIV, but early in the epidemic, these blood products were not routinely heat-treated. Some Blood Banks, thinking that HIV only caused AIDS in a small number of patients, decided the expense of heat-treating or destroying blood products was not justified. Studies show that hemophiliacs infected with HIV are more likely to have higher viral loads and clinical progression to AIDS than individuals without hemophilia. *See also* **Factor VIII.**

Hepatitis

Hepatitis is a condition of liver inflammation that may be caused by bacterial or viral infection, parasitic infestation, alcohol, drugs, toxins or transfusion of incompatible blood.

Hepatitis viruses, which can be sexually transmitted, represent a heterogeneous group of genetically unrelated viruses that target liver cells (hepatocytes), causing hepatitis. The hepatitis viruses are remarkably different in their physical structure, pathology, and epidemiology. And although hepatitis is an ancient disease, it has only been in recent years that these various viruses responsible for hepatitis have been recognized. Other viruses, such as herpesviruses, can infect the liver, but they are not classified as hepatitis viruses because they primarily target other organs.

Five categories of hepatitis virus have been identified, designated alphabetically as A to E. Each subtype of hepatitis belongs to a different viral family. Although these five viruses account for the majority of known cases of viral hepatitis, the possibility remains that other hepatitis viruses have not yet been identified. A new candidate human hepatitis virus has provisionally been identified and termed the "GB virus C" or "hepatitis G virus," and may be transmitted during blood transfusions. It was initially suspected of being the cause of liver disease in some patients who have acute or chronic hepatitis without evidence of infection with the other five viruses. However, this has not been confirmed in more recent studies, and at the genetic level it cannot be considered a variant of hepatitis C. To date, there is no evidence that this virus is sexually transmitted.

Hepatitis viruses in groups A through E can cause clinically overt acute hepatitis with noticeable jaundice. The specific viral type of hepatitis a patient has can only be diagnosed by serological tests showing specific viral antigens or antibodies. As is usual with antibody responses, IgM antibodies are formed in early infection, followed by IgG antibodies. IgM antibodies are typically present only during acute infection, whereas IgG antibodies often persist throughout life. The presence of viral antigens, viral RNA, or viral DNA is indicative of acute infection.

Hepatitis A, B, C, and D can all be sexually transmitted, with some viruses transmitted more efficiently than others. Hepatitis A, B, C, and D can all also be transmitted through other means.

Lemon, Stanley M., and Miriam J. Alter. "Viral Hepatitis." Chapter 26 in *Sexually Transmitted Diseases*. 3rd Edition. Edited by King K. Holmes, et al. New York: McGraw-Hill, 1999.

Hepatitis A (HAV)

Hepatitis A generally causes a mild form of hepatitis although it can cause acute hepatic (liver) failure.

Etiology

The hepatitis A virus is classified as an enterovirus belonging to the *Picornaviridae* family. Its virion is 27 nm in diameter and does not contain an outer envelope. HAV is composed of multiple copies of four nucleocapsid subunits. First reported in 1973, HAV causes symptoms 2–6 weeks after initial infection. Within 1–4 weeks after initial exposure, HAV can be detected in feces. The titers of HAV in feces are much higher than the HIV titers found in blood. HAV is primarily transmitted by

fecal-oral contact, with contaminated food and water sources responsible for most infections.

The hepatitis A virus is extremely stable, existing for long periods in feces, and can be found in shellfish inhabiting contaminated waters. HAV may be sexually transmitted, especially through anal-oral routes. HAV may also be transmitted by transfusion of contaminated blood products, but this is rare because viral antigen titers in the blood are only high during periods of acute illness. Studies show that HAV may also be transmitted among injection-drug users who share contaminated needles.

Epidemiology

The incidence of HAV has declined in developed nations during the last few decades, likely as a result of improvements in sanitation. In developing nations most HAV infections occur during childhood. In the United States, outbreaks in preschool day care facilities, especially those caring for children younger than the age of two, also play a significant role in HAV transmission. The majority of children infected with HAV do not develop jaundice and may not be recognized as having hepatitis.

Studies show a higher incidence of HAV infection among homosexual men when compared to heterosexual males. The risk of infection in this population is related to age and number of sex partners. Unlike other STDs, HAV infection confers immunity, and patients are never reinfected. Individuals with HAV are only infectious for a short time. The prevalence of previous HAV infection among the U.S. population is 33 percent.

Symptoms

HAV in adults can cause early symptoms of viral infection, including low grade fever, malaise, headaches, and muscle pain, followed by an acute episode of nausea, anorexia, vomiting, and diarrhea. Most children with HAV infection have very mild symptoms. Symptoms generally resolve within six weeks, although in rare instances HAV infection may trigger the onset of chronic autoimmune hepatitis. Some patients also have relapsing hepatitis, in which symptoms recur several months after the initial bout of HAV infection. Hepatitis A accounts for less than 10 percent of all cases of severe hepatitis. The mortality in acute HAV infection is less than 0.2 percent.

Diagnosis

Patients with HAV infection have abnormal liver function tests and evidence of jaundice, which demonstrates hepatitis. The specific viral cause relies on the demonstration of IgM antibodies to HAV (IgM HAV). These antibodies remain in the blood circulation for up to six months after the initial infection. Because IgG antibodies persist indefinitely, the IgG HAV test cannot be used to diagnose current infection.

HAV RNA	Seen in acute HAV infection
Anti-HAV	Seen at onset of HAV infection, persists for life
IgM Anti-HAV	Seen in recent HAV infection; persists for 4–6 mo

Treatment

Because hepatitis A runs its own course, treatment is generally directed at specific symptoms, for instance, anti-emetics for nausea. Drugs metabolized by the liver should be avoided or used with caution. Hospitalization may be necessary for patients who are dehydrated because of nausea and vomiting, or who have fulminant hepatitis A.

Prevention

Inactivated hepatitis A vaccines for both adults and children have been available since 1995 and are the most effective means of preventing HAV infection. For adults older than 17 years, two vaccines are administered six months apart. Vaccines are recommended for persons at increased risk, such as homosexual men and international travelers to regions endemic for HAV. A combined hepatitis A and B vaccine has been developed for adults. When administered on a zero, one, and six month schedule of three doses, the vaccine offers identical protection to that of the separate monovalent vaccines.

Post-exposure prophylaxis is also available. Immune globulin (IgG) in a dose of 0.02 mL/kg administered intramuscularly within two weeks after exposure is 80–90 percent effective in protecting against HAV infection. Vaccines to HAV administered more than 2 weeks after infection are not effective because it takes 2–4 weeks after immunization for immunity to develop. Persons who received at least one dose of hepatitis A vaccine one month or more before exposure to HAV do not need prophylactic IgG. Post-exposure prophylactic treatment with IgG is recommended for household and sexual contacts of persons with HAV.

Risk Factors

Risk factors include a high degree of susceptibility (individuals who have not been previously infected or immunized); men who have sex with men; sexual promiscuity or multiple sexual partners; injecting and non-intravenous drug use; and sexual practices that facilitate fecal-oral spread of the virus, including oral-anal intercourse and digital-rectal intercourse. Epidemics of HAV infection may occur in select communities, causing adding risk.

Centers for Disease Control and Prevention. *Sexually Transmitted Diseases Treatment Guidelines 2002.* Atlanta: U.S. Dept. of Health and Human Services, 2002.

Hepatitis B (HBV)

Hepatitis B, which was first reported in 1961, is a common sexually transmitted disease with potentially serious complications, including death. In the United States, HBV leads to an estimated 6,000 deaths annually.

Etiology

Unlike the other known hepatitis viruses, HBV has a DNA genome. It is classified as a hepadnavirus type 1 in the *Hepadnaviridae* family. The HPB virion is 42 nm in diameter, spherical in shape, with a lipid envelope. The intact virion is known historically as the *Dane particle*. Epitopes on the major surface protein of the virion are known as hepatitis B surface antigen (HbsAg). There are several variations of this antigen. The core of the virion is known as the hepatitis B core antigen (HbcAg). During acute infection HbsAg can be found in the blood circulation.

HBV is primarily transmitted by blood, although other body fluids can potentially transmit the virus. Exchanges of blood and other body fluids during intimate contact, perinatal-maternal transfer, blood transfusions and unsafe needles are all modes of transmission. The incubation period after viral exposure is usually two to three months.

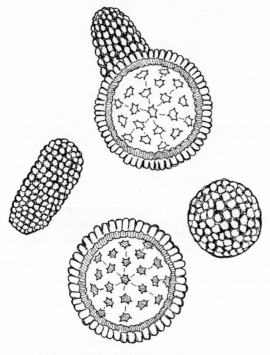

Hepatitis B virus and surface antigen components (Marvin G. Miller).

Epidemiology

In the United States, in the last decade approximately 30–60 percent of the estimated 200,000 annual new HBV infections were sexually transmitted. Worldwide, horizontal transmission to young children is probably the most common means of transmission of HBV. The exact mechanism is unknown but is probably due to unapparent open skin abrasions (percutaneous transmissions) that are exposed to saliva or blood.

Approximately one to six percent of adults infected with HBV develop chronic infections. These persons remain capable of transmitting HBV to others and they are at high risk for chronic liver disease, which may lead to cirrhosis of the liver and primary hepatocellular carcinoma (liver cancer). The risk for perinatal HBV infection in infants born to HBV infected mothers is 10–85 percent depending on the mother's hepatitis Be antigen (HbeAg) status. Even when not infected during the perinatal period, children of HBV infected mothers are at high risk for acquiring chronic HBV infection by person-to-person transmission during the first five years of life.

Symptoms

The incubation period from the time of exposure to the onset of symptoms is six weeks to six months. Approximately 15–20 percent of patients develop a transient illness during the prodromal or early acute stage of HBV infection. This syndrome is characterized by a reddened skin rash, joint pain and frank arthritis that may affect both large joints of the extremities and the proximal interphalangeal joints (between the fingers) of the hands. HBV infection can be self-limited or chronic. Symptoms of acute infection include fever, nausea, vomiting, anorexia, and muscle ache. Signs include jaundice of the eyes and skin and the presence of bile in the urine.

Approximately 90 percent of infected

infants, 60 percent of children younger than five years, and one to six percent of adults remain viremic (have evidence of viral antigens in their blood) and become chronic carriers for many years or for life. Although these patients often have few signs of acute infection, they are at risk for chronic active hepatitis, cirrhosis, or hepatocellular carcinoma. A rare but serious complication of HBV infection is acute fulminant hepatitis or fulminant hepatitis associated with chronic infection. Fulminant hepatitis results in massive hepatic necrosis (liver cell destruction) and has a high fatality rate. Fulminant hepatitis is often associated with HDV co-infection. Patients with chronic HBV infection may also develop a number of autoimmune syndromes, including polyarteritis nodosa, glomerulonephritis, and essential mixed cryoglobulinemia.

Hepatitis B can lead to cirrhosis of the liver. People with advanced hepatitis and cirrhosis often develop ascites, which are pockets of free fluid that accumulate in the abdomen, and generalized edema, which causes fluid to accumulate in the tissues causing swelling. Normally, the protein component albumin traps water and prevents fluid accumulation. A diseased liver cannot produce sufficient albumin and symptoms of fluid retention occur.

Diagnosis

The viremic phase is typically more prolonged than in hepatitis A, with HbsAg evident prior to the development of symptoms, and declining during clinical recovery. About 90 percent of all patients with acute HBV infection have detectable HbsAg when they first seek medical care. In addition, various serologic markers can be used in a hepatitis B profile that helps determine the stage of infection.

Hepatitis B surface antigen (HbsAb) is present in either acute or chronic infection. The presence of IgM antibody to hepatitis B core antigen (IgM anti–HBc) is diagnostic of acute HBV infection. Anti-

body to HbsAg (anti–HBs) is produced following a resolved infection and after immunization. The presence of HbsAG with a negative test for IgM anti–HBc is indicative of chronic HBV infection. The presence of anti–HBc (hepatitis B core antibodies) may indicate either acute, resolved, or chronic infection. The presence of HbeAg in an HbsAg positive individual suggests a high degree of infectivity. Conversion of HbeAg to anti–Hbe (the antibody to Hbe) in a patient with chronic hepatitis B generally signals a resolution of hepatocellular (liver cell) disease, although the clinical value of the HbeAg and anti–Hbe tests are uncertain.

HBV DNA	Seen in current HBV infection; once called Dane particle
HbsAg	Seen in chronic HBV infection; once called Australian antigen
HbcAg	Seen during HBV replication when HBV titers are high
Anti-HBs	Seen in past infection and in immunity from vaccines
Anti-HBc	Seen in recovery phase; with HbsAb seen in carriers
Total Anti-HBc	Seen in prior HBV infection
IgM anti–HBc	Seen for 4–6 months after recent HBV

Treatment

No specific therapy is available for persons with acute HBV infection. Treatment is supportive and intended to help reduce symptoms. Antiviral agents, such as alpha-interferon or lamivudine, are available for persons with chronic HBV infection.

In September 2002, the FDA approved Hepsera (adefovir dipivoxil) tablets for the treatment of chronic hepatitis B in adults with evidence of active viral replication and either elevations in the serum liver enzymes alanine aminotransferase (ALT) or aspartate aminotransferase (AST), or histologically active disease (active liver cell destruction). Hepsera slows the progression of chronic hepatitis B by interfering with viral replication and causing DNA chain termination after its incorporation into viral DNA. A stastically significant improvement in the degree of liver fibrosis was also observed in the patients using Hepsera. Major adverse effects associated with Hepsera include severe, acute exacerbation (worsening) of symptoms after discontinuation of Hepsera, and kidney toxicity. Response to treatment can be demonstrated by normalization of liver function tests, improvement in liver histology, and sero-reversion from HbeAg positive to HbeAg negative.

Alternative Medicine

Writing in *Sugars That Heal*, Dr. Emil Mondoa describes the use of glyconutrients to promote immune system healing. Although glyconutrients are not a substitute for conventional medical treatment, they are useful adjuncts to current treatment protocols. In one study, researchers treated 22 hepatitis B patients with the glyconutrient cordyceps for three months. The patients' blood work and symptoms improved. Ascites resolved in 70 percent of the patients, and the other patients exhibited improvement. In addition, immunoglobulin (antibody) levels declined, which is an important sign of recovery. A similar placebo-controlled study at the Shanghai Academy of Traditional Chinese Medicine and Pharmacology in Shanghai, China, noted similar results. Mondoa explains that liver recovery may be related to the increased levels of adenosine triphosphate (ATP), a form of stored energy, seen in cordyceps therapy. Mondoa advises that patients first consult their physicians before using cordyceps. The suggested dose is 3–9 grams of cordyceps extracts or Cs-4 daily in divided doses.

Mondoa also reports the use of reishi and maitake mushroom extracts to lower liver enzymes, enhancing the liver's detoxifying capabilities. In one study of maitake extract therapy in hepatitis B, about two-thirds of the patients exhibited decreased levels of the enzyme alanine transferase (ALT). The suggested dose is 3–9 grams of maitake extract daily in divided doses. Similar studies involved the use of reishi extract, also using 3–9 grams daily. However, reishi should be used with caution in patients with bleeding disorders or who are on blood thinners.

Prevention

Two products have been approved for hepatitis B prevention: hepatitis B immune globulin (HBIG), and hepatitis B vaccine. HBIG is prepared from plasma known to contain a high titer of anti–HBs and is used for post-exposure prophylaxis. The recommended dose of HBIG for children and adults is 0.06 mL/kg. The dose is 0.5 ml to prevent perinatal HBV infection among infants born to HbsAG positive mothers.

The hepatitis B vaccine uses HbsAg produced in yeast by recombinant DNA technology. The hepatitis B vaccine provides protection from HBV infection when used for both pre-exposure immunization and post-exposure prophylaxis. The two available monovalent hepatitis B vaccines for use in adolescents and adults are Recombivax HB, manufactured by Merck and Company, and Engerix-B, manufactured by SmithKline Beecham Biologicals. The dose varies by product and age of recipient, and is administered intramuscularly in the deltoid muscle. More than 90 percent of people receiving the full course of three doses develop long-lasting protection from HBV infection, and booster doses are not recommended.

A combined hepatitis A and B vaccine has been developed for adults. When administered on a zero, one, and six-month schedule of three doses, the vaccine offers identical protection to that of the separate monovalent vaccines.

The hepatitis B vaccine is recommended for all persons who attend STD clinics who have not been previously vaccinated. It is also recommended for persons with history of an STD; persons with multiple sex partners; persons who have had sex with an injection-drug user; sexually active men who have sex with men; household members of persons infected with HBV; persons on hemodialysis; persons receiving clotting factor concentrates; and persons having occupational exposure to blood. In addition, the hepatitis B vaccine should be offered to all persons who have not been previously vaccinated who receive services in drug treatment programs and long-term correctional settings.

Pregnancy

All pregnant women receiving STD services should be tested for HbsAg, regardless of whether they have been previously tested. If positive, this test result should be reported to state perinatal immunization or HBV prevention programs to ensure proper case management of the mother and appropriate post-exposure immunization of her at-risk infant. HbsAg-negative pregnant women seeking STD treatment who have not been previously vaccinated should receive hepatitis B vaccine, since pregnancy is not a contraindication to vaccination.

Perinatal transmission is also frequent following acute maternal HBV infection in the third trimester. The presence of maternal HbeAg is associated with an increased risk of viral transmission to the newborn. Intrauterine infection may occur, but most infections are suspected of occurring at the time of birth due to direct contact with the maternal blood circulation.

Risk Factors

Risk factors include unprotected sex, intravenous drug use, and sexual intercourse with persons infected with HBV. Risk factors for heterosexual transmission include having multiple sex partners (more than one partner in a six month period), or a recent history of an STD. Risk factors for infection among men who have sex with men include having multiple sex partners, en-

gaging in unprotected receptive anal intercourse, and having a history of other STDs.

HBV infection in HIV-infected persons is more likely to lead to chronic HBV infection. HIV infection can also impair the response to hepatitis B vaccine. Therefore, HIV-infected persons who are vaccinated should be tested for hepatitis B surface antibody 1–2 months after the third vaccine dose to tell if they have established immunity (a positive HbsAb test shows immunity). Those who do not show evidence of immunity should receive three more doses. If immunity is not established, they should be advised that they might remain susceptible to HBV infection. *See also* **Hepatitis** and **Hepsera**.

Centers for Disease Control and Prevention. *Sexually Transmitted Diseases Treatment Guidelines 2002.* Atlanta: U.S. Dept. of Health and Human Services, 2002.

U.S. Food and Drug Administration. *FDA Talk Paper* T02-36. "FDA Approves New Treatment for Chronic Hepatitis B." September 20, 2002.

Mondoa, Emil. *Sugars That Heal.* New York, Ballantine, 2001.

Hepatitis C (HCV)

The hepatitis C virus is one of the leading known causes of liver disease in the United States. It is a common cause of cirrhosis and hepatocellular carcinoma, as well as the most common reason for liver transplantation. Before the hepatitis C virus was identified, patients with hepatitis who tested negative for hepatitis A and B were said to have non–A and B hepatitis, which is now known to be hepatitis C in most cases. In the late 1980s, HCV was shown to be the cause of almost all cases of non–B post-transfusion hepatitis.

Etiology

HCV, which was first discovered in 1989, is an RNA virus belonging to the genus *Hepacivirus* of the *Flaviviridae* family and shares properties with other members of this family, including the yellow fever virus.

HCV is unique in that it causes a persistent, chronic infection in about 85 percent of individuals infected with the virus. The hepatitis C virion is about 30–60 nm in diameter and has a lipid envelope and a nucleocapsid core protein. Its replication cycle is not well known. Different strains of HCV with distinct genotypes have been identified, and genotype 1b strains appear to be more refractory to interferon therapy than non-1b strains.

Epidemiology

HCV is primarily transmitted by blood-to-blood contact, including transfusions of blood and blood products. HCV is the most common chronic bloodborne infection in the United States. An estimated 2.7 million persons are chronically infected, and more than two thirds of all infected persons are younger than 50. HCV accounts for approximately 15 percent of acute viral hepatitis cases within the United States, although it is the leading cause of chronic viral hepatitis and is present in more than 40 percent of all persons with chronic liver disease.

The highest prevalence of infection is found among those with substantial or repeated direct percutaneous (skin penetration) exposures to blood, including persons with hemophilia treated with clotting factor concentrates produced before 1987, and recipients of blood from HCV positive donors before 1992 when blood donor screening for HCV became mandatory.

Needle sharing in intravenous drug use represents the most commonly identified risk factor in the United States, accounting for more than 60 percent of all studied HCV infections. Hepatitis C may be sexually transmitted and represents approximately 15–20 percent of all cases. Now that blood products are screened, the risk of infection related to transfusion is low, representing less than one percent of all cases. Community-acquired or sporadic cases of hepatitis C in patients with no identifiable risk factor account for about 15 percent of cases. Maternal-neonatal transmission represents about four percent of cases, and another two percent of cases occur in health care workers due to needle stick injuries. The CDC reports that no association has been documented between HCV and military service, or HCV and exposures resulting from medical, dental, or surgical procedures; tattooing; acupuncture; ear piercing; or foreign travel.

Symptoms

The typical incubation period of HCV is from two to 12 weeks. Infections are usually clinically mild. Many patients remain free of symptoms and only about 25 percent of patients develop jaundice. The most common symptoms are fatigue and anorexia. Hepatitis C infection often progresses to chronic infection.

Chronically infected individuals remain in a chronic carrier state, since about 90 percent of apparently healthy blood donors with antibodies to HCV remain capable of transmitting HCV infection to transfusion recipients. In addition, approximately 50 to 60 percent of acute infections, even when they are clinically mild, lead to chronic hepatitis, as evidenced by elevated levels of the liver enzyme alanine aminotransferase (ALT) for more than one year. The risk of developing chronic disease persists for at least 20 years after infection.

The severity of chronic HCV infection can be determined by the ratio of the concentration of the enzyme aspartate aminotransferase to that of ALT. In studies, the AST/ALT was less than 1.0 in patients who had not developed fibrosis. In patients with cirrhosis, the ratio was 1.0 or greater. The AST/ALT ratio is not reliable in patients on antiviral therapy.

The percentage of patients who progress to liver cancer is unknown, although the prevalence of antibodies to HCV in patients with liver cancer is high. The course of chronic active hepatitis and cirrhosis in hepatitis C appears milder than that seen in alcoholic cirrhosis. Although the development of portal hypertension remains low, liver-related mortality is possible. Mortality associated with HCV infection is due to its unique ability to cause persistent chronic infection in most infected persons. This distinguishes HCV from other hepatitis viruses.

• PORPHYRIA CUTANEA TARDA—Porphyria cutanea tarda is a condition of heightened sun sensitivity and mechanical fragility. Skin lesions occur in sun-exposed areas or in areas sustaining even minimal trauma. The skin lesions may occur as erosions, pustular lesions, hypopigmentation, and hyperpigmentation. This condition may also cause excessive growth of facial hair.

Porphyria cutanea tarda results from decreased activity of the liver enzyme uroprophyinogen decarboxylase related to liver disease or from an inherited enzyme deficiency. This condition can occur in any type of hepatitis, but it is most often seen in hepatitis C. Treatment consists of avoiding all liver toxins, particularly ethanol, and in some cases anti-malarial medications are used.

Diagnosis

HCV is diagnosed by detecting either antibodies to HCV (anti–HCV) or by positive tests for HCV RNA. Anti-HCV is recommended for routine screening of persons without symptoms and should include use of both an EIA or CIA method and a supplemental antibody test, such as the recombinant immunoblot assay (RIBA) or NAT testing to confirm all positive results. The rate of false positive tests using EIA alone is 30–50 percent if used alone in populations with a low prevalence of HCV.

As of 2003, the AMPLICOR and COBAS AMPLICOR were the only FDA approved diagnostic NAT tests for HCV. NAT tests are able to diagnose active HCV infection because they measure HCV RNA. A negative test on a patient with a positive screening test for HCV antibodies would have to be further tested with an alternate screening test method such as RIBAS. Tests employing the reverse transcriptase polymerase chain reaction (RT-PCR) to detect HCV RNA may also be used, although this test has not yet been FDA-approved. NAT testing is able to detect earlier evidence of HCV and can detect potential system failures (false positive results) associated with antibody testing.

Certain situations exist in which the HCV RNA can be negative in persons with active infection if they have started producing anti HCV. As the anti–HCV titer rises, the level of HCV RNA typically declines, causing a transient period in which the HCV RNA test can be negative even in people who develop chronic infection. For this reason the HCV RNA test should not be used alone as a screening test for HCV infection.

Diagnosis of chronic HCV infection can be made by liver biopsy. Liver cirrhosis is generally diagnosed on the basic of clinical signs of portal hypertension and by various grading systems.

HCV RNA   Seen in acute HCV infection
Anti-HCV   Seen in current and past HCV infection

Treatment

Current approved therapy for HCV-related liver disease includes alpha interferon alone or in combination with the oral agent ribavirin for a duration of 6–12 months. Pegylated interferon plus ribavirin is the treatment of choice. Side effects of interferon include flu-like symptoms, headache, fatigue, myalgia, fever, chills, nausea, diarrhea, alopecia, injection site reaction, depression, and mood changes. Side effects of ribavirin include hemolytic anemia, cough, shortness of breath, itching, rash, insomnia, and teratogenicity (cancer risk in future children). In addition, interferon may trigger the development of autoimmune conditions, including type 1 diabetes and autoimmune thyroid disease. Interferon is contraindicated in persons with significant depression, cardiac failure or arrhythmias, low platelet count, or a low white blood cell count. Ribavirin is contraindicated in anemia and in renal failure.

The goals of antiviral therapy include viral eradication (disappearance of HCV RNA), normalization of liver enzymes, improved liver histology, and improved quality of life. The National Institutes of Health Consensus Development Conference Panel recommends limiting therapy to patients with persistently high ALT levels and who have tissue studies showing progressive disease. More information can be found at the National Institutes of Health Consensus Development Conference Panel Web site, http://consensus.nih. gov/cons/116/116cdc_intro.htm.

Persons who test positive for HCV should be advised to protect their livers from further harm by avoiding alcohol and any new medicines, including herbal products, without checking with their doctors. They should also be advised to receive hepatitis A and hepatitis B vaccinations if they are not immune. To reduce transmission to others, they should also be advised not to donate blood, body organs, other tissue, or semen, and not to share any personal items that may have blood on them, such as razors and toothbrushes.

Alternative Medicine

In *Sugars That Heal*, Dr. Emil Mondoa describes the use of glyconutrients to promote immune system healing. Unlike interferon, which has a number of adverse side effects, including immune system stimulation and risk of autoimmune diseases, glyconutrients cause the immune system to work more efficiently with a specific response to the particular challenge. Although glyconutrients are not a substitute for interferon compounds, they are useful adjuncts to current treatment protocols. In particular, Mondoa describes a shiitake mushroom extract, active hexose correlated compound (AHCC), as increasing survival time and quality of life of pa-

tients with liver cancer caused by hepatitis C. Although survival, blood work, and quality of life improved in the AHCC treated group, tumor recurrence did not decline. Mondoa recommends only using AHCC (using 3–4 grams daily in divided doses) after first consulting with one's personal physician.

Prevention

No vaccine for hepatitis C is currently available, and prophylaxis with immune globulin is not effective in preventing HCV infection after exposure. The use of universal precaution by health care workers and appropriate screening and testing of donor blood is intended to reduce or eliminate HCV infection. Persons seeking care in STD clinics or other primary-care settings should be screened for risk factors for HCV infection, and those with the following risk factors should be offered counseling and testing: illegal injection drug use, even once or twice many years ago; blood transfusion or solid organ transplant before July 1992; receipt of clotting factor concentrates produced before 1987; and long-term hemodialysis.

Pregnancy

The CDC reports that HCV positive women do not need to avoid pregnancy or breastfeeding, although children born to HCV-positive women should be tested for HCV.

Risk Factors

Risk factors for sexual transmission of HCV include exposure to an infected sex partner, increasing numbers of partners, failure to use a condom, history of another STD, heterosexual sex with a male intravenous drug user, and sexual activities involving trauma. The risk for men who have sex with men is the same as the risk for heterosexual partners. Other risk factors include illegal injection drug use, even once or twice many years ago; blood transfusion or solid organ transplant before July

1992; receipt of clotting factor concentrates produced before 1987; and long-term hemodialysis. Of all Americans with hepatitis C virus infections, about 12 to 15 percent have been incarcerated. Of all Americans with chronic hepatitis C virus infection, about 29 percent have been incarcerated.

Risk factors for progressive fibrosis and cirrhosis include longer duration of infection; persons older than 40 years of age; excess alcohol consumption; persistently elevated serum ALT levels; HIV co-infection; male gender; and absence of antiviral therapy.

Occupational Exposures

Persons who test negative for HCV following exposure should be reassured that they have not been exposed. Persons who test positive for HCV infection should be provided information regarding how to protect their livers from further harm.

Prison Population

Because of the rising number of cases of hepatitis C seen in individuals leaving the prison population, in January 2003, the CDC recommended that every state administer hepatitis C tests to all prison inmates with a history of injection drug use, which is a common route of transmission for this virus. Of the estimated 4.5 million people with hepatitis C in the United States, more than 30 percent are expected to pass through prisons and other correctional facilities. Of all Americans with chronic HCV infection, about 39 percent have been incarcerated at some time in their lives.

Precautions

Studies show that individuals with Hepatitis C who are co-infected with the HIV virus have a higher Hepatitis C virus viral load than persons without HIV. The viral load of patients co-infected with HIV is not affected by HAART therapy for HIV.

Centers for Disease Control. *Sexually Transmitted Diseases Treatment Guidelines 2002*. Atlanta: U.S. Dept. of Health and Human Services, 2002.

APHL Infectious Disease Conference, Denver, CO, March 2003. "Molecular Methods: Impact on Public Health Practice, from BT to STDs."
"Guidelines for Laboratory Testing and Result Reporting of Antibody to Hepatitis C Virus." *MMWR* February 7, 2003/52 (RR03); 1–16.
Mondoa, Emil. *Sugars That Heal*. New York: Ballantine, 2001.

Hepatitis D (Delta) Virus (HDV)

The hepatitis D or delta virus virion has a defective RNA genome in the sense that HDV requires a helper function from HBV for it to be infective. The lipid envelope of HDV contains hepatitis B surface antigen (HBsAg) while the core of the virus consists of the HDV RNA genome and hepatitis D antigen (HDAg). The RNA genome, which encodes HDAg, is single-stranded. HDV has some features in common with plant satellite viruses or viroids.

Discovered in 1989, HDV is a bloodborne virus. HDV is transmitted by exposure to virus-contaminated blood and is endemic among hepatitis B-infected patients in the Mediterranean region where it was first described. HDV infection occurs only in individuals with acute or chronic hepatitis B infection. HDV superinfection in chronic hepatitis B or in HDV infection in persons previously susceptible to HBV is associated with fulminant hepatitis and increased mortality.

Current studies show that the hepatitis D virus is probably sexually transmitted, since the incidence of HDV is higher among homosexual men with HBV than it is in intravenous drug users with hepatitis B. In epidemiological studies, the presence of antibodies to hepatitis D was found to be associated with an increased number of sex partners. Although sexual transmission of HDV is probably uncommon, infections associated with HDV have a higher incidence of mortality. The hepatitis B vaccine offers protection against HDV because HBV is necessary for HDV replication.

Hepatitis E (HEV)

Hepatitis E, a member of the *Caliciviridae* family, is similar to hepatitis A in that its primary mode of transmission is fecal-oral. However, HEV is not sexually transmitted and it has not been found to cause chronic infection. Outbreaks of hepatitis E have primarily occurred in developing countries with inadequate environmental sanitation. Epidemics of hepatitis E have been reported in India, Asia, Central America, and Africa due to the consumption of fecally contaminated water.

While HEV infection has a course similar to that of hepatitis A, infection with HEV during pregnancy is associated with a high mortality rate. Prevention in endemic areas primarily relies on the provision of clean water and avoiding uncooked food.

Hepsera

Hepsera (adefovir dipivoxil) is an antiviral drug approved by the FDA in September 2002, for the treatment of chronic hepatitis B in adults with evidence of active viral replication and either elevations in the serum liver enzymes alanine aminotransferase (ALT) or aspartate aminotransferase (AST), or histologically active disease (active liver cell destruction).

Hepsera slows the progression of chronic hepatitis B by interfering with viral replication and causing DNA chain termination after its incorporation into viral DNA. At week 48 of two randomized, double-blind, placebo-controlled studies, 53 percent of patients receiving Hepsera in one study and 64 percent of patients in the other study showed significant improvement in the liver inflammation caused by HBV compared to 25 percent and 35 percent of patients receiving placebo. A stastically significant improvement in the degree of liver fibrosis was also observed in the patients using Hepsera. Major adverse effects associated with Hepsera include severe, acute exacerbation (worsening) of symptoms after discontinuation of Hepsera (similar to the effects of other antiviral agents used for HBV), and kidney toxicity.

The drug's manufacturers caution that patients who discontinue Hepsera should be monitored for liver function at repeated intervals over a period of time. There is also a theoretical concern associated with Hepsera that HIV resistance could emerge in patients with chronic HBV who may have unrecognized or untreated HIV infection.

U.S. Food and Drug Administration. *FDA Talk Paper* T02-36. "FDA Approves New Treatment for Chronic Hepatitis B." September 20, 2002.

Herbal medicine

A variety of herbal products are used to reduce symptoms in patients with STDs. For best results these should be administered under the direction of a naturopath or herbalist working in conjunction with the primary physician. Many herbs interact with pharmaceutical preparations, and many herbs have their own side effects.

Because STDs result from infection with specific microorganisms, herbal medicine is generally not effective used as the sole therapeutic agent. Herbal medicine does offer complementary benefits. For instance, the herb milk thistle (*Silybum marianum*) is often used as a complementary agent to help prevent liver cell damage in patients with hepatitis, although retroviral agents are the primary therapy. *See also* **Choraphor.**

Herpes simplex virus

Herpes simplex is a viral infection that causes painful, recurrent blisters around the mouth or genitals. Herpes may also infect the skin around the rectum, the hands (especially the nail beds), and may be transmitted to other parts of the body, such as the surface of the eyes. Herpes sores do not usually become infected with bacteria, but some people with herpes also have other STD organisms, such as syphilis or chancroid, in the same ulcers. Genital herpes is a recurrent life-long viral infection.

Etiology

There are two basic serotypes of herpes: herpes simplex virus (HSV)-1 typically causes cold sores or fever blisters, while HSV-2 is usually responsible for genital blisters. However, HSV-1 can affect the genitals, and HSV-2 can affect the lips. Herpes simplex has two phases: an inactive or latent phase in which the virus remains in the body in a dormant state, and an active phase, in which the virus may cause signs and symptoms or become contagious.

Epidemiology

Genital herpes is very common, with an estimated one million new cases in the United States occurring each year. The CDC reported in 2002 that about 50 million people in the United States have genital herpes. About one in five Americans over age 12 have genital herpes, although most do not know it. Many of these people have mild or unrecognized infections but nevertheless shed virus intermittently in the genital tract.

Herpes can be transmitted through vaginal, anal, and oral sex, and can spread from the mouth to the genitals, or vice versa, during oral sex. It is most easily transmitted during outbreaks, and can be spread by affected individuals with or without blisters.

Symptoms

Symptoms of the initial (primary) outbreak occur four to seven days after infection. The first symptoms are usually itching, tingling, and soreness. This is followed by a patch of redness, followed by a group of small, painful blisters. The blisters break and fuse together to form circular sores. The sores, which are usually painful, become crusted after a few days. The manifestations of atypical urogenital HSV infections, which are gener-

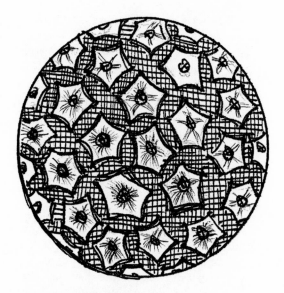

Herpes simplex virus (Marvin G. Miller).

ally not diagnosed unless an antibody test is done, include lower back pain, infrequent urination, aching lower limbs, and reddening of buttocks and thighs.

Symptoms of HSV-1 include fever blisters, cold sores, conjunctivitis, keratitis, and genital herpes. Symptoms of HSV-2 include tears in the skin of the genital region, jock itch, ill-defined discharge, blisters, and skin ulcerations. Urinating may be difficult, and walking may be painful. The sores generally heal after about 10 days but may leave scars. Lymph nodes in the groin are often enlarged and tender. The first outbreak is more painful, prolonged, and widespread than subsequent outbreaks (recurrences) and may be associated with fever and flu-like symptoms.

Neonatal Herpes

Neonatal herpes is one of the most serious outcomes of genital herpes. Estimates of the incidence of neonatal herpes range from one in 2500 to one in 20,000 live births. Since the greatest risk is in mothers experiencing a primary infection during pregnancy, diagnosis during pregnancy is critical. Most mothers of infants who acquire neonatal herpes lack histories of clinically evident genital herpes.

The risk for transmission to the neonate from an infected mother is high (30–50 percent) among women with histories of herpes who acquire genital herpes near the time of delivery. The risk is low (less than one percent) among women with histories of recurrent herpes at term or who acquire HSV during the second half of pregnancy. However, because the risk of recurrent herpes is higher than initial herpes during pregnancy, the risk of transmitting neonatal herpes remains high in mothers with recurrent herpes.

Infants exposed to HSV during birth, as documented by virologic testing or presumed by direct observation of lesions, should be followed carefully in consultation with a specialist. Some specialists recommend performing cultures of the mucosal surface to detect herpes before clinical signs develop. Some specialists recommend the use of acyclovir for infants born to women who acquired HSV near term, because the risk for neonatal herpes is high for these infants.

All infants with evidence of neonatal herpes should be promptly evaluated and treated with systemic acylovir. The recommended regimen for infants is acyclovir 20 mg/kg of body weight given intravenously every eight hours for 21 days for disseminated and central nervous system disease, or 14 days for disease limited to the skin and mucous membranes.

• NEONATAL CONJUNCTIVITIS—Neonatal herpes eye infections may affect one or both eyes, and the onset is generally within the first two weeks of life. Conjunctivitis or keratitis may occur alone or in neonates with skin lesions. Corneal lesions may lead to permanent corneal scarring and vascular disturbances. Approximately 70 percent of all neonatal herpetic infections, including ocular herpes, are caused by type 2 HSV. Topical antiviral treatment should not exceed seven days.

Diagnosis

Diagnosis of genital herpes is insensitive and non-specific. The typical painful multiple vesicular or ulcerative lesions are often absent in infected people. Up to 30 percent of first instances of herpes are caused by HSV-1, a condition less likely to be associated with recurrences. The type of HSV can influence treatment and counseling and it can be misleading.

The new guidelines recommend the use of type-specific serologic tests for HSV. Because people with herpes produce antibodies that can be detected in their blood within several weeks after infection, serologic tests for IgG immunoglobulin are now available and recommended for diagnosis. Until recently, commercially available tests were unreliable at distinguishing HSV-1 from HSV-2. However, two new type-specific tests are commercially available. Currently, HerpeSelect is the only laboratory-based type specific test. Pockit HSV-2 is a point of care assay available for HSV-2 and can be used in CLIA-approved medical facilities. Both measure antibodies to the glycoprotein G gene of HSV-1 and HSV-2. The sensitivity and specificity of these tests are greater than 96 percent when compared to Western blot tests. The Herpes Western blot test is considered the gold standard for herpes testing. Manufactured by the University of Washington, the Herpes Western blot is more than 99 percent specific and sensitive. For all antibody tests, the test is most effective when used at least 12 to 16 weeks following exposure.

Using newer antibody tests, researchers have found that by age 30 almost 25 percent of Americans have detectable HSV-2 antibodies. Only 10 to 20 percent of these individuals have a history of a classical HSV infection. Another 10–20 percent have totally asymptomatic disease (no symptoms) and 60–80 percent have an unrecognized or unapparent HSV infection.

The 2002 CDC guidelines recommending HSV-1 and HSV-2 antibody testing for anyone with suspicious symptoms or history suggestive of atypical or undiagnosed HSV infection; anyone diagnosed clinically who does not believe the diagnosis; anyone requesting or getting an STD screen or who is at risk for HIV infection; anyone whose partner has a genital HSV infection; and pregnant women with an atypical or unrecognized genital HSV-2 infections, or who are at risk of acquiring an HSV-1 or HSV-2 infection.

Pregnancy

Women with genital herpes outbreaks during pregnancy can pass the infection on to their newborn babies. This can result in death or severe, permanent disabilities, including brain damage. The risk of transmission of HSV-2 from an infected mother to a neonate is between 30 and 50 percent from women who acquire herpes around the time of delivery. The risk is low (less than one percent) for women with recurrent genital herpes. Even so, because genital herpes is so common and partners can reinfect one another, the risk is high.

CDC guidelines recommend counseling during the third trimester and careful examination of the patient for lesions at the time of delivery. Treatment for patients newly infected near the time of delivery varies with different practitioners. Some recommend acyclovir (400 mg twice daily) to try to prevent transmission, some recommend cesarean section and some recommend both. Pregnant women who are not infected should avoid intercourse with HSV-infected partners and they should avoid oral sex during the third trimester. The safety of systemic acyclovir, valacyclovir, and famicilovir therapy in pregnant women has not been established. Available data do not indicate an increased risk for major birth defects compared with the general population in women treated with acyclovir during the first trimester.

Treatment

Herpes cannot be cured, but medications can be prescribed that lower the number of outbreaks, make them less painful, and help blisters heal faster. Treatment is most effective if started early, usually within two days of the start of symptoms. Antiviral chemotherapy offers clinical benefits to most patients and is the main therapy used. Patients should also be counseled regarding disease transmission and prevention to prevent recurrences. The three antiviral medicines recommended for initial infections are valacyclovir, using 500 mg twice daily or 1,000 mg once daily for three days, acyclovir 400 mg orally three times daily for 7–10 days or 200 mg five times daily for seven to 10 days; or famciclovir 250 mg orally three times daily for 7–10 days. The CDC recommends the three day course of valacylovir.

A recent study found that acyclovir using 800 mg three times daily for two days had a significant effect on lesion duration, episode length, and viral shedding compared with placebo. This regimen was also found to increase the proportion of aborted episodes. All three antiviral agents are considered safe for use in immunocompromised patients (patients with immune deficiency syndromes, including HIV/AIDS) at the doses recommended for treatment of genital herpes.

Acyclovir may be administered orally to pregnant women with first episode genital herpes or severe recurrent herpes, and should be administered intravenously to pregnant women with severe HSV infection. Preliminary data suggest that acyclovir treatment late in pregnancy might reduce the frequency of cesarean sections among women with genital herpes by diminishing the frequencies of recurrences at term.

In November 2002, Lawrence Corey of the Fred Hutchinson Cancer Research Center, speaking at the 42nd Interscience Conference on Antimicrobial Agents and Chemotherapy, reported that the drug valacyclovir reduces HSV transmission in partners of individuals infected with HSV-2. Once daily valacyclovir markedly reduces the likelihood of sexual transmission to the uninfected partner. According to Corey, valacyclovir reduces transmission of HSV seroconversion by 50 percent and of symptomatic genital herpes by 75 percent.

• TREATMENT FOR POSTHERPETIC NEURALGIA—In the genital area, the virus initially infects the nerves in the skin. It then travels to the nerve roots near the spinal column, and then returns to the skin or mucous membranes. During the inactive phase the virus hides within the nerve roots. Before an outbreak, many people experience itching, tingling, or pain in the area where their recurrent lesions may develop. This warning system or prodrome can be very painful.

Treatment with either opioids (morphine derivatives such as codeine) or tricyclic antidepressants is reported to be effective in treating postherpetic neuralgia (pain) without causing cognitive impairment. In a randomized study at Johns Hopkins University, opiates such as controlled release morphine (91 mg) and methadone (15 mg) was superior to antidepressant therapy, such as nortriptyline or desipramine. Both were effective in relieving pain, but opiates did not affect any aspect of cognitive function, whereas tricyclics had a slight effect.

Risk Factors

Unprotected sex; condoms, when used properly, can prevent herpes infections. The 2002 CDC guidelines emphasize that HSV virus is shed constantly even when there are no signs or symptoms of infection. Results of several studies suggest that chronic stress can contribute to outbreaks. The conclusion from an analysis of this study published in the *Archives of Internal Medicine* suggests that persistent stressors and highest level of anxiety predicted genital herpes recurrence, whereas transient mood states, short-term stressors, and life change events did not. Short-term stressful life experiences and dysphoric mood states do not cause increased outbreaks.

Precautions

Recurrences can occur, especially in HSV-2 infections; patients should be advised that suppressive and episodic treatment is available to help prevent future outbreaks and shorten their duration. Individuals with herpes should inform current and future sex partners so they can receive treatment. Partners with symptoms should receive antiviral therapy. Partners without symptoms should be questioned about past symptoms, educated to recognize symptoms of infection, and offered serologic testing. Antiviral therapy is not recommended for persons who do not have clinical signs of infection.

It is important to differentiate HSV-1 from HSV-2, and newer blood tests are able to accomplish this easily. The ramifications of HSV-2 are very different from HSV-1. Crude antigen tests, which are very inexpensive, are still on the market and are not able to distinguish accurately HSV-1 from HSV-2. Tests for IgG immunoglobulin antibodies are very specific. The risk of women transmitting HSV-2 to uninfected men is about three percent and the risk of men transmitting HSV-2 to uninfected women is about eight percent.

Herpes has long been suspected of having a role in the HIV epidemic. A meta-analysis of 27 studies suggested that the risk of HIV acquisition was doubled in persons who were HSV-2 seropositive. One study in Africa found a five-fold greater risk of acquiring HIV in HSV-2 seropositive patients. Conversely, persons who are seropositive for both HIV and HSV-2 transmit HIV more efficiently and have an increased rate of HIV replication. Diagnosis and control of HSV in populations that are particularly susceptible to HIV may be a cost-effective HIV prevention measure. *See also* **Choraphor; Conjunctivitis; Herpes simplex virus (HSV)-1; Herpes simplex virus (HSV)-2;** and **Stress.**

Barclay, Laurie. "Valacyclovir Reduces HSV Transmission." *Medscape*, Nov. 11, 2002

Centers for Disease Control. *Sexually Transmitted Diseases Treatment Guidelines 2002.* Atlanta: U.S. Dept. of Health and Human Services, 2002.

Cohen, Frances, et al. "Persistent Stress as a Predictor of Genital Herpes Recurrence." *Archives of Internal Medicine*, Nov. 8, 1999, 2430–2436.

Sexually Transmitted Diseases Fact Sheet. Quest Diagnostics Incorporated, 2002.

Herpes simplex virus (HSV)-1

HSV-1, which is also known as human herpesvirus-1 or HHV-1, is one of the etiologic agents responsible for genital herpes. The presence of antibodies to HSV-1 can indicate either orolabial (oral or vaginal) or anogenital (anal or genital) infection.

Symptoms

HSV-1 infection may cause primary conditions of gingivostomatis (fever blisters, cold sores), conjunctivitis/keratitis, herpetic whitlow, herpetic encephalitis, genital herpes, and neonatal herpes. Recurrent infections of HSV-1 include herpes labialis, herpetic whitlow, herpetic encephalitis, and genital herpes. However, more than 95 percent of cases of recurring genital herpes are caused by HSV-2. HSV-1 reactivates more effectively in the facial nerves. Here it causes fever blisters or herpes labialis (herpes of the lips). *See also* **Herpes Simplex Virus** and **HERPEVAC Trial for Women**.

Herpes simplex virus (HSV)-2

HSV-2, which is also known as human herpesvirus-2 or HHV-2, is the primary etiologic agent responsible for genital herpes. The presence of antibodies to HSV-2 indicates anogenital infection. HSV-2 is also the most common cause of neonatal herpes, causing up to 70 percent of all neonatal herpes infections. HSV-2 is also responsible for most incidences of neonatal conjunctivitis caused by the herpes virus.

Epidemiology

Genital herpes is common in the United States, with 45 million people ages 12 or older infected with HSV-2. HSV-2 is more common in women, occurring in one of every four women, and in one of five men. This may be due to male to female transmission being more efficient than female to male transmission.

Risk Factors

Living in communities with a high incidence of STDs, illicit drug use, poverty with less access to health care, unprotected sex.

Symptoms

Most people with HSV-2 are not aware of their infection. However, if signs and symptoms occur during the first episode, they can be quite pronounced. The first episode generally occurs within two weeks after the virus is transmitted, and the sores typically heal within two to four weeks. Patients may also develop a second crop of sores during the primary episode and flu-like symptoms, including fever and swollen glands. However, most people with HSV-2 never develop sores, or they have mild signs that they mistake for insect bites or a rash. Most people with a first episode of genital herpes can expect to have several symptomatic recurrences a year (typically four or five). These recurrences are usually most noticeable during the first year.

Symptoms tend to recur in the same or adjacent areas because the virus persists in nearby pelvic nerves and reactivates to reinfect the skin during recurrences.

Diagnosis

The POCkit HSV-2, which is a point-of-care test, and the HerpesSelect-2 methods can be used for diagnosis. Both false positive and false negative results can occur. Therefore, repeat testing with a different test methodology is recommended for confirmation. *See also* **Herpes Simplex Virus.**

Herpesviruses (Herpesviridae)

More than 100 different herpesviruses have been identified as members of the family Herpesviridae. Of these, at least eight types are known to infect humans. Herpesviruses are classified as alpha, beta, and gamma herpesviruses according to their host range, cytopathology, and molecular strictures. Typical herpesvirus virions consist of four components: 1) an outer envelope with surface projections; 2) a tegument between the envelope and nucleocapsid (capsule surrounding the nucleus); 3) a nucleocapsid, approximately 100 nm in diameter with 162 capsomers; and 4) a core consisting of a fibrillar spool in which the DNA is wrapped.

The alpha human herpesviruses (alpha HHVs) include: 1) herpes simplex viruses types 1 and 2 (HSV-1, HSV-2, which are also known as human herpesvirus types 1 and 2 [HHV-1, HHV-2]) and 2) varicella-zoster virus (VZV, which is also known as HHV-3 and is the virus that causes chicken pox and Marek's disease virus, a cancer-causing or oncogenic virus found in chickens). Alpha herpesviruses have a relatively short reproductive cycle, destroy infected cells quickly, and are capable of remaining dormant (latent) in sensory nerve ganglia.

The beta human herpesviruses include: 1) human herpesvirus-6 (HHV-6); 2) human herpesvirus-7 (HHV-7); and 3) human cytomegalovirus or CMV, which is also known as herpesvirus-5. Both HHV-6 and HHV-7 infect and replicate in CD4+ lymphocytes and are associated with the rash exanthema subitum or roseola.

Gamma herpesviruses include Epstein-Barr virus (EBV or HHV-4) and human herpesvirus 8 (HHV-8). Both EBV and HHV-8 are lymphotrophic, meaning that they target specific white blood cells known as lymphocytes. HHV-8 is associated with

Kaposi's sarcoma and is sometimes called Kaposi's sarcoma-associated herpesvirus.

Diseases caused by herpes viruses are generally mild and self-limited in healthy people, although they may be severe in individuals who have suppressed immune function. Herpes can cause cold sores, fever blisters, and also blisters in the genital area (genital herpes).

Herpes viruses differ from other viruses in that they have a double-stranded DNA genome ranging in size from 125,000 to 250,000 base pairs; they also have a capsule, an amorphous layer of viral proteins called the tegument, and a lipid bi-layer envelope containing viral glycoproteins. They also express a large number of viral enzymes, destroy cells that they productively infect, and are able to establish latent infections in an infected host (they're able to stay dormant). The pathology of herpes virus infections depends on viral replication and associated cytotoxicity and on their capacity to cause latent infections. Latent infections can be converted to productive infections by means that have not yet been clearly identified.

The family of Herpesviridae can be divided into three major subfamilies: alpha herpesviruses, such as VZV, HSV-1 and HSV-2 that can infect rapidly and infect a number of different cells; beta herpesviruses, such as CMV, HHV-7, and HHV-7 that replicate slowly and infect a restricted number of cell types, which often become enlarged; and gamma herpesviruses, such as HHV-8 and EBV, which infect beta lymphocytes. Gamma herpesviruses replicate relatively slowly and some viruses in this subgroup are associated with malignancies.

Except for HSV-1 and HSV-2, which are closely related to one another, most herpesviruses are more closely related to animal viruses than other human viruses. Human herpes viruses are endemic and transmission usually requires physical contact. Often, the person shedding the virus is free of symptoms.

Herpes viruses are DNA viruses. Infection begins when the virus attaches to a susceptible cell. Viral glycoproteins in the virion envelope bind to components of the host cell surface that allow viral penetration. The viral genome is then delivered to the infected cell nucleus and viral genes are transcribed into the host cell. Viral DNA is replicated into the infected cell. *See also* **Choraphor; Cytomegalovirus; Epstein-Barr virus; Herpes simplex; Herpes simplex-1; Herpes simplex-2; Human herpes virus;** and **Human herpes virus-8.**

HERPEVAC Trial for Women

Beginning in November 2002, the HERPEVAC Trial for Women represents the phase III clinical trial of a novel prophylactic genital herpes candidate vaccine. The study is being conducted by GlaxoSmithKline Biologicals in conjunction with the National Institute of Allergy and Infectious Diseases. The double-blind randomized placebo-controlled trial will study 7550 women, aged 18 to 30, free of Herpes Simplex Virus Types 1 and 2. The objective of the study is to assess vaccine efficacy against genital herpes disease and infection. In previous phase III trials of men and women ages 18 to 45, 73 percent of the subjects, all of whom had partners with genital herpes, remained free of the disease after receiving the vaccine.

The vaccine contains a piece of outer coat of herpes virus called a glycoprotein. It also has an adjuvant, containing aluminum, as well as another ingredient derived from bacterial cell walls. Together, the glycoprotein and the adjuvant "prime" the immune system so that it is able to attack the virus more quickly.

Stanberry, Lawrence. "Glycoprotein-D-Adjuvant Vaccine to Prevent Genital Herpes." *New England Journal of Medicine*, Nov. 21, 2002; 347:1652–1661.

High-Risk HPV DNA Test

The High-Risk HPV DNA Test, manufactured by Digene Corporation, was approved by the FDA in March 2003, to be used as a screening tool for human papillomavirus (HPV) infection in conjunction with the pap smear. The High-Risk HPV DNA Test, which had previously been approved for diagnosing HPV infection, is performed by collecting cells from the cervix. The test detects DNA of the 13 high-risk types of HPV most likely to result in cervical cancer. Women who have normal Pap test results and a negative HPV DNA test are at very low risk (0.2 percent) of developing cervical cancer. Women with an abnormal Pap test and a positive HPV test are at higher risk (six to seven percent or greater) of developing cervical cancer if they are not treated.

The HPV DNA test is not intended as a substitute for a regular Pap test, nor is it intended to screen women under 30 who have normal Pap tests. Although the rate of HPV infection in this group is high, most infections are short-lived and not associated with cervical cancer. *See also* **Human papillomavirus.**

High-Risk Insurance Pool

The High-Risk Insurance Pool is a state health insurance program that provides coverage for individuals who are denied coverage due to a pre-existing condition or who have health conditions that would normally prevent them from purchasing coverage in the private market.

Highly active antiretroviral therapy (HAART)

Highly active antiretroviral therapy is a highly effective treatment protocol for HIV. HAART employs a combination of multiple antiretroviral drugs to reduce viral load to undetectable levels while maintaining or increasing levels of CD4. HAART is effective in a number of patients, although it can cause side effects that prohibit its use in some people.

The main goal of HAART is to achieve long-lasting suppression of HIV viral replication. A secondary goal is to help repair the immune system, and studies show that partial, but not complete, recovery of host immunity does occur, most noticeably an increase in CD4 counts, which occurs in almost all individuals who experience complete suppression of viral replication. The increase in CD4 count correlates with a reduced incidence of opportunistic infections.

Studies show that HAART therapy is most effective when initiated at the time of seroconversion. The institution of effective HAART during the early stages of HIV infection results in a higher level of immune system repair compared with treatment started during chronic infection. Patients treated in the early course of HIV infection usually no longer require prophylactic antibiotics following effective HAART therapy. This evidence of immune system repair can be seen in the observation of immune reconstitution syndromes that occur following the use of HAART. These syndromes cause a heightened clinical manifestation of infection, indicating improved immune function.

The usual HAART regimen combines three or more different drugs, such as two nucleoside reverse transcriptase inhibitors (NRTIs) and a protease inhibitor, two NRTIs and a non-nucleoside reverse transcriptase inhibitor (NNRTI), or other combinations. This allows for HIV replication to be halted at different steps of its replication cycle. These treatment regimens have been shown to reduce the HIV viral load to undetectable levels. *See also* **Acquired immune deficiency syndrome** and **Retrovirus replication**.

Hispanics

The U.S. has a large and growing Hispanic population that is heavily affected by the HIV/AIDS epidemic and also HPV infection with related cervical cancer. The CDC reports that in 2000, Hispanics represented 13 percent of the U.S. population, but accounted for 19 percent of the total number of new U.S. AIDS cases reported that year. The AIDS incidence rate per 100,000 population among Hispanics in 2000 was three times the rate for white, but lower than the rate for African-Americans. The CDC reports that transmission related to substance abuse continues to be a significant problem among Hispanics living in the United States, especially among those of Puerto Rican origin.

Histoplasmosis and penicilliosis

Histoplasmosis and penicilliosis are fungal infections that may occur as opportunistic infections in people infected with HIV.

Etiology

Histoplasmosis is caused by the dimorphic fungus, *Histoplasma capsulatum*, which is endemic in the Mississippi and Ohio river valleys of North America and also certain parts of Central and South America and the Caribbean. The mycelial (filamentous fungal) form of histoplasmosis is found in the soil and is particularly associated with bird roosts and caves. Penicilliosis is caused by the dimorphic fungus, *Penicilium marneffei*, which is endemic in Southeast Asia, especially Northern Thailand and southern China.

Epidemiology

Both histoplasmosis and a similar disorder, penicilliosis, cause disseminated infection in 20–30 percent of patients who have AIDS and reside in endemic areas. Sporadic infections also occur among HIV positive migrants from and visitors to these areas. Infection results when spores are inhaled and become lodged in lung tissue. The spores are then converted to the pathogenic yeast form at body temperature.

Symptoms

Usually, the immune system limits acute infection to a mild respiratory illness. However, patients with HIV infection develop disseminated disease, either due to reactivation of previously acquired infection or a progressive acute infection. The most common symptoms in both disorders are fever and weight loss, which occur in about 75 percent of patients. Respiratory symptoms (cough, shortness of breath) occur in about half of all cases. Patients with both disorders may also have local or generalized lymph node enlargement, enlarged spleen, skin lesions and oral ulcers. Skin lesions are more likely to occur in penicilliosis than histoplasmosis. Gastrointestinal ulcers may occur and cause gastrointestinal pain and bleeding. From five to 10 percent of patients develop an acute septic shock-like syndrome that includes hypotension and blood clotting disorders (disseminated coagulopathy or DIC).

Diagnosis

Imaging studies of the chest show diffuse nodular infiltrates in about half the cases of histoplasmosis and penicilliosis. Otherwise, chest films are normal. Patients who develop septic shock may have anemia, neutropenia, low platelet counts, and elevated liver enzymes.

Diagnosis is usually made by fungus culture or by tissue examination of bone marrow aspirate, lavage fluid, or biopsy specimens from lung or skin lesions. Blood cultures are positive in more than 90 percent of patients. Antibody tests for *H. capsulatum* are positive in 70–80 percent of patients. Tests are also available to detect *H. capsulatum* antigen in blood and urine. Serologic tests are not yet available for diagnosing penicilliosis.

Treatment

Both conditions are treated initially with amphotericin B for one to two weeks until there is an improvement in symptoms, followed by itraconazole, using 200 mg orally every 12 hours. Since relapse is common, long-term suppressive therapy with itraconazole may be warranted.

History of AIDS *see* AIDS history of; White, Ryan; Ryan White Comprehensive AIDS Resources Emergency Act

History of STDs *see* STD, history

History of syphilis *see* Syphilis history

HIV *see* Human immunodeficiency virus

HIV blood tests

In the U.S. individuals must be informed of the nature of the HIV test as well as its limitations before they can be tested for HIV. In some states, written consent must be given before the test is performed. HIV testing is recommended and should be offered to all persons who seek evaluation and treatment for STDs.

Blood tests for the presence of HIV-1 and HIV-2 antibodies using the enzyme-linked immunosorbent assay (ELISA) method and Western blot methods remain the primary methods for the detection of HIV infection. The sensitivity and specificity of these tests is reported to be greater than 99 percent in patients who have converted and are producing antibodies against HIV.

However, because antibodies to HIV are usually not detected for at least six to eight weeks after infection, and sometimes as long as six months, antibody detection tests fail to detect early infection. Health care providers are advised that individuals with symptoms of acute retroviral syndrome should be tested with nucleic acid methods. These tests are able to diagnose acute early infection because they detect HIV proteins, such as HIV RNA and DNA. These proteins are signs of active infection.

False positive HIV antibody test results may occur and be caused by cross-reacting antibodies, technical error, or other medical conditions. Therefore, positive ELISA tests for HIV antibody must be confirmed by another technology, such as the Western blot test. HIV antibodies can be detected in both serum and urine. Tests are also available for detecting HIV-1 and HIV-2 immunoglobulin G (IgG) antibodies, which can be demonstrated in seminal fluid and vaginal secretions.

Tests are available for detecting HIV DNA, HIV RNA, the p24 antigen, and HIV-1 core protein encoded by the gag gene. The p24 antigen is expressed shortly after acquisition of the HIV-1 virus, and antibody to p24 forms shortly thereafter. Assays to detect p24 antigen in serum and cerebrospinal fluid are also available using an ELISA technique. The p24 antigen also reappears or increases in HIV-1 infected individuals during the period of transition to AIDS. The p24 antigen test, which has not been FDA approved as a diagnostic test, is seldom performed since the advent of the newer nucleic acid tests for HIV-1 RNA and DNA.

When HIV enters human cells, the HIV-1 viral RNA is converted into a complementary strand of cDNA by the enzyme reverse transcriptase. These DNA molecules then integrate into the host cell's DNA genome, becoming the proviral form of HIV-1. After RNA translation and the production of new virions, HIV-1 RNA is released into the blood circulation. HIV-1 DNA can be detected by nucleic acid amplification tests, employing several different technologies. The DNA-PCR test, which is a polymerase chain reaction test, is highly reliable for detecting HIV-1 subtype B, which is the most common type observed in North America.

Tests that measure HIV-1 RNA or viral load became available in 1996. These tests are seldom used as a diagnostic aid, although they are widely used to evaluate response to therapy in HIV-1 infection. Tests for viral load are considered superior to CD4+ counts for evaluating prognosis in HIV infection. Three methods of quantitatively measuring HIV-1 RNA are available, including the RT-PCR assay, the branched DNA assay, and the nucleic acid sequence-based amplification technique. These methods appear to have equivalent specificity and sensitivity.

Serum HIV genotype and phenotype assays are also available to help in determining optimal treatment and antiretroviral drug resistance by identifying specific disease strains.

Home based and rapid tests for HIV are also available. Because these tests only measure HIV antibodies, they can miss early infections. They are also subject to operational error and misinterpretation.

Because antiretroviral therapy has been found to be most successful when used in the early stages of infection, when HIV-1 viral RNA load is low, patients suspected of infection with HIV should be tested for p24 antigen, HIV-1 RNA or HIV-1 DNA.

Because maternal HIV antibody can be passed through the placenta, it is not a good predictor of neonatal HIV infection. Placentally-transferred HIV antibodies, which can stay in the infant's circulation for up to 12 months, do not cause HIV infection.

For this reason, HIV-1 RNA, HIV-1 DNA, or p24 antigen are recommended for the diagnosis of HIV infection in neonates. Cord blood samples should not be used, and positive test results should be confirmed with repeat testing using a separate blood sample. PCR tests for proviral HIV DNA are the most commonly used tests for diagnosing neonatal HIV infection, although tests may not be positive for two weeks and sometimes not until the age of three months. For this reason, more often, the test for HIV RNA is used, although it has not been FDA approved as a diagnostic test and rare false positive results can occur. Tests for HIV-1 culture are available and were once considered the gold standard for HIV diagnosis, but they are seldom used today because they are time consuming and results are not available for 2–4 weeks.

The CDC recommends that initial counseling should be provided to individuals who test positive for HIV. This counseling should occur in the form of a personal session when results are provided and should include behavioral, psychosocial, and medical evaluation as well as monitoring services. Patients may also require assistance with making reproductive choices, gaining access to health services, and confronting possible employment or housing discrimination. *See also* **HIV-1 DNA; HIV-1 RNA; HIV DNA; p24; Enzyme-linked immunosorbent assay (ELISA); HIV home tests; Rapid HIV tests; Seroconversion;** and **Western blot test.**

HIV Center for Clinical and Behavioral Studies

The HIV Center for Clinical and Behavioral Studies, with offices at the New York State Psychiatric Institute and Columbia University in New York City, was established in September 1987. The center is supported by a comprehensive center grant from the National Institutes of Health as well as by many individual grants. The HIV Center has a commitment to serve underserved, often neglected, inner-city populations (including the HIV-infected) and to develop innovative research that emphasizes the social context of vulnerability and risk. Since its inception, the HIV Center has forged productive community and clinical partnerships, contributing to pre-vention efforts in the international arena, addressing issues of policy and ethics, and providing a unique multidisciplinary training environment. A number of special programs investigate adolescent STDs, HIV-positive populations, and HIV/STD prevention.

HIV Cost and Services Utilization Study (HCSUS)

HCSUS is a study using a national sample representative of the adult U.S. population infected with HIV and receiving ongoing care. The study found significant variation in service utilization and receipt of medication. Women were more likely than men to use the emergency department and be hospitalized, and less likely to have received antiretroviral therapy including a protease inhibitor or non-nucleoside reverse transcriptase inhibitor by early 1998.

HIV disease

During the initial infection with HIV, when the virus comes in contact with the mucosal surface and finds susceptible T cells, lymphoid tissue is the first site of truly massive viral replication. This leads to a burst of massive viremia (presence of virus in the blood circulation), with wide dissemination of the virus to lymphoid organs.

The resulting immune response intended to suppress the virus is only partially successful and some virus escape. Eventually, this results in high viral turnover that leads to immune system destruction. HIV disease is characterized by a gradual deterioration of immune functions. During the course of infection, CD4+ T lymphocytes are disabled and killed, and their numbers progressively decline.

HIV DNA

HIV DNA refers to the proviral form of HIV that occurs as host cells become infected with HIV. Proviral DNA can be tested in the blood as an early disease marker to detect acute HIV infection in persons who have not yet seroconverted (formed antibodies against HIV).

HIV home tests

HIV home tests were designed to encourage patients to undergo HIV-1 testing in a more confidential and convenient manner. The first FDA approved kit, the Home Access kit, allowed patients to lance their fingers, place a drop of blood on the reagent card and mail it to the company. The Home Access test uses an ELISA and immunofluorescent assay on the dried blood sample. The patient can call a toll-free number providing the number of the reagent card so confidentiality is assured. If results are positive or indeterminate, the caller is transferred to a counselor regarding the results. Sensitivity and specificity of the Home Access test approaches 100 percent.

HIV mutation

The HIV virus has the ability to mutate, changing its DNA code. Up to dozens of different strains of HIV can be found in one individual infected with HIV. The ability to mutate keeps neutralizing antibodies from eradicating HIV and it thwarts efforts to create a vaccine against it.

California scientists, in a team led by Douglas Richman, a virologist and physician with the Veterans Affairs San Diego Health Care System and the University of California, San Diego School of Medicine, have provided the first detailed look at how human antibodies may actually drive HIV to mutate, allowing the HIV virus to escape detection by the immune system.

Patients infected with HIV rapidly develop specific antibodies against the virus. Normally, antibodies help fight against infection and help neutralize infectious agents. However, these researchers have found that antibodies to HIV exert a strong selective pressure on the virus. This, in turn, causes the virus to mutate continually in an effort to avoid antibody attack.

Using sophisticated new technology made by ViroLogic, a company based in San Francisco, the scientists were able to clone HIV virus taken from the plasma of patients infected with HIV. They genetically combined the cloned virus with a gene that makes luciferase, the same light-emitting enzyme found in fireflies. The glowing enzyme helped the scientists track the viral replication.

Studies showed that most patients developed HIV antibodies within a few months after infection. These antibodies continually changed their activities to keep in pace with the ever-changing HIV virus. That is, the antibodies changed their protein structure to keep up with the protein changes in the outer coating of the virus. However, the antibodies always stayed a step behind the viral replication, keeping the antibody from neutralizing the virus.

"The Mutation of HIV." *Proceedings of the National Academy of Sciences,* March 18, 2003.

HIV-1

The major subgroups of the HIV retrovirus are HIV-1 and HIV-2. The extraordinary variability of the HIV virus, caused by its ability to mutate rapidly, has led to the development and geographical distribution of distinct groups and subgroups. The HIV-1 subtype can be further subdivided into major (M), outlier (O), and N groups. Group M primarily occurs in North America and Western Europe. Group O strains have traditionally been seen in West African countries, although rarely O strains are seen in the United States and Europe. The first Group N HIV-1 strain, which is very rarely seen, was found in Cameroon in 1998.

Group M is further subdivided into subgroups (clades) A–J. The HIV-1, subtype or clade B of Group M, is most commonly seen in North America and Western

Europe. This clade is responsible for nearly all HIV/AIDS infections in the United States. Tests for HIV-1 viral load in the United States primarily detect group M, subtype B, although some of the newer assays, such as the LCx HIV RNA assay, have been modified to detect group O HIV-1 also. *See also* **Human immunodeficiency virus** and **Acquired immune deficiency syndrome**.

HIV-1 Group M subtypes

Group M subgroup of HIV-1 can be further subdivided into subgroups (clades) A–J. The clade or subtype B of Group M HIV-1 is most commonly seen in North America and responsible for nearly all HIV/AIDS infections in the United States. Subtypes or clades A and C are found predominantly in Africa, whereas subtype E occurs in Thailand, and other M clades are found primarily in Africa and Asia.

HIV-1 Group O

HIV-1 group O HIV-1 strains have been primarily detected in West African countries, although strains have also been found in Europe and the United Strains.

HIV-1 RNA

Soon after entering a host cell, the HIV virus integrates HIV RNA into the host cell. The enzyme reverse transcriptase converts RNA into a complementary strand of DNA, cDNA. These DNA molecules then integrate into the host cell's DNA genome, becoming the proviral form of HIV. After gene translation and the production of new HIV virions, RNA is released into the host's blood.

HIV-1 RNA can be detected as early as two weeks after infection, and in most instances it can be detected within four weeks after infection. In early infection, HIV-1 RNA can be as high as 20 million copies/ml. At the time of seroconversion, which can occur from four weeks to three months after infection, viral load drops rapidly. The presence of symptoms does not appear to correlated with viral load, although patients who have symptoms at the time of seroconversion generally have higher viral loads 6–12 months after seroconversion.

Tests are available to measure HIV-1 RNA. Tests for HIV-1 viral load in the United States primarily detect group M, subtype B, although some of the newer assays, such as the LCx HIV RNA assay, have been modified to detect group O HIV-1 as well.

Tests that measure HIV-1 RNA or viral load are seldom used as a diagnostic aid, but they are extremely helpful in measuring response to therapy in HIV-1 infection because they measure the degree of HIV replication. Tests for viral load are considered superior to CD4+ counts for evaluating prognosis in HIV infection. Three methods of quantitatively measuring HIV-1 RNA are available: the RT-PCR assay; the branched DNA assay; and the nucleic acid sequence-based amplification technique. These methods appear to have equivalent specificity and sensitivity.

The typical course of plasma HIV RNA in HIV infection includes an early viral explosion with high levels of HIV RNA occurring shortly after infection and increasing for one to two months. As the immune system is activated, plasma HIV levels fall rapidly. Within 6–9 months, a dynamic equilibrium between cell infection, viral replication and CD4+ T lymphocyte levels occurs. The amount of HIV RNA levels off to a plateau known as the setpoint. Virus may remain at this level or gradually increase over time. The higher the setpoint level of HIV RNA, the greater the chance of disease progression.

The U.S. Department of Health & Human Services in conjunction with the International AIDS Society has developed specific recommendations for the use of the plasma HIV-1 RNA test. These agencies recommend that baseline levels of HIV-1

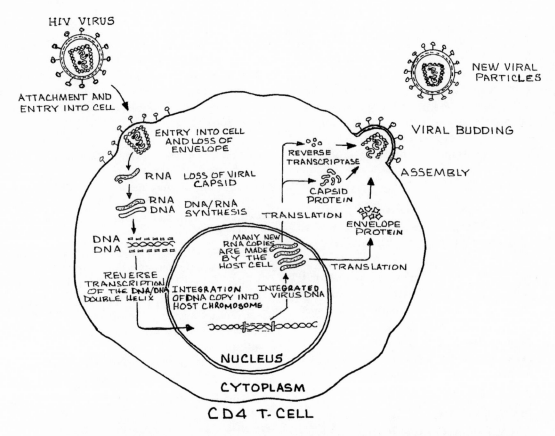

CD 4 T-Lymphocyte infected with human immunodeficiency virus (HIV) (Marvin G. Miller).

RNA along with CD4+ counts should be performed before starting antiretroviral therapy. The goal of therapy is to reduce HIV-1 to below detection levels. Available tests can measure HIV-1 RNA as low as 50 copies/ml. A one to two-log reduction of HIV-1 RNA is expected within 4–8 weeks after starting therapy, and the viral load should become undetectable within 16 to 24 weeks.

Higher baseline levels of HIV-1 RNA (levels higher than 100,000 copies/ml) are associated with less dramatic responses to therapy. Lower initial viral loads are associated with a greater chance of successful anti-retroviral therapy. Several studies have shown differences in the viral load of men and women, after controlling for CD4+ count and other variables. In general, women usually have a higher baseline viral load. Babies infected in utero were

found to have a significantly higher median viral load within the first month of life compared to babies infected closer to the time of delivery.

The guidelines recommend performing viral load tests within one month after starting or changing therapy, followed by monthly tests until levels are undetectable. Afterwards, tests should be performed at 2–3 month intervals. *See also* **HIV blood tests** and **Seroconversion**.

HIV RNA

Patients with acute HIV infection generally begin to produce detectable blood levels of HIV RNA shortly after infection. HIV-1 RNA, which is responsible for the AIDS epidemic, can be detected as early as two weeks after infection, and in most instances it can be detected within four weeks after infection. In early infection, HIV-1 RNA can be as high as 20 million copies/ml. HIV RNA or viral load is primarily used to determine response to antiretroviral therapy. *See also* **HIV-1 RNA** and **HIV viral load test**.

HIV-2

HIV-2 is a subtype of the human immunodeficiency virus. HIV-2 and HIV-1 are the causative agents of acquired immune deficiency syndrome (AIDS). HIV-2 was first identified in 1986 in an AIDS patient in West Africa and appears to be less pathogenic than HIV-1. Rates of heterosexual and mother-to-child transmission of HIV-2 are low, and the clinical picture in HIV-2 is primarily one of latent or slow-developing infection rather than overt AIDS. However, there are reports of superinfection and recombination occurring in patients with both HIV-1 and HIV-2, and as the disease advances, infection with HIV-2 increases.

HIV-2 is primarily seen in Africa, but serological tests for HIV antibodies usually are capable of detecting antibodies to both HIV-1 and HIV-2. Tests for HIV-1 alone show some cross-reactivity for HIV-2, but overall tests for HIV-1 antibodies generally do not detect HIV-2 antibodies. West African nations with a prevalence of HIV-2 of more than one percent in the general population include Cape Verde; Cote d'Ivoire (Ivory coast); Gambia; Guinea-Bissau; Mali; Mauritania; Nigeria; and Sierra Leone. Other African countries with a prevalence of HIV-2 greater than one percent include Angola and Mozambique. Other West African countries reporting HIV-2 are Benin, Burkina Faso, Ghana, Guinea, Liberia, Niger, Sao Tome, Senegal, and Togo.

The first case of HIV-2 infection in the U.S. was diagnosed in 1987. In 1998, the CDC reported 79 HIV-2 infections in the United States. 52 of these individuals were born in West Africa, one in Kenya, seven in the United States, two in India and two in Europe. The region of origin was not known for 15 of those infected, although four of them had a malaria-antibody profile consistent with residence in West Africa. AIDS defining conditions had developed in 17 of these individuals, and eight had died at the time of this report. Statistics on HIV-2 may be low because reporting of HIV-2 infection differs from state to state.

Because the incidence of HIV-2 infection is low in the United States, the CDC recommends that routine patients only be tested for HIV-1, although blood donors should be tested for both HIV-1 and HIV-2 to reduce the possible risk of transmission. Persons at risk for HIV-2 include those having sex partners from a country where HIV-2 is prevalent or whose sex partners are infected with HIV, people who share needles with a person from a country where HIV-2 is endemic or who have HIV-2, and people who received a blood transfusion in a country where HIV-2 is endemic. People should also be tested for HIV-2 if they have an illness that suggests HIV infection or who have Western blot results with certain indeterminate patterns. Since 1992, all U.S. blood donors have been tested for antibodies to both HIV-1 and HIV-1.

HIV-2 subgroups

Because of its ability to mutate rapidly, the HIV virus has formed a number of different subgroups. HIV-2 has five distinct subgroups (A–E) that have been defined. Evidence for superinfection and recombination has also been documented for HIV-2.

HIV viral load test

The HIV-1 viral load level measures the levels of HIV RNA circulating in an infected person's blood. Tests can measure HIV RNA over the range of 50–750,000 copies per ml and detect Group M subtypes A–G of the virus. The AMPLICOR HIV-1 MONITOR test by Roche Diagnostics is the only FDA approved test as of January 2003, for detecting levels as low as 50 copies/ml. With the prevalence of non–B subtypes increasing worldwide, the ability to measure low levels of other subtypes is crucial for HIV patient care.

Measuring viral load levels is an important part of assessing an infected patient's prognosis and response to drug therapy. This helps in making choices regarding optimal therapy. Studies indicate that lowering plasma HIV RNA below 50 copies per ml is a strong indicator of viral suppression.

Studies show that viral load is likely to be increased in both adults and children who are co-infected with oncogenic strains of cervical human papillomavirus, *Pneumocystis jiroveci*, cytomegalovirus, Mycobacterium avium complex (MAC), *plasmodium falciparum*, oral *Candida*, or HHV-8 even if they have not yet developed Kaposi's sarcoma. *See also* **HIV Blood tests** and **HIV-1 RNA**.

HIV/AIDS Bureau (HAB)

The HIV/AIDS Bureau is a department within the Health Resources and Services Administration (HRSA) of The U.S. Department of Health & Human Services that is responsible for administering the Ryan White CARE Act.

HIV/AIDS Dental Reimbursement Program

The HIV/AIDS Dental Reimbursement Program within the Health Resources and Services Administration HIV/AIDS Bureau's Division of Community Based Programs assists with uncompensated costs incurred in providing oral health treatment to individuals with HIV.

HIV/AIDS surveillance data

The CDC tracks the progression of HIV/AIDS, the behaviors that place people at risk, HIV-related knowledge, and testing behaviors in an effort to provide communities with the most complete and timely information possible about ongoing and emerging trends. More information on surveillance is available at http://www.cdc.gov/hiv/surveillance.htm.

Ho, David

Head of the Aaron Diamond AIDS Research Center in New York City, Ho received the *Time* magazine Man of the Year for AIDS award in 2000 for discovering protease inhibitors. Protease inhibitors work by disabling the protease enzyme necessary for viral replication of HIV in AIDS. Ho also established that the use of multiple antiviral agents at early stages of AIDS can prolong life.

Hoffman, Erich (1868–1959)

A scientist specializing in the study of syphilis, Hoffman, along with Fritz Schaudinn, isolated and identified *Treponema pallidum* as the infectious agent of syphilis in 1905.

Homosexual

Homosexual is a term of, relating to, or characterized by a tendency to direct sexual desire toward individuals of one's own sex. *See also* **Lesbians** and **Men who have sex with men (MSM)**.

Housing Opportunities for People with AIDS (HOPWA)

Housing Opportunities for People with AIDS is a program administered by the U.S. Department of Housing and Urban Development (HUD) that provides funding to support housing and related services for low income persons with HIV/AIDS and their families. Since 1992, HOPWA has assisted thousands of individuals who face severe challenges in meeting personal, medical, and housing costs during their illness with assistance to avoid homelessness and with access to medical and other care. HOPWA is the only federal housing program that provides comprehensive, community-based housing for people with HIV. Funding for HOPWA is approximately $258 million a year and provides services to 105 jurisdictions in 34 states.

HOPWA funds are awarded as grants from one of three programs: the HOPWA Formula Program, the HOPWA Competitive Program, and HOPWA National Technical Assistance. Through the formula program, HUD distributes 90 percent of HOPWA funding directly to cities and states with high AIDS caseloads. Caseload data is based on AIDS surveillance information from the Centers for Disease Control and Prevention (CDC), for cumulative AIDS cases and area incidence. Cities with a population of more than 500,000 and at least 1,500 cumulative cases are eligible for the formula grants. States with more than 1,500 cumulative AIDS cases (in areas outside cities eligible to receive HOPWA funds) are also eligible for formula grants. One-quarter of the formula funds are awarded to metropolitan areas that have a higher than average per capita incidence of AIDS.

Ten percent of HOPWA funding is available on a competitive basis to projects of national significance in areas that do not receive formula funds. Technical assistance funds are awarded to HOPWA grants project sponsors to strengthen their operations and managements. This ultimately benefits patented HOPWA applicants.

Communities may use HOPWA funds to develop a broad range of housing, including emergency shelter, shared housing, apartments, single room occupancy (SROs), group homes, and housing combined with supportive services. Grantees may also use HOPWA funds for a variety of housing-related expenses, supportive services, and

program development costs, such as housing information and resource identification; purchase, rehabilitation, conversion, lease and rental housing; new construction for SROs and community residences; meeting mortgage and utility payments; operating costs; technical assistance; administrative expenses; and supportive services (such as health care, health services, chemical dependency treatment, nutritional services, case management, and help with daily living). Each household receiving rental assistance or living in housing funded under the program pays rent in the amount of 30 percent of its adjusted income.

As the number of HIV/AIDS cases continues to grow, the number of jurisdictions eligible for HOPWA funding grows as well. Each year, new jurisdictions become eligible for formula grants based on caseload increases.

For more information on the HOPWA competition, see Housing Opportunities for Persons with Aids (HOPRA) http://www.hud.gov/progdesc/hopwaa.cfm and HIV/AIDS Housing at http://www.hud.gov/offices/cpd/aidshousing/.

HTLV-1 *see* Human T-cell lymphotropic virus-I

HTLV-II *see* Human T-cell lymphotropic virus-II

HTLV-III *see* Human T-cell lymphotropic virus-III

Human Growth Hormone (HGH)

Human growth hormone is a peptide hormone secreted by the anterior pituitary gland in the brain. HGH enhances tissue growth by stimulating protein formation. A recombinant (genetically engineered) form of HGH, called Serostim, has been approved by the FDA as a treatment for AIDS wasting syndrome.

Human herpesvirus-8 (HHV-8)

The human herpes virus-8, which was first discovered in 1994, is considered the etiologic agent in Kaposi's sarcoma (KS). HHV-8 is also known as KS-associated herpesvirus. Recent studies show HHV-8 to be a gamma-2 sublineage of the Gamma-herpesvirinae subfamily, making HHV-8 the first human gamma-2 herpesvirus to be identified. This species has a particular affinity for human lymphocytes.

Human herpesviruses of the first six subtypes are commonly seen in man, but the prevalence of HHV-8 is not as well known. Studies show that HHV-8 may be found in up to 25 percent of the normal population, although it is only associated with disease in patients with Kaposi's sarcoma and in a subset of AIDS-related cases of non–Hodgkin's lymphomas, including body cavity lymphoma, Castleman's disease, and primary effusion lymphoma. KS only occurs in people with severely damaged immune systems, including persons with advanced AIDS and persons on immunosuppressant medications. Data from the Multicenter AIDS Cohort Study also show that individuals infected with HHV-8 did not develop KS until they were also infected with HIV.

Serological tests for antibodies to HHV-8 cannot differentiate active from past infection or exposure. Many studies suggest that HHV-8 is a sexually transmitted virus. A study from the University of Washington showed that HHV-8 is spread through saliva, and that deep-kissing was linked to HHV-8 infection. *See also* **Body cavity lymphoma; Kaposi's sarcoma;** and **Primary effusion lymphoma.**

Seattle Treatment Education Project, Epidemiology of HHV-8. University of Washington Virology Research Center. Seattle, 2002.

Human herpesviruses

The human herpesviruses, including the Epstein-Barr virus, are commonly found in humans, with nearly all people infected by early childhood with one of the first six human herpesviruses discovered (HHV1-HHV-6). Herpes simplex 1 and 2 represent the first two alpha herpesviruses discovered. They are also known as HHV-1 and HHV-2. Varicella-zoster, which causes chicken pox, is HHV-3. Epstein-Barr Virus (EBV) is also known as HHV-4, and human cytomegalovirus is also known as HHV-5. Both HHV-6 and HHV-7 appear to be widely spread through the population and are both related to the skin rash exanthema subitum. HHV-7 is also associated with roseola and is known to cause febrile illness in infants.

The prevalence of HHV-8, discovered in 1994, is unknown. HHV-8 is associated with Kaposi's sarcoma and other non–Hodgkin's lymphomas in patients who are severely immune suppressed. *See also* **Cytomegalovirus; Epstein-Barr virus; Herpesviruses;** and **Human herpesvirus-8.**

Human immunodeficiency virus (HIV)

The Human immunodeficiency virus is the infectious agent in AIDS. HIV, including HIV-1 and HIV-2, represents a specific class of retroviruses that impairs immune system function because of its predilection to destroy human lymphocytes. HIV is a lentivirus or lentoretrovirus belonging to the family of retroviruses. Originally called LAV by its discoverers, scientists at the Institut Pasteur, HIV was initially called HTLV-3 by the American scientist Robert Gallo, who mistakenly identified it as a human T-cell leukemia virus. *See also* **Acquired immune deficiency syndrome; HIV blood tests; HIV-1; HIV-2; HIV DNA; HIV RNA; Lentiviruses;** and **Retroviruses.**

Human leukocyte antigens (HLA)

HLA antigens are marker molecules on the surface of white blood cells that identify cells as "self" and prevent the immune system from attacking them. Specific HLA antigens are associated with a propensity to develop certain diseases, particularly autoimmune diseases. HLA antigens also play a role in determining how severely someone will respond to certain foreign antigens.

Human neutrophil proteins 1–3 *see* Alpha defensins

Human papilloma virus (HPV)

The human papillomavirus is responsible for a number of different conditions, including anal warts, genital warts, pre-cervical cancer, and cervical cancer. Studies also suggest that HPVs may play a causative role in cancers of the anus, vulva, vagina, and penis, and some cancers of the oropharynx (the middle part of the throat that includes the soft palate, the base of the tongue, and the tonsils). Written reports of genital and anal warts date back to the first century A.D. The link between these warts and viruses was first discovered in about 1910. However, it was not until the 1970s that the carcinogenic changes attributable to HPV became known.

These viruses are called papillomaviruses because of their ability to cause warts, or papillomas, which are benign (noncancerous) tumors. HPV may also cause no symptoms. In the majority of cases, the virus is present silently in the skin and goes away spontaneously within three to six months. Unlike the Herpes simplex virus, HPV does not persist throughout one's lifetime after infection. Some HPVs, such as HPV-6 and HPV-11, are referred to as low-risk viruses because

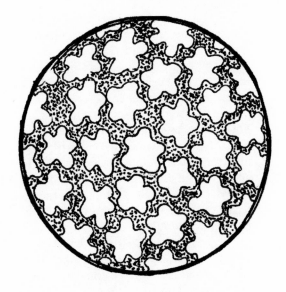

Human papillomavirus (HVP) (Marvin G. Miller).

they rarely lead to cancer. The high-risk viruses for cancer, in descending order of frequency are types 16, 18, 45, 31, 33, 52, 58, 35, 39, 51, 56, 59, 68, 73, and 82, and have been linked with cancer in both men and women. Probably-high risk types include types 26, 53, and 66. These high-risk HPVs cause growths that are usually flat and nearly invisible. Both low and high risk HPVs can cause the growth of abnormal cells, but generally only the high-risk types of HPV may lead to cancer.

Etiology

The etiologic agent is the human papillomavirus, of which there are more than 100 different types or strains. The types are numbered in order from the first identified, with type 1 being the first type identified. Nearly 35 different types of HPV cause genital and anal warts. About 12 different strains are known to cause cervical cancer. Recent studies show that nearly all, if not all, cases of cervical cancer are caused by HPV. HPV has an affinity for squamous epithelial cells, which form most tissue and mucous membranes. HPV infected epithelium has a characteristic prickle cell layer (fish-scale appearance known as acanthosis).

Types suspected of causing anal, penile, vulvar, vaginal, and cervical cancer include types 16, 18, 31, 33, and 35. These types are also found occasionally in visible genital warts, and have been associated with squamous cell carcinoma in situ, bowenoid papulosis, Erythroplasia of Queyrat, or Bowen's Disease of the genitalia. HPV types 6 and 11 have been associated with conjunctival, nasal, oral, and laryngeal warts, and also with visible genital warts and invasive squamous cell carcinoma of the external genitals. Patients with HPV may be infected with multiple strains.

The Los Alamos National Laboratory maintains an HPV sequence database, which contains annotated records for each unique papillomavirus type.

The HPV virus is readily transmitted when warts are present, but it can also be transmitted by people without symptoms, as well as by people who are unaware that they have the virus. HPV may also be transmitted from mother to child during vaginal delivery, in which case the infant may develop warts on the vocal chords that may show up months to years after delivery.

Epidemiology

Readily contagious, HPV infects from one half to two-thirds of sexually active people at some time in their lives. It is considered to be the most rapidly spreading viral STD. About 20 million Americans are infected with HPV and 5.5 million new cases of HPV are reported each year in the United States. A quarter of these infections occur in teenagers.

Symptoms

All warts on the body are caused by HPV. Genital warts, primarily condyloma acuminata, are usually caused by low-risk HPV strains. Strains that cause warts do not cause cancer. Most women with high-risk HPV strains do not develop warts. Instead they develop latent infections, that is, the virus is present within the tissues, but does not cause symptoms. When another illness or stress taxes the immune system, the body may respond to the latent virus, and symptoms may then occur. Latent viral infections can also disappear over time. High-risk types of HPV may cause cervical cell changes, including pre-cancer and cancer. (See the description of cervical precancer below in this entry.)

In women warts may appear on the vulva, in the vagina, or on the cervix. In 66 percent of women, warts appear on the vulvar region, including the vaginal opening (introitus), labia majora, and labia minora. The next most common area in women is the vagina. Women with vulvar warts have an even chance of having the virus in the cervix.

In men, genital warts may appear on the penis and scrotum. In both men and women, warts may also commonly appear on the perineum and in the anal area and in the mouth. Intra-anal warts are predominantly seen in patients who have had receptive anal intercourse. Warts in the perianal area can occur in patients who do not have a history of anal sex. Female partners of men who develop squamous cell carcinoma in situ of the genitalia are at high risk for cervical abnormalities.

Subclinical Genital HPV Infection

Subclinical genital HPV infection is a term often used to refer to manifestations of infection in the absence of genital warts, including situations where infection is detected on the cervix by Pap test, colposcopy, or biopsy; on the penis, vulva, or other genital skin by the appearance of white areas after application of acetic acid; or on any genital skin by a positive test for HPV.

Subclinical genital HPV infection occurs more frequently than visible genital warts among both men and women. Subclinical infection of the cervix is most commonly diagnosed by Pap screening with the detection of squamous intraepithelial lesions. The application of a three to five percent solution of acetic acid usually turns HPV infected genital mucosal tissue a whitish color. Acetic acid application is not a specific test for HPV infection, and this procedure is not recommended, but some experienced clinicians find this test useful for identification of genital warts.

Diagnosis

Warts appear a few days to a few weeks after exposure, although the incubation period is variable, making it sometimes difficult to determine the source of the infection. They start as an irritation or itching, then progress to a red bump that appears irregular and pebbly with pointed ends. Young warts are pale and have the classic pointed surface. As they grow older they arise from skin tissue and take on its pigment. In mucosal surfaces, they appear purple because of their partially visible blood vessel supply. Diagnosis of genital warts can be confirmed by biopsy, although biopsy is only necessary if diagnosis is uncertain, for instance, if patients do not respond to treatment.

The human papillomavirus can be seen in Pap smears, and in urine and respiratory smears where it causes epithelial cells to be enlarged and hyperchromatic with smudgy chromatin, and sharply outlined perinuclear cavitation.

A definitive diagnosis of HPV infection is based on detection of viral nucleic acid (DNA or RNA) or capsid protein, using nucleic acid amplification methods, such as polymerase chain reaction (PCR) tests. Pap-test diagnosis of HPV does not always correlate with detection of HPV DNA in cervical cells, although diagnosis with the Thin-Prep Pap test is more specific. Performed in conjunction with the new High-Risk DNA test, the Thin-Prep is an effective screening tool for HPV infection and cervical cancer risk.

In March 2003, the FDA approved the HC2 High-Risk HPV DNA test manufactured by Digene Corporation for use as an HPV screening test. The HC2 test, which is performed on cells collected from the cervix, can identify 13 of the high-risk types associated with the development of cervical cancer. The HPV DNA test does not test for cancer, but for the presence of HPV viruses that may cause cervical cancer if left untreated. The HC2 test was approved in 2000 for testing women who had abnormal Pap test results.

With the new approval, the HC2 test can be used in conjunction with the Pap test for women over age 30 to screen for HPV infection. It should be used along with the Pap test, a complete medical history, and an evaluation of other risk factors to help physicians determine appropriate follow-up. The HPV DNA test is not intended to substitute for regular Pap screening, nor is it intended to screen women under 30 who have normal Pap tests. Although the rate of HPV infection in the younger age group is high, most infections are short-lived and not associated with cervical cancer.

Treatment

The primary goal of treatment is the removal of symptomatic warts and removal of pre-cancerous tissue related to HPV. Treatment of genital warts includes freezing, chemical treatment, and surgery, which are described in the entries for Condylomata acuminata and genital warts. In most patients, treatment can induce wart-free periods. Untreated, visible genital warts may resolve spontaneously, remain unchanged, or increase in size or number. The CDC reports that no evidence indicates that either the presence of genital warts or their treatment is associated with the development of cervical cancer. Complications include depressed or hypertrophic scars, and rarely disabling chronic pain syndromes. In patients with recurrences, some doctors use interferon alpha as a preventive measure.

Treatment for anal warts includes cryotherapy with liquid nitrogen, surgical removal, or an 80 to 90 percent trichloroacetic acid or bichloroacetic acid application. The acid is applied only to the warts and allowed to dry. A white residue remains. If excess residue remains, the area may powdered with baking soda or talcum power. Liquid soap can also be used to remove excess acid residue. This treatment can be used weekly if needed. Treatment for warts occurring on the rectal mucosa should be managed in consultation with a specialist.

Treatment for oral warts includes cryotherapy with liquid nitrogen or surgical removal. In the absence of squamous intraepithelial cell changes, treatment is not recommended for subclinical genital HPV infection diagnosed by colposcopy, biopsy, or the detection of HPV by laboratory tests. Treatment for cervical precancer associated with HPV is described at the end of this section.

Risk Factors

Factors influencing the development of warts from HIV infection include diabetes and immune suppression related to cancer, HIV infection, lupus, or pregnancy. Other risk factors for developing HPV include age, chronic illness, smoking, antibiotic use, steroids, and the presence of other STDs. Having one to four sexual partners in the last one to four years causes a 12-fold increase in developing HPV and being 20 to 29 years of age causes a fivefold risk of contracting HPV. Having other STDs increases the risk of developing HPV infection.

One's response to HPV depends on one's immune system health. Epidemiological studies have shown that only a small fraction of women infected with high-risk strains of HPV will eventually progress to high grade lesions and cervical cancer. Risk factors for developing high grade lesions include long-term use of oral contraceptives, having more than two children, and smoking. Other risk factors for HPV and cervical cancer include beginning sexual intercourse at an early age (especially age 16 and younger) and having many sexual partners. The CDC recommends avoiding

sex with anyone who has genital sores or unusual growths in the genital area or the anus. Several studies show that some people may also have immune system genes that cause them to be more susceptible to infection with certain strains of HPV.

Women attending STD clinics have five times the risk of developing HPV related cervical cancer than women attending family planning clinics. The cervical Pap test is an effective, low-cost screening test for preventing invasive cervical cancer. Increased risk is seen in women who do not have annual Pap smears, although after three consecutive normal Pap smears, future screening tests may be performed less frequently. Vaccines for HPV-16 and HPV-18 are currently undergoing clinical trials.

Precautions

Condoms, while offering protection, are of limited use in preventing HPV spread, since the condom covers only the penis. The exposed skin of the scrotum can also carry the virus. With new partners, condoms are associated with only a 35 percent reduction in transmission rates. However, the use of latex condoms is associated with a lower rate of cervical cancer. Recurrence of genital warts is likely, usually within the first three months after treatment. Sex partners of individuals with HPV benefit from counseling although treatment for patients without symptoms is not recommended.

Patients with HIV or who are immunosuppressed may not respond as well to therapy for genital warts, and they may have more frequent recurrences after treatment. Squamous cell carcinomas arising in or resembling genital warts may occur more frequently among immunosuppressed persons, thus requiring biopsy for confirmation of diagnosis. Because of the increased incidence of anal cancer in HIV infected homosexual men, screening for anal squamous cell changes is recommended by some experts.

Pregnancy

Common treatments for genital warts including imiquimod, podophyllin, and podofilox should not be used during pregnancy. Because genital warts can proliferate during pregnancy, surgical removal is recommended. HPV types 6 and 11 can cause respiratory papillomatosis in infants and children. The route of transmission (transplacental, perinatal, or postnatal) is not clearly understood. The preventive value of cesarean section is also unknown and not recommended solely to prevent transmission of HPV to the newborn. Cesarean delivery may be indicated for women with genital warts if the pelvic outlet is obstructed or if vaginal delivery would result in excessive bleeding.

Cervical Precancer (CIN)

The cervix is the mouth of the womb, located at the top of the vagina. The cervix is covered by squamous epithelial cells and it is lined by mucus-producing cells called columnar epithelial cells. These outer and inner layers of tissue meet at the squamocolumnar junction (SCJ). The cells at the SCJ are highly influenced by estrogen levels and are constantly changing. This constant change makes these cells susceptible to invasion by HPV. In this area, CIN (also known as dysplasia) and cancer are most likely to develop.

The location of the SCJ also changes its location on the cervix at different times and enlarges during pregnancy. When HPV attacks these cells it deactivates certain proteins that control cell division. This is the initial step in the development of cervical pre-cancer. Only a minority of women develop CIN that persists. CIN may progress to cervical cancer or it may go away on its own without treatment. These abnormal cells are seen on Pap smears, and on the thin-layer Pap test, the DNA of HPV can also be detected.

Diagnosis can be made using the Pap smear, colposcopy and biopsy. There are 3 grades of CIN. Grade 1 indicates that precancerous cells are seen only in the outer one-third of the epithelium. The lesion is called CIN 1 (mild). If the cells reach to the middle third of the epithelial, the lesion is called CIN 2 (moderate). If the cells involve the entire thickness of the cervical epithelial layer, the lesion is called CIN 3 (severe). CIN 3 is also referred to as *carcinoma in situ*. Studies of patients with mild cervical dysplasia over the years show that these cells returned to normal in 62 percent of cases. Today, however, most cases of CIN related to HPV are treated to prevent progression to cervical cancer.

In the Bethesda System used to grade Pap tests in the United States, precancerous conditions are divided into low-grade and high-grade squamous intraepithelial lesions (SILs). Squamous cells are thin, flat cells that cover internal and external surfaces of the body, including the tissue that forms the surface of the skin, the lining of the hollow organs of the body, and the passages of the genital, respiratory, and digestive tracts.

Some systems refer to abnormal cell changes by using the terms ASCUS, HSIL, ASC-H, and LSIL. ASCUS stands for atypical squamous cells of undetermined significance. HSIL stands for high-grade squamous intraepithelial cell lesions. LSIL stands for low-grade squamous intraepithelial cell lesions. ASC-H refers to atypical squamous cells, and cannot exclude HSIL. Patients with ASC-H have a 24–49 percent chance of having HSIL.

Laboratory research at the National Cancer Institute has indicated that HPVs produce proteins known as E5, E6, and E7. These proteins interfere with the cell functions that normally prevent excessive cell growth. For example, HPV E6 interferes with the human protein p53, which normally suppresses tumor growth. Researchers are studying ways to interrupt the process by which HPV affects cell growth and leads to cancer.

Treatment of CIN

Treatment is aimed at destroying abnormal cells in a specific area. This allows for a return of healthy cell growth. Treatments include: surgical removal of tissue, freezing (cryosurgery), laser treatment, and cutting tissue with an electrically wired loop, or loop electrosurgical excision procedure (LEEP).

Cryosurgery, laser therapy, and LEEP all have a success rate of about 90 percent and have few complications. Patients undergoing these treatments have a 10 percent chance that precancerous conditions may return, especially in patients who initially had severe dysplasia (CIN 3).

• CRYOTHERAPY—destroys the top layer of the cervix by turning the water inside cells into ice crystals, destroying the cells. Nitrous oxide or carbon dioxide are used to cool a two-inch metal circle to -196°C for nitrogen and -78.5°C for carbon dioxide. The cold metal probe is placed against the cervix until ice crystals form outside the probe circle. Cryotherapy may cause a fine watery discharge that may persist for 2 to 4 weeks after the procedure.

• LASER TREATMENT—With laser treatment, a laser beam is positioned with the aid of a colposcope so that neighboring tissue is not injured. Laser is particularly effective for excising areas of tissue too large for cryotherapy to treat successfully. Laser therapy can also be used to remove a section of tissue that can be further examined by a pathologist.

• LOOP ELECTROSURGICAL EXCISION PROCEDURE (LEEP)—can be used for both diagnosis and treatment in one visit, eliminating the need for biopsy. A loop of wire with electrical current is used to remove a circle of tissue containing the abnormal cells. The lesion can then be cauterized to prevent bleeding. The procedure is performed under local anesthesia and has a low rate of complications. Recurrence after LEEP is low, ranging from two to four percent. A pathologist can study removed tissue, making this procedure a form of conization, a method that was once used to obtain cervical biopsy specimens. *See also* **Anal intraepithelial neoplasia; Bethesda System; Condyloma acuminata; Genital warts; Pap smear;** and **Squamous intraepithelial lesions.**

Centers for Disease Control. *Sexually Transmitted Diseases Treatment Guidelines 2002.* Atlanta: U.S. Dept. of Health and Human Services, 2002.
Human Papillomaviruses and Cancer, Cancer Facts, National Cancer Institute, Oct. 15, 2002.

Human T-cell lymphotropic virus (HTLV)

The human T-cell lymphotropic virus is a retrovirus. HTLV-I, the first subtype of HTLV discovered, was found to cause disease in humans in 1979. HTLV is a single-stranded RNA virus that replicates by producing complementary cDNA, which is a proviral intermediate, with the help of reverse transcriptase, a viral enzyme. HTLV is found throughout the world, with prevalence and subtype varying significantly in different geographic regions. HTLV can be transmitted sexually, through parenteral administration of blood and blood products, and through intravenous drug use. In the United States, blood donors are screened for both HTLV-I and HTLV-II to prevent transfusion-related transmission.

HTLV-associated diseases include infective dermatitis, persistent lymphadenopathy, and infant death in children. In adults, associated diseases include: adult T-cell leukemia/lymphoma; myelopathy; infective dermatitis; uveitis; arthritis; infiltrative pneumonitis; invasive cervical cancer; and small cell carcinoma of the lung. *See also* **Adult T-cell leukemia/lymphoma (ATL); Human T-cell lymphotropic virus (types I and II);** and **Tropical spastic paraparesis/HTLV-1 associated myelopathy.**

Human T-cell lymphotropic virus-I (HTLV-I)

The human retrovirus HTLV-1 was first isolated in 1979 from an African-American patient with cutaneous T-cell leukemia. This finding represented the culmination of a lengthy search for human retroviruses. Initially, HTLV-I was only associated etiologically with adult T-cell leukemia/lymphoma (ATL), a disease first described in 1977 in Japan. Other diseases associated with HTLV-I have since been described, including tropical spastic paraparesis/HTLV-I-associated myelopathy (TSP/HAM), infective dermatitis, and various inflammatory syndromes.

Etiology

The etiologic agent in HTLV-I infection is the human retrovirus HTLV-I. Although the precise mechanism for entering host cells is not fully known, HTLV-I primarily targets CD4+ T lymphocyte cells, which is the same target as that of the HIV virus. HTLV-I is transmitted through sexual intercourse, transfusion of blood products, and intravenous drug use. It is known to occur among married couples and commercial sex workers as well as homosexual and bisexual men. There appears to be a lower transmission of the virus from women to men, evidenced by the fact that the prevalence rate is higher in women. HTLV-1 is the only retrovirus known to be the etiologic agent of human cancer. HTLV-1 transforms T-cells in vitro.

Epidemiology

HTLV-1 is distributed at low endemic rates throughout the world, but there are specific populations in which HTLV-I has greater prevalence. Geographic clustering of HTLV-I was first documented in southern Japan and the surrounding villages, where up to 30 percent of the population may be infected. The virus prototype originating in Japan is termed cosmopolitan because it is also found in other parts of the world, including Africa and the Caribbean. HTLV-I is rarely seen in the rest of Asia and is largely absent in mainland China, Taiwan, Korea, and Vietnam. Melanesia, however, has a very high prevalence rate, particularly in New Papua New Guinea. High rates are also seen in Australian aborigines and in some areas of the Solomon Islands as well as Central America and South America. HTLV-I has been found in Caribbean migrants to the United States and the United Kingdom. Blood donors in the United States have rates of HTLV-I/HTLV-II infection of 0.43 per 1,000 donors.

In all areas studied the rate of HTLV-I prevalence begins in adolescence and levels off in males at about age 40 years. In women, the prevalence rate continues to rise with age. This may be a consequence of reactivation of immunologically silent infections combined with continued exposure through sexual contact. Mother-to-child transmission may account for up to 15 percent of all infections. HTLV-I has been found in breast milk, and breast-feeding is thought to account for the majority of mother-to-child infections. Early infection may increase the risk for adult T-cell leukemia.

Symptoms

Symptoms of HTLV-I infection are variable, as are the clinical conditions that may result from HTLV-I infection. HTLV-I infection may cause a condition of infective dermatitis, which primarily occurs in children; adult T-cell leukemia/lymphoma (ATL), a neurological condition of tropical spastic paraparesis/HTLV-I associated myelopathy (HAM/TSP); polymyositis of skeletal muscle; large joint polyarthropathy, an arthritic condition primarily occurring in the elderly; infiltrative pneumonitis; and the autoimmune eye disorder uveitis. Children with infective dermatitis frequently develop staphylococcal and streptococcal infections, and they may go on to develop adult T-cell leukemia/lymphoma in later life.

HTLV-I infection may cause subclinical and clinical immunosuppressive effects that cause susceptibility to certain parasitic and bacterial infections, including

Strongyloides stercoralis and *Mycobacterium tuberculosis*. In Japan, HTLV-I infection has been reported to cause an AIDS-like illness. Co-infection with HTLV-I and HIV-I is associated with shortened survival, although this may be a consequence of increased sexual exposure and the presence of multiple HIV strains. Adult T-cell leukemia/lymphoma and tropical spastic paraparesis are described in separate entries in this book.

Diagnosis

Serology tests are used to diagnose HTLV-I infection. Screening assays, primarily using enzyme-linked immunoabsorbent assay (ELISA) methods, detect HTLV infection. A more specific test, such as polymerase chase reaction (PCR) DNA amplification techniques, are then used to determine the precise subtype (HTLV-I or HTLV-II).

Treatment

Diseases caused by HTLV-I infection are difficult to treat. Consequently, HTLV-I associated disease has a poor prognosis. Despite multiple chemotherapeutic regimens, most patients with ATL die within six months of diagnosis. New therapies using monoclonal antibodies offer promise but are not readily available. HTLV-I diseases associated with inflammation, such as uveitis and HAM/TSP, are generally treated with corticosteroids.

Precautions

The CDC recommends counseling for persons infected with HTLV-I, and it provides guidelines for counseling. These recommendations include measures to limit sexual and maternal-to-infant viral transmission. For seropositive mothers, the CDC recommends limiting breastfeeding to the first three to six months of life. The effectiveness of condoms in preventing HTLV-I infection has not been proven, but condoms are recommended for preventing viral transmission. The blood supply in the United States and Japan is now screened for HTLV-I and HTLV-II. Positive units are discarded.

Risk Factors

Risk factors include unprotected sex, multiple sexual partners, the presence of other STDs, especially syphilis and gonorrhea, and commercial sex work. Intravenous drug use is also a risk factor, although it is more likely to transmit HTLV-II infection. *See also* **Adult T-cell leukemia/lymphoma** and **Tropical spastic paraparesis**.

Cleghorn, Farley, and William Blattner. "Human T-cell Lymphotropic Virus and HTLV Infection." Chapter 19 in *Sexually Transmitted Diseases*. 3rd Edition. Edited by King K. Holmes, et al. New York: McGraw-Hill, 1999.

Human T-cell lymphotropic virus-II (HTLV-II)

HTLV-II, discovered in 1982, was the second human T-cell lymphotropic virus to be discovered. Consequently, much less is known about it, although it has not been unequivocally associated with any human disease. Studies of serum (liquid portion of blood) from known United States drug users from the 1960s have demonstrated the presence of HTLV-II in every sample tested.

The prevalence of HTLV-II is thought to range from 10 to 15 percent of the population. Unusually high rates of seropositivity in older groups of intravenous drug abusers in the United States have been linked to the sharing of injection equipment. Sexual transmission of HTLV-II has been difficult to determine because of the high rate of intravenous drug users present in most epidemiological studies. The diseases caused by HTLV-II are also difficult to ascertain, but case reports suggest that infection may cause degenerative neurologic, hematologic (changes in blood cells), and infectious diseases.

Human T-cell lymphotropic virus III (HTLV-III)

The human T-cell lymphotropic virus or HTLV is a class of retroviruses associated with leukemia and lymphoma in man. Mistakenly thinking that the AIDS virus was an HTLV virus, Robert Gallo gave it the name HTLV-III. Gallo claimed to have isolated HTLV-III from a pooled mix of cells collected from different AIDS patients. It was later discovered that this isolate was contaminated with a strain of LAV, the AIDS virus first isolated by scientists at the Institut Pasteur. While taking credit for discovering the AIDS virus, Gallo used the isolate he called HTLV-III as the basis for the first American AIDS tests manufactured by Abbott Laboratories and other American companies. The virus was later renamed and christened human immunodeficiency virus (HIV).

Hydroxyurea

Hydroxyurea is an inexpensive prescription drug used for the treatment of sickle-cell anemia and some forms of leukemia, which has been used experimentally for the treatment of HIV. Its potential safety and effectiveness for treatment of HIV have not been established, and clinicians should be aware of important safety precautions regarding its use. Hydroxyurea does not have direct antiretroviral activity. However, it inhibits the cellular enzyme ribonucleotide reductase. This results in reduced intracellular levels of deoxynucleoside triphosphates (dNTPs) that are necessary for DNA synthesis. For the most current information about the use of hydroxyurea in HIV treatment regimens, see the "Guidelines for Use of Antiretroviral Agents in HIV-Infected Adults and Adolescents," available at http://www.hivatis.org/.

Glossary of HIV/AIDS-Related Terms. 4th Edition. HIV/AIDS Treatment Information Service, 2001.

Hypergammaglobulinemia

Hypergammaglobulinemia is a condition of abnormally high blood levels of immunoglobulins. Hypergammaglobulinemia is common in HIV infection and also occurs in a number of other diseases.

Hyperglycemia

Hyperglycemia is a condition of high blood glucose, which is often seen in patients with diabetes. Hyperglycemia, new onset diabetes mellitus (type 1 diabetes), diabetic ketoacidosis (high blood ketone levels), and exacerbation of existing diabetes mellitus have all been reported in patients receiving protease inhibitors for treatment of HIV infection.

Hyperlipidemia

Hyperlipidemia is a condition of increased blood lipids (cholesterol and triglycerides). This condition can lead to cardiovascular disease and pancreatitis (inflammation of the pancreas) and may occur as a side effect of HAART therapy. In clinical studies, all protease inhibitors have been shown to cause hyperlipidemia.

Hyperthermia

Hyperthermia is a condition of elevated body temperature. The induction of hyperthermia (with temperatures up to 108°F) has been used as a dangerous experimental treatment for HIV infection on the theory that this temperature kills free HIV and HIV-containing cells. One method for accomplishing this is by passing patient's blood through an external heater. This is called extracorporeal whole body hyperthermia and is not a recommended therapy.

Hypogonadism

Hypogonadism is a deficiency in the secretory activity (hormonal production and secretion) of the ovaries and testes. Prior studies have shown that 45 percent of patients with AIDS and 27 percent of HIV-infected patients without AIDS have subnormal testosterone levels. Testosterone replacement therapy is recommended for men with low or low-normal levels. Testosterone is an anabolic steroid that may restore nitrogen balance and lean body mass in HIV patients with wasting syndrome.

Immune deficiency syndrome

Immune deficiency syndrome is a collective term used to describe a variety of different congenital or acquired conditions that cause diminished immune system function. The immune system has two primary defense mechanisms: the B lymphocyte system of cells that control antibody production or humoral immunity; and the T lymphocyte system that responds to a variety of intracellular organisms causing cellular immunity.

Immune system deficiency can be caused by decreased levels of immunoglobulins, the proteins used in antibody production. Immunoglobulin deficiencies cause diminished antibody production and result in recurrent infections, particularly of the lungs and sinuses. Deficiencies of T cells cause recurrent or persistent infections with opportunistic organisms, including *Pneumocystis jiroveci* and Epstein Barr virus. These infections are uncommon in a normal host, but may be seen in people with diminished numbers of T cells. This may be caused by immunosuppressant medications or infection with the HIV virus.

Diminished numbers of white blood cells known as phagocytes or neutrophils permit recurrent or chronic cutaneous and deep-seated bacterial and fungal infections, including abscesses, pneumonias, and periodontitis. Deficiencies of immune system chemicals known as complement may also cause repeated sinus and pulmonary infections.

Assessment of immune function begins with immunoglobulin levels, complement levels, and a complete blood count. If HIV infection is suspected in children younger than 18 months, tests for HIV antibodies may be falsely negative due to the inability of the immature immune system to produce antibodies efficiently. Tests for HIV RNA are more appropriate.

A clinical history of recurrent opportunistic infections suggests an abnormality in T cell function. A test for delayed-type hypersensitivity (DTH) can be used to evaluate response to recall antigens. The DTH response provides an in vivo window of cell function in response to previously encountered antigens such as tetanus toxins. Failure to respond may reflect T cell dysfunction. In suspected T cell dysfunction, the blood can be tested for T cell levels and cytokine levels. In susceptibility to Mycobacterium avium complex, abnormalities of protein components of specific cytokine receptors may be responsible.

Fleisher, Thomas. "Evaluation of Suspected Immunodeficiency." *Medical Laboratory Observer*, February 2003.

Immune (idiopathic) thrombocytopenic purpura (ITP)

ITP is an autoimmune mediated condition in which the body produces antibodies directed against platelets, a component of blood necessary for normal clotting. ITP is very common in persons infected with HIV.

Immune system

The immune system is a complex network of organs and cells that work together to protect people from infection and cancer. The key players of the immune system are white blood cells known as lymphocytes, which originate in the bone marrow.

Healthy immune systems work efficiently, helping people heal when they encounter infectious agents. The immune system has two primary defense mechanisms: the B lymphocyte system of cells that controls antibody production or humoral immunity; and the T lymphocyte system that responds to a variety of intracellular organisms causing cellular immunity.

White blood cells known as T lymphocytes circulate through the blood watching for foreign particles or antigens, such as bacteria, viruses, pollen, and toxins. When T lymphocytes encounter foreign antigens, they enlist the aid of other white blood cells known as B lymphocytes. The B cells help in producing specific antibodies against these antigens from proteins known as immunoglobulins. Antibodies attack and destroy the specific antigens that caused their production. When the immune system recognizes cancerous cells, cytotoxic T lymphocytes destroy these cells, preventing malignant growth.

The immune system also releases certain chemicals known as cytokines and complement that modulate how severely people react to foreign antigens. These chemicals may also cause symptoms such as fever and inflammation, signs that the immune system is trying to combat infection or injury. *See also* **Lymphocytes**; **B Lymphocytes**.

Immunogen (Remune)

Immunogen, developed by Immune Response Corporation, was one of the first HIV therapeutic vaccines to undergo clinical trials. In May 1999, a data and safety monitoring board ordered an end to clinical trials, stating that the vaccine was seen to produce no discernible effect on either survival or viral load.

Immunosuppression

Immunosuppression (bone marrow suppression) is a condition of immune system suppression caused by decreased numbers of circulating white blood cells. Because white blood cells originate in the bone marrow, immunosuppression is also referred to as bone marrow suppression. Immunosuppression can result as a side effect of various medications, known as immunosuppressant agents (primarily anticancer and antiviral drugs including AZT), and it can be caused by a number of diseases and conditions of immune deficiency. Immunosuppression is characterized by a low white blood cell count, commonly referred to as leukopenia, and decreases in red blood cells and platelets. Such cell reductions can cause anemia, bacterial infections, and spontaneous or excess bleeding.

Infants with STDs

Infants may acquire STDs transmitted in utero or during passage through the birth canal. Specific neonatal infections are discussed in the specific disease entries. *See also* **Pediatric AIDS** and **Pediatric STDs**.

Infection

Infection refers to the condition caused by the establishment of an infective agent in or on a suitable host. Infections generally occur in various stages, including a prodrome stage that occurs soon after exposure to an infectious agent but before overt infection develops.

In overt infections symptoms generally peak, although patients may be asymptomatic, showing no symptoms of infection. Overt infections occur during the primary immune response to the offending microorganisms. In persistent infections, patients exhibit poor specific immunity to the organism and have symptoms of chronic active or inactive microbial infection.

Patients with latent infections are generally symptom-free, with occasional periods of relapsing reactivation. In latent infections, patients have adequate immunity. At this time patients may be carriers. In the carrier state, patients are capable of infecting others even when they do not have symptoms of disease.

Systemic infection refers to poor systemic immunity and the ability of the microorganism to disseminate throughout the body, affecting multiple organs and tissues. Parainfectious syndromes occur as a result of aberrant inflammatory changes directed against microbes and infected tissues. These occur as the immune system tries to fight infection. Postinfection syndromes occur to certain autoimmune responses that may develop as a result of infection, such as Reiter's syndrome and Guillain-Barré syndrome.

Peter, James B. *Use and Interpretation of Tests in Infectious Disease.* 4th Edition. Santa Monica, CA: Specialty Laboratories, 1994.

Infectious agents

Infectious agents are bacteria, viruses, fungi, and related microorganisms that are capable of causing infection in humans.

Infectious diseases

Infectious diseases are diseases that are caused by infectious organisms. Tests used to diagnose infectious diseases include direct cultures from patient exudates or by serological (blood) tests that show the presence of infectious organisms, their DNA particles, or the antigens or antibodies that result from infection with these organisms.

Infectious mononucleosis (mono)

Infectious mononucleosis, or "mono," is also known as "the kissing disease."

Etiology

The primary etiologic agent in mononucleosis is Epstein-Barr virus (EBV). Primary EBV infection in children usually does not cause symptoms. In adolescents and adults, acute EBV infection causes infectious mononucleosis. EBV accounts for about 90 percent of all cases of mononucleosis. Herpesviruses, particularly cytomegalovirus (CMV), can cause infectious mononucleosis in 10 percent of all cases. EBV is generally transmitted through saliva and kissing in adolescents. Infection with CMV is usually initiated by contact of virus with cells of the throat or the genital tract or by transfusion of contaminated blood. EBV is known to infect white blood cells known as B lymphocytes located in the salivary glands.

Epidemiology

Approximately 70–80 percent of all cases occur in individuals between the ages of 15 to 30. Slightly more males than females are affected. Doctors estimate that 50 of every 100,000 Americans develop symptoms of mononucleosis annually, although the rate in college students is reported to be several times higher.

Symptoms

Symptoms generally occur from 2 to 7 weeks after exposure. Symptoms can vary in severity and last from several days to several months. In most cases, however, symptoms disappear within 1–3 weeks.

Early symptoms, which may be vague, include headache, fatigue, chills, puffy eyelids, loss of appetite, pharyngitis, fever, swollen lymph nodes, tonsillitis, difficulty swallowing, and enlarged spleen. Rarely, rash may occur, and the liver may be affected, causing jaundice. CMV infection is likely to cause immune system suppression as evidenced by a low WBC count.

Illness is generally more severe in adults older than 30. In young children, symptoms are generally mild, with sore throat the most frequent complaint.

Diagnosis

The most common test for EBV infection is the rapid slide test (Monospot) that detects heterophile antibody agglutination. The heterophile antibody response is detectable at some point during infectious mononucleosis in approximately 95 percent of non–Asian adolescents and adults, and can be detected for several months after acute infection in some instances. Heterophile antibodies are not specific for EBV but represent a larger antibody group that includes other antibodies similar to EBV.

Enzyme immunoassay (EIA) methods for EBV are more specific, although the test is more expensive and time-consuming. Rapid EIA methods are available but less reliable and are associated with a significant number of false positive results. In the acute phase of the disease, IgM and IgG antibodies are produced against EBV early antigens (EA), followed by viral capsid antigens (VCA) and nuclear antigens (EBNA). Thus, either the presence of IGM VCA antibodies or IgM/IgG EA antibodies with low or absent EBNA antibodies is indicative of current or recent infection. Assaying for these antibodies is also helpful in distinguishing patients with reactivation or latent infection from recent infection. Viral cultures of throat swabs can be used to diagnose CMV infection.

Treatment

Infectious mononucleosis is usually self-limited and does not entail recommended specific therapy. Treatment is generally palliative and directed at relieving symptoms such as sore throat. Ibuprofen is often recommended to reduce fever, chills, headache, and muscle pain. Treatment with high doses of the antiviral agent acylovir stops viral replication in infected cells but does not reduce symptoms. Corticosteroids are helpful in reducing symptoms, but because of potential side effects they are only used in extreme situations. Antibiotics have no effect on viral infections and should not be prescribed, unless a co-existing infection, such as a streptococcal throat infection, develops.

Infertility

Infertility is a condition characterized by the inability to reproduce. Infertility can be caused by infection with a number of STDs, such as Chlamydia, that cause pelvic inflammatory disease or urethritis.

Informed consent

Informed consent refers to the permission granted by a participant in a research study or before certain treatments and diagnostic procedures after receiving comprehensive information regarding the study, treatment, or procedure. This is a signed statement of trust between the institution providing the service and the person who is receiving the service or participating in the study.

Injecting drug use *see* Intravenous drug use

Institut Pasteur

The Institut Pasteur in Paris is the premier scientific research institute in France. Named in honor of Louis Pasteur, the top floor houses Pasteur's original living quarters.

In January 1983, the Pasteur scientist Francoise Barré detected a new human retrovirus called LAV, and later renamed HIV, in cultured blood cells from a patient with symptoms of AIDS. The patient, Frédéric Brugière, was described in an early *Science* article as a homosexual with more than 50 partners per year. Brugière traveled in many countries, including North Africa, Greece, and India, and had been known to visit New York City in 1979. LAV suspensions were subsequently isolated from two other French patients. The scientists Luc Montagnier, Jean-Claude Chermann, Francoise Brun, and Willy Rozenbaum were part of the team responsible for identifying LAV as the AIDS virus.

The American researcher Robert Gallo,

after contaminating a cell suspension with LAV provided by the Institut Pasteur for research purposes, renamed the isolate and tried to take credit for the discovery of the virus, later named HIV. The contributions of the French were not recognized until 1987, when they were allowed to share in the royalties of American HIV tests. In 1994, agreeing to cede the French some $6 million in future patent royalties, the U.S. Department of Health & Human Services (HHS) formally recognized the Pasteur as having first discovered HIV. In 1994 HHS also acknowledged that a virus provided by the Institut Pasteur was used by National Institute of Health scientists and used in the American HIV test manufactured in 1984.

Institute of Medicine

The Institute of Medicine of the National Academy of Sciences was founded in 1970 as a nonprofit agency that offers science-based advice on matters of biomedical science, medicine, and health. The institute provides a public service by working outside the framework of government to ensure scientifically informed analysis and independent guidance.

Integrase

Integrase is an enzyme that plays a vital role in the process of HIV infection. Integrase is essential for inserting HIV genes into a host cell's normal DNA. Integrase operates after reverse transcriptase has created a DNA version of the RNA form of HIV genes present in virus particles. Substances that inhibit integrase are being studied as potential therapies for HIV infection.

Interferon (IFN)

Interferon is one of the immune system antiviral proteins known as cytokines that helps modulate the immune response. Interferon-alpha is released during the immune response by virally infected cells, which strengthen the defenses of neighboring cells. Interferon interferes with the ability of viruses to multiply. A manufactured version of IFN-alpha (IFN-α) is an FDA-approved treatment for Kaposi's sarcoma, hepatitis B and hepatitis C. Brand names include Roferon and Intron A.

Interferon gamma is a cytokine synthesized by immune system cells (natural killer or NK cells and CD4 cells). IFN gamma activates macrophages and helps orient the immune system to a mode that promotes cellular immunity.

Interleukins

Interleukins compose a large group of glycoproteins that acts as cytokines. Interleukins are secreted by and affect many different immune system cells.

Interleukin-2 (IL-2)

IL-2 is an immune system chemical known as a cytokine, which is produced during the immune response.

International travel

The increased incidence of international travel in the last several decades has contributed to the spread of many STDs that were once endemic to only certain areas. International travel also contributed to the rapid spread of global AIDS and the current pandemic.

Intravenous drug use

Some infectious agents responsible for STDs are blood-borne, that is, they are transmitted through blood. Intravenous drug use is a significant cause of blood-borne infection. Up to 60 percent of all cases of hepatitis C and 36 percent of all cases of HIV/AIDS are caused by intravenous drug use. Up to 75 percent of all HIV/AIDS in women can be related to intravenous drug use. Other STDs that can be transmitted by intravenous drug use include gonorrhea, hepatitis A, hepatitis B, HTLV-II, cytomegalovirus, and syphilis.

The CDC, in its 1998 guidelines for treatment of sexually transmitted diseases, recommends that intravenous drug users 1) enroll or continue on drug-treatment programs; 2) never share injection equipment (needles and syringes) that has been used by another person; 3) obtain clean needles if they're available in the community (drug paraphernalia laws vary in different states); 4) and disinfect needles and syringes with bleach and water if equipment is shared. This does not sterilize the equipment or guarantee that HIV is inactivated. However, for intravenous drug users, thoroughly and consistently cleaning injection equipment with bleach should reduce the rate of HIV transmission when equipment is shared.

Isolate

An isolate refers to a virus that has been isolated or extracted from an infected cell in laboratory studies by transmission to a previously uninfected cell. Isolated and transmitted to a distinct cell line, the viral isolate can be studied and used for the production of antibodies used in diagnostic tests. Isolates are also used in the production of vaccines.

Isolates also refer to the growth of pure bacterial or viral strains that have been taken from patient exudates or body fluids, inoculated onto culture media, and successfully grown. These isolates can be further studied to show their various identifying properties and to demonstrate resistance or susceptibility to various antimicrobial agents. *See also* **Culture and sensitivity.**

Isosporiosis

Isosporiosis is a rare intestinal infection similar to crytosporidiosis that is caused by the protozoan parasite *Isospora belli.* Protozoa represent a class of single-cell or-

ganisms that includes ameoeba, trypanasomes, paramecium, and sporozoans. Isopora is a sporozoan protozoa. Isosporiosis develops in individuals with suppressed immune systems and is considered an AIDS-defining illness. An enteric disorder, isosporiosis is endemic in Central and South America, Southeast Asia, and Africa in both healthy and immunocompromised individuals.

In the United States, *I. Belli* infection has been reported in less than 0.5 percent of AIDS patients. In Africa and Haiti isosporiosis is seen in 15 percent of patients with AIDS. The generalized use of prophylactic trimethoprim-sulfamethoxazole for *P. jiroveci* pneumonia has led to a large decrease in the prevalence of this disease. Specific treatment includes a regimen employing both trimethoprim and sulfamethoxazole. Pyrimethamine is used in patients who cannot tolerate sulfa medication.

Joint United Nations Programme on HIV/AIDS (UNAIDS) *see* UNAIDS

Kaposi's sarcoma (KS)

Kaposi's sarcoma is a vascular neoplasm or tumor of uncertain tissue origin occurring primarily in patients infected with the HIV virus. Kaposi's sarcoma also occurs in uninfected persons, especially patients who are immunosuppressed. KS primarily affects skin and mucosa and less commonly lymph nodes, lungs, and the gastrointestinal tract.

KS was originally described by Moritz Kaposi in 1872. Patients with KS, at that time primarily men older than 40, developed cutaneous red-blue skin nodules on their extremities. The name Kaposi's sarcoma, however, did not come into use until 1912. The precise classification of KS remains controversial, with the cell of origin primarily recognized as vascular.

Etiology

Epidemiologic studies show that the human herpesvirus 8 (HHV-8) is the etiologic agent of KS.

Epidemiology

Traditionally, KS primarily occurred as skin lesions, although approximately 10 to 20 percent of patients, mostly older men of Mediterranean and Jewish origin, developed a more aggressive form of KS with internal organ involvement. Since the emergence of AIDS, higher proportions of KS patients with internal organ development have been described in Uganda. Among African children, the aggressive form of KS is usually seen. KS primarily occurs in homosexual males who contracted HIV through sexual contact in contrast to patients who contracted HIV as a result of blood transfusion. This led researchers to speculate that a sexually transmitted infectious agent caused KS.

In industrialized countries, KS is over 2000 times more common in people who have HIV infection than in the general populations. KS develops in up to 21 percent of patients with AIDS. At highest risk are homosexual or bisexual men, whereas intravenous drug use is associated with a lower risk

Symptoms

Kaposi's sarcoma associated with HIV infection, with a disseminated pattern involving internal organs, is primarily seen in the United States. KS typically appears as pink or purple to dark brown painless spots, plaques, tumors, or nodules on the surface of the skin or oral cavity. However, lesions may be itchy, painful, disfiguring, or interfere with local function, and they may be dark purple or hyper-pigmented in patients with darker skin. Other symptoms include lymphedema (edema or swelling due to poor lymphatic drainage), particularly of the face, genitalia, and lower extremities. The lymphedema may be out of proportion to the skin disease and may also be related to the release of other immune system chemicals such as cytokines.

KS can also occur internally, especially in the intestines, lymph nodes, and lungs. Pulmonary involvement is life-threatening. KS may spread and also attack the eyes. Symptoms can be very mild to severe. Oral cavity KS occurs in approximately 35 percent of patients and is the initial site of disease in about 15 percent of patients. Lesions typically affect the roof of the mouth and gums. More than 50 percent of patients with skin disease also have gastrointestinal (GI) lesions, particularly affecting the stomach and duodenum. GI lesions rarely cause symptoms, although they may cause bowel malabsorption or obstruction, and, rarely, bleeding. Pulmonary involvement is also common. In 20 percent of cases, pulmonary lesions may occur in the absence of skin lesions. Symptoms of pulmonary involvement include shortness of breath, fever, cough, blood-tinged vomiting, and chest pain.

Diagnosis

Diagnosis is generally confirmed by skin biopsy. Tissue studies show atypical spindle-shaped KS cells. A number of studies have demonstrated that the HHV-8 virus and also HIV-*tat* genetic material can be found in KS lesions. HHV-8 has also been demonstrated in saliva and nasal secretions and in the cells of healthy blood donors, suggesting that transmission through blood products may be possible.

Treatment

No specific therapy has been shown to cure KS or prolong survival. However, the results of two randomized clinical trials indicated that the choice of chemotherapy is doxorubicin-based regimens, including doxorubicin with bleomycin and vinblastine. Preliminary evidence suggests that the KS cell line can be inhibited by human intra-lesional injections of chorionic gonadotropin (hCG), a hormone that rises in pregnancy. Other therapies used include vinblastine, vincristine, idarubicin, angiostatic drugs such as pentosan polysulfite, taxol, and retinoic agents. Corticosteroid therapy induces the development of KS and worsens pre-existing KS lesions. The antiretroviral agents didanosine and zalcitabine are beneficial and do not cause myelocyte (white blood cells of the granulocytic line) cell suppression.

KOH prep

The KOH prep is a laboratory test used for the detection of yeast and other fungal elements. The test is performed on skin or vaginal scrapings, although specimens from genital discharges may also be tested.

Laboratory tests

Laboratory tests are used to diagnose STDs and in some cases to monitor therapeutic response. Most tests for STDs include culture techniques to identify the causative organisms of disease or antibody tests, which determine exposure to specific tests. Tests employing nucleic acid amplification (NAT) techniques are also used to detect the presence of DNA specific for infectious organisms.

In patients on retroviral therapy, HIV viral load or quantitative HIV-1 RNA is measured to see if the therapy is effective. CD4+ T cell counts are used to monitor signs of immune system recovery. Some diseases and also some drugs used to treat STDs can also affect other organs. In these cases, blood tests are used to monitor the function of various organs. For instance, liver enzymes are often tested, with higher concentrations of liver enzymes indicating more severe liver disease.

LAI

LAI, which is also known as IIIB or LAV (lymphadenopathy-associated virus), is an

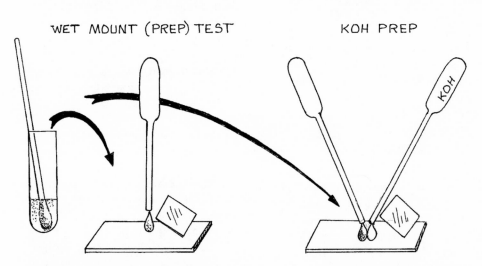

WET MOUNT (PREP) TEST   KOH PREP

① USING A COTTON-TIPPED SWAB COLLECT A VAGINAL SECRETION OR A URETHRAL DISCHARGE.

② PLACE SWAB IN A STERILE TEST TUBE CONTAINING 0.5 mL OF NORMAL SALINE.

③ EXAMINE SPECIMEN IMMEDIATELY UNDER A MICROSCOPE.

ONE DROP OF SUSPENDED SPECIMEN IS ADDED TO ONE DROP OF 10% KOH

EXAMINE SPECIMEN IMMEDIATELY

KOH HELPS TO DIFFERENTIATE BETWEEN YEAST AND RED BLOOD CELLS.

Wet mount and KOH prep tests (Marvin G. Miller).

HIV-1 isolate used in HIV vaccine development. LAI belongs to clade B, the clade from which most HIV-1 found in the U.S. and Europe belongs.

Lamivudine (Epivir, 3TC)

Lamivudine is a nucleoside analog reverse transcriptase inhibitor drug with fewer toxic side effects than other drugs of its class. 3TC has been approved in combination with AZT for the treatment of progressive HIV disease. The use of suboptimal or inappropriately low doses of lamivudine results in the fast development of HIV strains with resistance to lamivudine. This can occur within two weeks of failed therapy.

Laryngeal papilloma *see* Human papillomavirus (HPV)

LAV

LAV or lymphadenopathy-associated virus was the name first given to the AIDS virus by its discoverers, scientists at the Institut Pasteur in Paris. The name of the AIDS virus was later changed to HIV, human immunodeficiency virus.

Lee, Jong Wook, MD

Appointed in 2003, Dr. Jong Wook Lee of South Korea heads the World Health Organization (WHO). The former head of the United Nations' Stop Tuberculosis Program, Lee's focus is on reducing AIDS and epidemics of infectious disease related to poverty and inequalities in medical services for the poor.

Legal issues

The legal system plays an important role in STD prevention. State laws regulate and often fund STD screening, treatment, and prevention programs, and determine which STDs are reportable. State laws also govern partner notification programs, and determine if the willful transmission of certain STDs is a criminal offense. State laws are also responsible for funding of syringe exchange programs and for preventive services available to prison inmates.

Laws also protect the rights of people with disabilities and sickness to work and to receive health benefits and insurance. The organization Lambda Legal provides services to people with HIV/AIDS and to people who are gay. For more information see www.lambdalegal.org.

Lentiviruses

Lentiviruses (slow viruses) are a subtype of the retrovirus family. Usually occurring in animals, HIV is the only lentivirus known to affect humans. Lentiviruses typically take years to cause symptoms of disease. Rather than causing cancer, the outcome of most retroviruses, lentiviruses cause a chronic infection with a long incubation followed by chronic immunosuppression or central nervous system disease.

Animal lentiviruses include Visna virus, which infects sheep; equine infectious anemia virus, which infects horses; simian immunodeficiency virus (SIV) that infects non-human primates; and caprine arthritis-encephalitis virus, which infects goats. The discovery of HIV-1 in 1983 was followed by the discovery of SIV, feline lentivirus (FIV), and a second bovine lentivirus (Jembrana disease virus). Animal lentiviruses cause a spectrum of symptoms ranging from mild infection to frank immunodeficiency. As in HIV infection, the response to lentivirus infections varies among individual hosts. The young of all species, including humans, are more prone to lentiviral disease, and often manifest degrees of disease that do not occur in adults.

The lentivirus is exclusively transmitted via body fluids. Lentiviral infections are generally characterized by an initial period of intense viral replication, which may cause acute disease. This phase is generally followed by viral persistence, with the possibility of organ-specific disease in the area of viral replication, usually followed by chronic or late disease. All lentiviruses can affect the function of neurons, the primary cells of the brain, causing neurological symptoms. Lentiviral infection is often associated with abnormal blood cell counts. In HIV infection, these abnormalities may result in severe clinical disease. The lungs and gastrointestinal system are also frequently affected by lentiviral infection.

Lesbians *see* Women who have sex with women

Lesions

Lesions are abnormal structural changes in organs or tissues due to injury or disease. Lesions may occur in the form of raised or flat papules or nodules or as open sores.

Leukopenia

Leukopenia is a condition in which the number of leukocytes (white blood cells) circulating in the blood is abnormally low. Leukopenia usually results from a decreased production of new cells (bone marrow suppression) in conjunction with various infectious diseases, as a reaction to various drugs or other chemicals, or in response to irradiation.

Lifestyle factors

Lifestyle factors play an important role in both susceptibility to infection and the healing process. Intravenous drug use, unprotected sex, cigarette smoking, multiple sex partners, the use of recreational drugs, and inadequate diets all have detrimental effects on immune system health and add to the risk of developing infectious disease.

Lipoatrophy

Lipoatrophy is a condition of facial wasting related to subcutaneous fat loss in the cheeks and temples resulting in a bony or emaciated facial appearance. Lipoatrophy can be mild or severe and occurs as a consequence of treatment, affecting 20 to 40 percent of all people on antiretroviral drug therapy. People with facial wasting have reported psychological disturbances related to their changed appearance, including depression, anxiety, social isolation, reduced confidence and self-worth, and lack of sexual interest. Depression, which is common in HIV infection, may be severely increased as a result of lipoatrophy. Changes in appearance may also contribute to stress and anxiety and make it difficult to protect HIV status confidentiality.

The psychological distress related to lipoatrophy may have a negative impact on adherence to drug therapy. Several studies show NRTIs, and d4T (Zerit) in particular, are likely to involve higher rates of facial wasting.

Biotech Industry S.A., a pharmaceutical company in Luxembourg, is reported to market a product made from polyacetic acid (New-Fill) to correct lipoatrophy. Applied topically, it has long been used in reconstructive surgery and as an ingredient in surgical sutures. Although not yet FDA-approved in the United States, it has been approved in Europe for aesthetic correction of scars and wrinkles. New-Fill was also approved in Mexico in 2000.More information on New-Fill can be obtained at www.new-fill.com.

Cheonis, Nicholas. "New Fill to Treat Facial Wasting." *Bulletin of Experimental Treatment for AIDS.* Spring 2002.

Lipodystrophy

Lipodystrophy (also known as buffalo hump, protease paunch, pseudo–Cushing's syndrome, or Crixivin potbelly) is a condition of abnormal body fat redistribution that often occurs in HIV/AIDS patients as a result of antiretroviral drug therapy, particularly when protease inhibitors and NRTIs are used. Lipodystrophy manifests itself as fat wasting of the extremities, buttocks, and face (lipoatrophy), or it may cause central fat accumulation, including visceral adiposity, enlargement of breasts (gynecomastia), increased neck circumference, increased fat pads on the upper back (buffalo humps) and deposits of fat on the skin surface known as lipomas.

Lipodystrophy symptoms involve the loss of the thin layer of fat under the skin, making veins seem to protrude. The face and limbs may appear wasted, although accumulates of fat occur on the abdomen, both under the skin and within the abdominal cavity, or between the shoulder pads. Women may develop narrowed hips and enlarged breasts.

Most people with lipodystrophy have accompanying disorders of glucose and lipid metabolism. People with facial wasting and other forms of lipodystrophy have reported psychological disturbances related to their changed appearance, including depression, anxiety, social isolation, reduced confidence and self-worth, and lack of sexual interest.

In an article in the *Journal of Acquired Immune Deficiency Syndromes*, Dr. Marie Gelato of the State University of New York at Stony Brook reports that a diabetes drug that boosts insulin sensitivity, rosiglitazone (Avandia), might also be helpful to HIV patients with insulin resistance and lipodystrophy. Very small limited trials with eight HIV-positive patients showed an improvement in insulin resistance in many of the patients and benefits to lipodystrophy in that patients showed an increase in peripheral fat and a decrease in visceral fat. *See also* **Lipoatrophy**.

Gelato, M.C., et al. "Improved Insulin Sensitivity and Body Fat Distribution in HIV-Infected Patients Treated with Rosiglitazone: A Pilot Study." *Journal of Acquired Immune Deficiency Syndromes*, Oct. 1, 2002, 31(2):163–170.

Liver disease

Liver diseases are conditions in which the hepatic liver cells or components of the biliary transport system are injured. Individuals infected with HIV-1, the causative agent of AIDS, or hepatitis B virus (HBV) are at increased risk of death from liver disease. Individuals infected with both viruses are at highest risk.

In one study reported in *The Lancet* in 2002, the liver mortality rate was 1.1/1,000 (person-years) and was higher among men with HIV-1 and hepatitis B (14.2/1,000) than among those with one disorder. Among co-infected individuals, liver-related mortality was highest with lower nadir (point of lowest level) CD4-plus counts, and rose twice as high after 1996, when antiretroviral combined therapy (HAART) was introduced. Researchers concluded that individuals co-infected with both HIV and HBV with low DC4-plus nadir counts are at increased risk for liver-related mortality.

Los Alamos National Laboratory (LANL)

The LANL in New Mexico maintains an STD database containing the nucleotide sequence for most responsible organisms.

Lymphadenopathy syndrome

The condition of lymphadenopathy syndrome is a precursor to AIDS. This syndrome is also considered a marker for HIV infection. In lymphadenopathy syndrome, the lymph nodes remain enlarged for a period of weeks or months as the immune system makes its initial response to infection with the HIV virus. This syndrome is frequently associated with flu-like symptoms including muscle pain, sore throat, and headache. Lymphadenopathy syndrome was formerly known as AIDS Related Complex or ARC. *See also* Acute Retroviral Syndrome in the entry on **Acquired Immune Deficiency Syndrome**.

Lymphocytes

Lymphocytes are white blood cells that have a mononuclear nucleus. Lymphocytes are the key players of the immune system and work to protect people against infection. There are several different classes of lymphocytes, including T cells, B cells, cytotoxic lymphocytes, natural killer cells, and killer cells. T lymphocyte cells guard the body against infectious and toxic agents, whereas B cells are directly involved in antibody production. There are two primary subtypes of T lymphocytes: CD4+ helper T cells and CD8+ suppressor T cells. *See also* **CD4+ T lymphocytes** and **CD8+ T lymphocytes.**

Lymphogranuloma venereum

Lymphogranuloma venereum is a sexually transmitted disease caused by infection with *Chlamydia trachomatis*, a bacterium that grows within cells. Lymphogranuloma venereum is caused by other strains of Chlamydia trachomatis than those that cause urethritis and cervicitis.

Epidemiology

Lymphogranuloma venereum mostly occurs in tropical and subtropical areas and is uncommon in the United States.

Symptoms

Symptoms typically emerge between three to 12 days after infection. A small, painless, fluid-filled blister develops usually on the penis or in the vagina. The blister usually becomes ulcerated and quickly heals, often without being noticed. After the blister heals, lymph nodes in the groin on one or both sides may become enlarged and tender. The skin covering the infected area usually becomes warm and red. If left untreated, openings (sinuses) may cover the skin covering the lymph nodes. These openings discharge pus or bloody fluid. Although they usually heal, they may leave a

scar and recur. Other symptoms include fever, malaise, headache, joint pain, loss of appetite, vomiting, back pain, and a rectal infection that results in a discharge of bloody pus.

With prolonged or repeated episodes, the lymphatic vessels may become obstructed, causing tissue to swell. Rectal infection may cause scarring, which may cause a narrowing of the rectum.

Diagnosis

Diagnosis is based on the characteristic symptoms and can be confirmed by a blood test that identifies antibodies against *Chlamydia trachomatis.*

Treatment

Early diagnosis and treatment, such as oral doxycylcine, erythromycin, or tetracycline, used for three weeks, results in rapid healing. After treatment, patients should have a follow-up visit to ensure that the infection has been cured. Sexual partners should be notified so that they can receive treatment.

Lymphoid interstitial pneumonitis (LIP)

LIP is a type of diffuse pneumonia that affects 35 to 40 percent of children with AIDS. LIP, which is considered an AIDS-defining illness in children, causes hardening of the lung membranes involved in absorbing oxygen.

LIP often occurs in conjunction with PHL. PHL is a focal pulmonary disorder related to an infiltration of lymphocytes into lung tissue. PHL-LIP initially causes nodular infiltrates that may progress to an illness characterized by chronic cough and a progressive lowering of blood oxygen level (hypoxemia) that causes a typical clubbing of the fingers similar to what is seen in the initial ascent to high altitudes. PHL has an association with the Epstein-Barr virus (EBV). Children with PHL-LIP frequently show high titers of EBV antigen.

Other symptoms include enlarged lymph nodes and salivary glands. PHL-LIP is associated with a higher survival rate in children compared to that caused by *Pneumocystis jiroveci* infection. Conditions of PHL-LIP are less likely to cause fever and lowered respiration. PHL-LIP often improves with antiretroviral therapy either as a direct result of EBV eradication or from immune system improvement. *See also* **Pulmonary lymphoid hyperplasia.**

Lymphoid organs

Lymphoid organs are sites of increased immune system activity, particularly in the germinal centers, which act as traps for invading organisms. Lymphoid organs include tonsils, adenoids, lymph nodes, spleen, thymus, and other tissues.

Lymphoma

Lymphoma is a cancer of the lymphoid tissues. Lymphomas are often described as being large cell or small cell types, cleaved or non-cleaved, or diffuse or nodular. Different types of lymphoma are associated with different prognoses. Lymphomas are also referred to by the organs where they are active, such as CNS lymphoma, which affects the central nervous system. The lymphomas most often associated with HIV infection are called non–Hodgkin's or B-cell lymphomas. In these types of cancers, certain cells of the lymphatic system grow abnormally, divide rapidly, and grow into tumors. *See also* **Cutaneous lymphoma** and **non–Hodgkin's lymphoma.**

Macrophage-Tropic Virus

The macrophage-tropic viruses are HIV strains that preferentially infect macrophages, rather than T helper cells, in cell culture experiments. These viruses readily fuse with cells that have both CD4 and CCR5 surface molecules, whereas they fail to fuse with cells expressing only CD4. These isolates are the main strains found in patients during the symptom-free stage of HIV disease.

Male reproductive organs

Male reproductive organs function to produce sperm and pass it to the female. This system consists of two testes glands that lie in the scrotum sac outside the body, a sperm duct to transport the sperm, and a penis to transfer sperm into the female.

Maternal-infant transmission

STDs can be transmitted from mother to child during childbirth and through breastfeeding. According to the CDC, the rate of maternal to child HIV transmissions has fallen sharply from 2,500 infections in 1992 to 300–400 infections annually by 2002. Worldwide, maternal-infant transmission

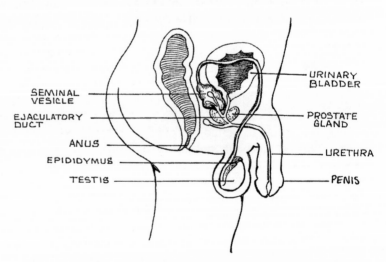

Male reproductive organs (Marvin G. Miller).

accounts for most of the cases of HIV infection in children. *See also* **Pediatric AIDS** and **Pediatric STDS**.

Medicaid *see* Centers for Medicare and Medicaid Services (CMS)

Medicaid Spend-down

Medicaid spend-down is a process whereby an individual who meets the Medicaid medical eligibility criteria but has income exceeding the financial eligibility ceiling may "spend down" to eligibility level. Spend-down is accomplished by deducting accrued medical related expenses from countable income. Most state Medicaid programs offer an optional "medically needy" eligibility category for these individuals.

Medical records

Medical records are the reports of all diagnostic procedures, physical examinations, medication records, and treatment records of patients. By law, patients and their designated caregivers have the right to access medical records. Medical records are protected by medical privacy laws. *See also* **Health Insurance Portability Privacy Act (HIPPA)**.

Medicare *see* Centers for Medicare and Medicaid Services (CMS)

Mega-HAART (multi-drug rescue therapy)

Mega-HAART are salvage or rescue regimens containing six or more antiretroviral drugs for patients who have had previous treatment and drug failure. Patients with multiple antiretroviral drug expo-

sures and failures are unlikely to be infected with virus resistant to all rescue regimen drugs.

Men who have sex with men (MSM)

Some men who have sex with men (MSM) are at high risk for HIV infection and other viral and bacterial STDs. Although the frequency of unsafe sexual practices and reported rates of bacterial STDs and incidental HIV infection has declined substantially in MSM in the last few decades, increased rates of infectious syphilis, gonorrhea, and chlamydial infection in the last few years indicate that the risk of STD development in MSM is still of grave concern. Preliminary surveillance data show the rate for HIV infection among MSM is also rising in some parts of the country, indicating higher frequencies of unsafe sex.

The underlying behavioral changes considered responsible for this rise in STDs are related to effects of improved HIV/AIDS therapy on quality of life and survival, lack of understanding regarding the side effects and failure rate of antiretroviral drug therapy, "safer sex" burnout, and in some cities, adverse trends in substance abuse.

The Centers for Disease Control STD prevention guidelines recommend that MSM should be screened at least annually for HIV serology if they have been HIV negative; they should be screened annually for syphilis. MSM should also be annually screened using a urethral swab or urine for gonorrhea, and chlamydia using sensitive NAT testing methods. In addition, men with oral-genital exposure should have pharyngeal culture for gonorrhea as well as a rectal gonorrhea and chlamydia culture if they have had receptive anal intercourse.

MSM should be vaccinated against hepatitis A and B if they have not been previously vaccinated. Men who are at highest risk (multiple sex partners or having sex in conjunction with illicit drug use or whose sex partners participate in these activities) should have more frequent screening (e.g., at 3–6 month intervals).

Centers for Disease Control and Prevention. *Sexually Transmitted Diseases Treatment Guidelines*, 2002. Atlanta: U.S. Dept. of Health and Human Services, 2002.

Metronidazole (Flagyl)

Metronidazole is an antibiotic used in the treatment of certain STDs, including Trichomonas and bacterial vaginosis. Used orally, metronidazole may cause a slight metallic taste, gastrointestinal disturbances, nausea, and headache. Intravaginal microgels are better tolerated, but are more expensive than oral preparations.

Microbicides

Microbicides are agents (usually chemicals or antibiotics) that destroy microbes. Research is being carried out to evaluate the use of rectal and vaginal microbicides to inhibit the transmission of STDs, including HIV. The main HIV prevention tools (condoms; reducing the number of sexual partners; and treatment of reproductive tract infections), are not feasible for many women worldwide. Women often have limited ability to get their male partners to use condoms due to social, cultural, and economic gender inequalities.

Microbicides in the form of gels, creams, or suppositories have shown promising results in clinical trials. Microbicidal candidates work by either killing or inactivating infectious agents; blocking fusion of the organism to its potential host cell; inhibiting post-fusion activity; and enhancing the natural defense mechanisms of the vagina.

Some of the most promising candidates include Savvy (C31G), which has shown effectiveness in killing HIV and a number of pathogens; Carraguard; topical tenofovir (Viread); and Emmelle. Phase III trials are difficult to conduct because they can only be conducted in developing countries with a high incidence of sexually transmitted HIV and other STDs. *See also* treatment section of the entry for **Acquired immune deficiency syndrome.**

Microsporidiosis

Microsporidiosis is an opportunistic intestinal infection that causes diarrhea and wasting in persons with HIV infection.

Etiology

Microsporidiosis results from several different species of the intracellular protozoal parasite microsporidia, which belong to the *Microspora* family. Five distinct genera have been reported in humans: *Enterocytozoon, Encephalitozoon,* Septata, and smaller occurrences of *Pleistophora* and *Nosema*.

Epidemiology

Microsporidia are obligate protozoans that have been described as infecting every major animal group, especially insects, fish, and mammals. They are important agricultural parasites in commercially important insects, fish, laboratory rodents, rabbits, fur-bearing animals, and primates. Microsporidiosis has recently been seen in increasing numbers in individuals infected with HIV. Infection is thought to occur through ingestion of spores from contaminated food products.

Symptoms

The intestine is by far the most common site of microsporidiosis in HIV infected patients, and 90 percent of cases are caused by *Enterocytozoon bieneusi*. Diarrhea of variable intensity between patients is the most frequent symptom. It may be accompanied by abdominal pain, cramps, and nausea. The liver and gall bladder may also be affected and rarely the urinary tract is affected. *Nosema corneum* and *Encephalitozoon* hellem have been reported in corneal infection or keratoconjunctivitis.

Diagnosis

Diagnosis is made by isolation of the organisms from stool, urine, sinus mucus, and bronchoalveolar lavage. Isolation has replaced biopsy as the initial diagnostic procedure in many laboratories. The specific identification of microsporidian species has classically depended on microscopic examination. PCR techniques as well as staining techniques are available for the identification of microsporidia in biological samples.

Treatment

There is no proven completely effective treatment of *E. bieneusii*, although albendazole, using 400 mg every 12 hours, may decrease the number of bowel movements without clearing the parasite. Fumagilin, used in veterinary medicine, is a potential antiparasitic drug.

Risk factors

In HIV infection, microsporidiosis generally occurs when CD4+ T cell counts fall below 100 cells/mm^3.

Military

Since World War II the U.S. armed forces have made an effort to help protect soldiers from STDs, primarily by distributing condoms, offering hepatitis vaccines, and through education. The military forces report that incidences of HIV had declined by about 30 percent in 2002 primarily as a result of educational programs. Under Defense Department rules, everyone in the military must have at least one hour of HIV education annually. In the mid–1980s, when little was known about HIV, infected people were forced to resign. Since 1990, HIV-positive people are allowed to remain in the military unless they develop AIDS. In a report from Capt. Glenn A. Schnepf of the National Naval Medical Center in Bethesda, MD, of the 900–1,000 persons in the military who are infected with HIV, only 4–8 percent are likely to leave the service because of AIDS. In the United States, the rate of HIV infection in the military is about 10 percent lower than in the general population.

Fields, Helen. "Military sees drop in HIV." *The Monterey Herald,* Nov. 19, 2002.

Minorities

The Institute of Medicine has reported that minorities in the United States receive inferior healthcare and treatment. This leads to poorer health and increased susceptibility to infectious diseases. *See also* **Health Disparities Initiative and Healthy People 2010.**

Minority AIDS Initiative (MAI)

The Minority AIDS Initiative is a national U.S. Department of Health & Human Services initiative that provides special resources to reduce the spread of HIV/AIDS and improve health outcomes for people living with HIV disease within communities of color. The Minority AIDS Initiative was enacted to address the disproportionate impact of HIV in such communities that were formerly referred to as the Congressional Black Caucus Initiative because of the Black community's role in its development.

Minority disparities initiative *see* Health disparities initiative

Mitochondrial Toxicity

Mitochondrial toxicity or dysfunction is a possible side effect of certain anti–HIV drugs, primarily NRTIs, that results in mitochondrial damage. This damage can cause symptoms in the heart, nerves, muscles, pancreas, kidney, and liver, and can cause abnormal results in some laboratory tests. Some of the conditions related to mitochondrial toxicity include myopathy; peripheral neuropathy; pancreatitis; thrombocytopenia (a condition of low platelets, which are blood components needed for clotting); anemia; and neutropenia. Mitochondrial damage can lead to lactic acid accumulation (lactic acidosis) and a condition of fatty liver. It may also contribute to lipodystrophy.

Mobilincus vaginitis

Mobilincus vaginitis is not an STD but it frequently occurs in women under treatment for STDs. Mobilincus occurs when there is overgrowth of bacteria belonging to the *Mobilincus* family. Small amounts of *Mobilincus* species normally inhabit the vagina. Overgrowth causes vaginitis.

Etiology

Mobilincus curtisii and *Mobilincus mulieris* are the cause of mobiluncus vaginitis.

Epidemiology

Mobilincus vaginitis is caused by the use of antibiotics used to treat other infections. Antibiotics including metronidazole used to treat bacterial vaginosis are a common cause.

Symptoms

Symptoms include a profuse white glistening discharge similar to vanilla yogurt. The discharge may be foul-smelling but not irritating and may easily be confused with yeast infection.

Diagnosis

Diagnosis is difficult because Mobilincus are too small to be seen on electron light microscopy, and they are impossible to culture. The pH of the vagina is elevated, and a whiff test is positive. The wet prep examination using a phase contrast lens shows numerous motile curved rods. The absence of normal flora such as lactobacilli suggest mobiluncus in patients treated with antibiotic therapy who are not responding to treatment for other causes of vaginitis.

Treatment

Although Mobilincus species are resistant to metronidazole, they may respond to higher and longer doses. Clindamycin used orally or intravaginally may also be effective. For difficult infections, a week-long course of intravenous ampicillin and gentamicin may be required.

Molluscum contagiosum (MCV)

Molluscum contagiosum is a benign skin condition that may occur as a sexually transmitted skin disease usually causing one or more small raised lesions or bumps. MCV was first described in 1817, and named molluscum for the footed edge of the lesion and contagiosum for the milky or transparent appearance of the lesion, which can express a milky fluid.

Etiology

The infectious agent is the molluscum contagiosum virus, which is considered a member of the poxvirus family.

Epidemiology

Molluscum may be sexually transmitted and spread by skin-to-skin contact or by direct contact with lesions. It may also be transmitted from inanimate objects such as towels and clothing that has been in contact with lesions. MCV transmission has also been associated with swimming pools and sharing baths with an infected person. Because it is often self-limiting, accurate statistics for the number of people infected are not available. Since the 1970s an 11-fold increase of MCV has been reported, and five to 18 percent of patients with HIV are reported to be infected.

Symptoms

Symptoms can occur within one week after exposure although the average incubation is 2–3 months. Lesions usually occur on the exterior surface of the thighs, buttocks, groin, and lower abdomen of adults, and rarely on the external genitals and anal region. Children, who may become infected through casual contact, typically develop lesions on the face, trunk, legs, and arms. MCV lesions typically are waxy flesh colored, gray-white, yellow or pink with a red base, emerging as small bumps, which can develop into larger sores over several weeks. Lesions may cause itching and typically last for two years, although they may resolve within two weeks or persist for as long as four years.

Diagnosis

Diagnosis is usually made by direct examination in which the characteristic pearly appearance of the lesion is diagnostic. A gram stain test will show changes in infected cells. Examining lesion samples with an electron microscope shows that the lesions consist of focal areas of overgrown epithelial cells surrounding cyst-shaped globules, which are filled with small elementary molluscum bodies. MCV may also be seen in gynecological samples or skin scrapings. In cytology studies, molluscum bodies appear as dense, homogeneous, eosinophilic round to oval intracytoplasmic (within the cell cytoplasm) inclusions found in squamous epithelial cells.

Treatment

MCV usually heals spontaneously, but lesions may need to be removed to reduce persistent self-infection and transmission to others. Treatment generally consists of surgical excisional curettage and expression of the lesion core by direct pressure. Lesions can also be treated with podophyllin, canthanridin, phenol, silver nitrate, trichloroacetic acid, or iodine, or with cryotherapy (freezing). Lesions may recur, but it is unclear if this is from a reinfection or from reactivation of a latent infection.

Pregnancy

Infection with MCV does not appear to affect the outcome of pregnancy, and no cases of maternal-fetal transmission have been reported.

Risk Factors

Risk factors include skin-to-skin or sexual contact with an infected person and contact with prostitutes; latex condoms or barriers for anal or oral sex are effective for preventing MCV. Condoms may protect the penis or vagina from infection but do not protect against contact with other areas, such as the scrotum or anal area.

Complications

The most frequent complication of infection is a condition of molluscum dermatitis, which occurs one to five months after the onset of lesions. It is characterized by a sharply bordered patch of eczema about 3–10 centimeters in size, which surrounds an individual lesion. The eczema clears as the lesion heals. When this reaction occurs on the eyelid it may cause conjunctivitis. Corneal changes similar to that of trachoma may also appear. In people with HIV, MCV is often a progressive disease.

Monilia *see* Candidiasis

Mononeuritis multiplex (MM)

MM is a rare type of neuropathy (nerve damage or inflammation) that has been described in patients with HIV infection. It may occur in the early period of the infection, when it has a more benign outcome, or late in infection, when it is more aggressive, leading to progressive paralysis and death in some patients. It has been suggested that MM is related to multifocal cytomegalovirus (CMV) infection.

Mucopurulent cervicitis (MPC)

Mucopurulent cervicitis is a condition of cervical inflammation characterized by a purulent (containing or consisting of pus) or mucopurulent (containing both mucus and pus) discharge visible in the endocervical canal or on an endocervical swab specimen collected during a cervical examination. Some specialists also diagnose MPC on the basis of easily induced cervical bleeding. Patients may be free of symptoms or they may have an abnormal vaginal discharge or vaginal bleeding, particularly bleeding after intercourse.

MPC can be caused by *Chlamydia trachomatis* or *Neisseria gonorrhoeae*, although in most cases neither organism can be isolated. Patients with MPC should be tested for these infectious agents with sensitive NAT testing. Patients with positive results are treated with antibiotics. In patients with negative results but who are suspected of having gonorrhea or chlamydia, antibiotic treatment is also recommended.

Multicenter AIDS Cohort Study (MACS)

The Multicenter AIDS Cohort Study, which was initiated in 1983 through the National Institute of Allergy and Infectious Diseases (NIAID), is an ongoing prospective study of the natural and treated histories of HIV-1 infection in homosexual and bisexual men. MACS studies, which include the effectiveness of the new antiretroviral therapies, are conducted at sites located in Baltimore, Chicago, Pittsburgh, and Los Angeles. Data from MACS is available to scientists and statisticians who study AIDS. For more information and to enroll, see http://www.statepijhsph.edu/macs.html.

Mutations

Mutations are changes that occur in DNA. Mutations occur as changes to the amino acid molecules of DNA. Some viruses, such as polio, do not mutate quickly. This enables researchers to produce effective vaccines that specifically target DNA. The virus influenza A, on the other hand, mutates quickly, and a new vaccine must be produced each year. HIV mutates very quickly. Therefore, an individual infected with the virus does not harbor one, but many, variants of the AIDS virus.

Mycobacterium avium-complex (MAC)

Mycobacterium avium-complex (MAC) is a group of "atypical" mycobacteria that has been identified in severely immunocompromised patients, including patients with AIDS.

Etiology

About 98 percent of the isolates found in MAC are *M. avium* (usually serovars or types 1, 4, and 8) and the remainder include strains of *M. intracellulare*. Because *M. avium* and *M. intracellulare* are difficult to distinguish, they are referred to collectively as MAC. *M. avium* are widely present in the environment and can be isolated from water, soil, dust, and air. They can also be found in sputum or stool specimens from normal individuals. Human-to-human infection has not been reported. Most infections occur from environmental sources. Typical MAC pulmonary infections are indistinguishable from tuberculosis on the basis of clinical presentation.

Epidemiology

MAC occurs in 40 percent of patients with AIDS in North America.

Symptoms

The gastrointestinal tract and lymph nodes are the organs most often affected by MAC, although in AIDS patients, infection is usually disseminated throughout the body. Infections of the intestinal tract usually occur as part of disseminated infection, which presents with fever, night sweats, abdominal pain, watery diarrhea, steatorrhea (fatty stools), and malabsorption of nutrients.

The characteristic findings seen in MAC infection of AIDS patients include severely decreased lymphocyte counts, anemia, reduction of circulating helper-T cells, skin test anergy, and polyclonal hypergammaglobulinemia (increased gamma globulin levels). These findings differentiate MAC from Whipple's disease, a condition that has similar clinical and radiographic features.

Diagnosis

The diagnosis of MAC infection was traditionally based on stool culture and tissue studies of small bowel biopsy specimens. Stool culture is no longer considered specific, since it can represent colonization rather than infection. Diagnosis can also be made from cultures taken from normally sterile sites such as bone marrow, lymph node, or liver. Recently, blood tests for the antibody against the antigenic glycopid G1-ai, which is present in the MAC cell wall, became available. This test is highly sensitive for the diagnosis of MAC disease. Furthermore, high serum IgM titers against G1-ai imply that MAC disease is active. MAC can also be diagnosed with blood tests using non-radiometric DNA probes or nucleic acid amplification techniques.

Treatment

Multi-drug therapy used for life has been found to decrease bacteremia (blood infection) and reduce symptoms. The usual treatment protocol includes a combination of clarithromycin using 500 mg twice daily along with ethambutol, using 15 to 25 mg/kg daily with or without ciprofloxacin, using 750 mg twice daily, and rifabutin, using 300 mg daily. An alternate regimen includes azithromycin, using 500 mg daily, and ethambutol, using 15 to 25 mg/kg daily with or without ciprofloxacin (750 mg twice daily) and rifabutin (300 mg daily). Clofazimine may be used in place of rifabutin and ciprofloxacin in alternate drug protocols.

Rifabatin leads to significant drug interactions because of the way it is metabolized by the liver. It should be used cautiously, with appropriate dose adjustments when used with fluconazole or protease inhibitors, especially ritonavir and indinavir.

Prophylactic treatment for AIDS patients with CD4+ lymphocytes < 50 cells/mm^3 includes clarithromycin, using 500 mg twice daily, azithromycin (1200 mg weekly), or possibly rifabutin (300 mg daily). Prophylactic treatment is used to decrease the frequency of disseminated disease and improve survival. The CDC 2002 treatment guidelines for MAC take HAART therapy into consideration, stating that when CD4+ T cell counts have increased to greater than 200 cells/mm^3 for three months or more, MAC prophylaxis can be discontinued. Prophylactic treatment for disseminated MAC can also be discontinued in patients with CD4+ T cell counts > 100 cells/mm^3 for six months or greater in response to HAART if the patient has completed 12 months of MAC therapy and has no symptoms or signs attributable to MAC.

Risk Factors

The major risk factor for MAC is a severely suppressed immune system, with CD4 lymphocyte counts of 75 cells per cubic millimeter of blood or less, or previous opportunistic infections, especially cytomegalovirus (CMV) disease.

Centers for Disease Control and Prevention. *Guidelines for Preventing Opportunistic Infection among HIV-Infected Persons 2002*. Atlanta: U.S. Dept. of Health and Human Services, 2002.

Mycobacterium tuberculosis
see **Tuberculosis**

Mycoplasma

Mycoplasma are small microorganisms without cell walls that differ from bacteria and viruses. *Mycoplasma genitalis* is reported to be a risk factor for HIV.

Myopathy

Myopathy is a condition of progressive muscle weakness. Myopathy may arise as a toxic reaction to AZT therapy or as a consequence of HIV infection.

NAAT *see* Nucleic acid amplification (NAT, NAAT) tests

NAT *see* Nucleic acid amplification (NAT, NAAT) tests

NAT tests *see* Nucleic acid amplification (NAT, NAAT) tests

National AIDS Hotline

Operated by the U.S. Department of Health and Human Services, this service is available everyday, 24 hours a day. The hotline provides confidential HIV/AIDS information, referrals to hospitals, clinics, testing and counseling sites, legal services, educational and support groups, and service agencies. Information is available in both English (1-800-342-AIDS) and Spanish (1-800-344-7432). More information on the hotline is available at http://www.ashastd.org/nah/.

National Cancer Institute (NCI)

The National Cancer Institute is a division of the National Institutes of Health. The NCI has an extensive virology division and actively studies STDs with viral origins.

National Center for Complementary and Alternative Medicine (NCCAM)

NCCAM is a division of the National Institutes of Health that conducts clinical trials to evaluate the safety and efficacy of specific alternative and complementary medical preparations and procedures used for specific diseases.

National Institute of Allergy and Infectious Diseases (NIAID)

NIAID is a branch of the National Institutes of Health that conducts and supports research to study the causes of allergic, immunologic, and infectious diseases, and to develop better means of preventing, diagnosing, and treating illnesses. NIAID is responsible for the federally funded, national basic research program in AIDS. For more information see http://www.niaid.nih.gov/.

National Institutes of Health (NIH)

The National Institutes of Health is a multi-institute agency of The U.S. Department of Health & Human Services. NIH is the federal focal point for health research. It conducts research in its own laboratories and supports research in universities, medical schools, hospitals, and research institutions throughout the country and abroad. For more information see http://www.nih.gov.

National Plan to Eliminate Syphilis in the United States

In October 1999, the Centers for Disease Control and Prevention (CDC), in collaboration with other federal programs, initiated this plan in an effort to eliminate syphilis in the United States. Syphilis elimination is defined as the absence of sustained transmission, with a goal of less than 1,000 new cases annually, which is less than 0.4 per 1000,000 persons. Another goal is to increase the number of syphilis-free counties to 90 percent by 2005.

However, 2001 experienced a slight overall increase in reported cases of primary and secondary syphilis compared to 2000. In New York City, after a steady decline for 10 years, the number of reported cases of primary and secondary syphilis more than doubled from 117 new cases in 2000 to 282 new cases in 2001. The increase was primarily seen in homosexual men.

The number of cases of syphilis in 2001 overall showed a decline among women and non–Hispanic Blacks. The data suggest that efforts to reduce syphilis in women and non–Hispanic Blacks appear effective and should continue, although efforts to prevent and treat syphilis among men who have sex with men need to be improved.

MMWR. Nov. 1, 2002: 51(43): 971 and *MMWR* Sep. 27, 2002: 51(38): 853-856.

NCCAM *see* National Center for Complementary and Alternative Medicine

Needle piercings *see* Body piercings

Needle sharing

Contaminated needles account for up to 60 percent of all cases of hepatitis C and 36 percent of all cases of HIV/AIDS. It is estimated that injection drug use accounts for 920 million to 1.68 billion injections annually in the United States. In 1999, needle exchange programs provided 19 million sterile syringes.

Despite a ban on federal funding for syringe and needle exchange programs, many states provide these programs, and some states have amended their drug paraphernalia and prescription laws to allow pharmacy sales of syringes and needles. Since Connecticut reformed its drug paraphernalia and prescription laws to allow pharmacy sales in 1992, needle sharing among intravenous drug users dropped by 40 percent.

Polls of intravenous drug users show that up to 75 percent of drug users are aware that hepatitis and HIV can be transmitted through contaminated needles. About 50 percent of those polled admit to having shared needles within the last 12 months. Studies also show that infection with AIDS in up two two-thirds of children and three-fourths of women infected are either directly or indirectly related to intravenous drug use. *See also* **Syringe exchange programs.**

Centers for Disease Control and Prevention. *HIV/ AIDS, Sexually Transmitted Diseases and Tuberculosis Prevention News Update.* August 13, 2002.

Needle sticks

More than 800,000 accidental needle sticks occur in U.S. hospitals annually. Accidental sticks involving patients with hepatitis and HIV infection pose the most risk, especially when the needles are hollow-bore, allowing them to hold significant quantities of blood. Additional risk factors include needle sticks involving needles that have been placed directly into veins or arteries, needle sticks involving deep puncture wounds, and needle sticks from patients with end-stage AIDS or hepatitis.

Through December 1999, the CDC had

received reports of 56 health care workers in the United States with documented, occupationally acquired HIV infection, of whom 25 have developed AIDS in the absence of other risk factors, primarily as a result of needle stick injuries. The United States General Accounting Office, in a November 2000 report on occupational safety, estimates that about 69,000 needlesticks in hospitals can be prevented annually through the use of needles with safety features. Using CDC data, the GAO estimates that this may prevent at least 25 new cases of hepatitis B infection annually and 16 new cases of hepatitis C infection. The reduction in the number of HIV infections could not be estimated.

With the implementation of universal precautions, widespread use of latex gloves, and improved blood collection with self-sheathing or retractable systems, and safer needle disposal devices, the incidence of needle stick injuries has been greatly reduced, although not all hospitals have implemented these changes. The risk of healthcare related needle sticks continues to exist. As a provision of the Ryan White Care Act, healthcare workers and emergency medical workers have access to post-exposure testing and prophylactic treatment if warranted. *See also* **Occupational exposures**.

Occupational Safety: Selected Cost and Benefit Implications of Needlestick Prevention Devices for Hospitals. Washington, D.C.: U.S. General Accounting Office, 2000.

NEF (*nef*)

NEF is one of the regulatory genes of HIV. Three regulatory genes, *tat, rev,* and *nef*, and three so-called auxiliary genes (*vif, vpr, and vpu*) contain information necessary for the production of proteins that control HIV, such as the ability to infect a cell, produce new copies of itself, or cause disease.

Neisser, Albert (1855–1916)

The scientist Albert Neisser isolated *Neisseria gonorrhoeae*, establishing it as the causative agent of gonorrhea in 1879.

Neonatal

Neonatal refers to the first six weeks of life after birth. Infants younger than six weeks are called neonates.

Neonatal AIDS *see* Pediatric AIDS and Acquired immune deficiency syndrome

Neuropathy

Neuropathy is a general term to describe a number of disorders involving damage, destruction, or inflammation of nerves. Symptoms range from a tingling sensation or numbness in the toes and fingers to paralysis. It is estimated that 35 percent of persons with HIV disease have some form of neuropathy. *See also* **Acquired immune deficiency syndrome** and **Peripheral neuropathy**.

Neurosyphilis

Neurosyphilis is a condition of syphilitic infection of the central nervous system. Neurosyphilis can occur during any stage of syphilis. A patient with syphilis who has clinical evidence of neurologic involvement, such as cognitive dysfunction, motor or sensory deficits, ophthalmic or auditory symptoms, cranial nerve palsies, and symptoms or signs of meningitis should have a lumbar puncture and examination of the cerebrospinal fluid.

Syphilitic uveitis or other ocular manifestations frequently accompany neurosyphilis. Patients with ocular manifestations should be treated following the recommended CDC guidelines for neurosyphilis that are included with the syphilis entry. *See also* **Syphilis**.

Neutropenia

Neutropenia is an abnormal decrease in the number of neutrophils (the most common type of white blood cells, also known as granulocytes) in the blood circulation. The decrease may be relative or absolute. Neutropenia may occur in HIV infection or it may be caused by a number of different drugs.

Nongonococcal urethritis

Nongonococcal urethritis refers to a condition of urethritis which is not caused by *Neisseria gonorrhoeae*. Other organisms responsible for urethritis include *Chlamydia trachomatis*, *Ureaplasma urealyticym*, *Trichomonas vaginalis*, or herpes simplex virus. Chlamydia is responsible for about 50 percent of all cases of nongonococcal urethritis.

Non-Hodgkin's lymphoma (NHL)

NHL is a lymphoma made up of B cells and characterized by nodular or diffuse tumors that may appear in the stomach, liver, brain and bone marrow of persons infected with HIV. After Kaposi's sarcoma, NHL is the most common opportunistic cancer in persons with AIDS. Systemic NHL represents 80 percent of all cases, and the remaining 20 percent are primary central nervous system lymphomas (PCNSL) and a small number of body cavity lymphomas.

Etiology

The origin of HIV-related NHL is unknown, although some of their characteristics are understood. In the initial stage, the host is predisposed because of his immune system suppression, chronic antigenic stimulation by HIV, deregulation of cytokines, and often EBV infection. These conditions favor development of B cell proliferation, which occurs as a persistent generalized lymphadenopathy.

Classification of Systemic NHLs

Systemic NHLs are described as large-cell lymphomas (G group); large-cell im-munoblastic lymphoma (LCIBL, H group); and small non-cleaved cell lymphoma (J group) equivalent to Burkitt's type lymphoma. Some lymphomas may be of intermediate grade. In addition, B-cell CD30+ anaplastic large-cell (ALCL) may occur.

Symptoms

A distinguishing feature of NHL is the widespread extent of disease at initial presentation and the frequency of B-cell related symptoms, including fever, night sweats, and weight loss of more than 10 percent of the normal body weight. At diagnosis, 75 percent of patients have advanced disease, with frequent involvement of extranodal sites, most often the central nervous system, bone marrow, gastrointestinal tract, and liver, although any site may be affected.

Approximately 20–40 percent of patients have infiltration of the meninges covering the spinal cord, and 65 percent have brain infiltration noted at autopsy. The gastrointestinal tract is involved in 10–40 percent of cases, and multiple sites may be involved. Bulky disease can be observed in the anorectal region, particularly in homosexual men. Symptoms of PCNSL, which usually occurs in very advanced HIV disease, include lethargy, confusion, and personality changes.

Diagnosis

Diagnosis is made by tissue studies of biopsy specimens, including fine needle aspiration samples.

Treatment

No optimal therapy has been defined, although the use of combination therapy is considered essential. Most clinicians favor regimens such as methotrexate and leucoverin with rescue-bleomycin-doxorubicin-cyclophosphamide-vincristine and dexamethasone with or without antiretroviral therapy. *Pneumocystis jiroveci* is reported to occur in 12–20 percent of patients, even with the use of prophylactic therapy. Colony stimulating factors are being studied for their use in NHL. Survival time ranges from 4–6 months in patients with active disease and 15–20 months for patients with NHL that is in remission. Patients with a low CD4+ count and a previous AIDS diagnosis have a median survival time of three months.

Non-nucleoside reverse transcriptase inhibitors (NNRTIs)

NNRTIs, a class of antiretroviral drugs commonly referred to as non-nukes, work by stopping HIV production. NNRTIs work by directly binding onto the enzyme reverse transcriptase within a CD4+ cell and preventing the conversion of HIV RNA to DNA. Unlike the NRTIs, the NNRTIs have no activity against HIV-2 infection. As non-competitive inhibitors of reverse transcriptase, their antiviral activity is additive or synergistic with most other antiretroviral agents. In the order of FDA approval, from first to last, the early NNRTIs include nevirapine (Viramune); efavirenz (Sustiva); and delaviridine (Rescriptor).

Non-Progressors

Non-Progressors is a term used to describe the one to two percent of individuals infected with HIV early in the AIDS epidemic who have never developed AIDS or HIV related illnesses, have not had antiretroviral therapy and have CD4+ T cell counts of 600 cells/mm^3. This group has been well studied for any physiological changes that could provide natural resistance. Researchers have found that members of this subgroup have high levels of alpha defensin proteins. Additional data suggest that the phenomenon of non-progression is associated with the maintenance of the integrity of the lymphoid tissues and with less virus trapping in the lymph nodes than is seen in other individuals living with HIV. *See also* **Alpha defensins.**

Nonoxynol-9 (N-9)

N-9 is the most common spermicide used in the United States. As a spermicide, N-9 has a very high failure rate, with failure in one of every four women using spermicide contraception alone. N-9 does not offer protection against most STDs, and its use has been associated with the development of genital ulcers, increasing the risk of HIV transmission. The CDC does not recommend using condoms with N-9, since they are no more effective than other lubricated condoms and they have a shorter half-life and higher cost.

Nucleic acid amplification (NAT, NAAT) tests

Nucleic acid testing is used to identify specific nucleic acid profiles (DNA) of infectious agents such as *Chlamydia trachomatis, Neisseria gonorrhoeae,* Hepatitis B, and HIV. Nucleic acid amplification tests are more sensitive than traditional culture techniques and are the preferred detection method for STDs. In NAAT, the DNA of bodily specimens, such as blood, vaginal swabs, or urine, is amplified many times and examined to see if the DNA characteristics of specific organisms can be detected. Because intact organisms are not required for detection, specimen integrity and preservation are not as critical as in other methodologies. The CDC recommends that specimens that test positive by NAAT testing must be confirmed with a NAAT method that uses a different platform, because amplification can lead to contamination, causing false positives.

Nucleoside/nucleotide analog reverse transcriptase inhibitors (NRTIs)

NRTIs, the first class of antiretroviral drugs to be discovered, are commonly called nukes. NRTIs, whose chemical structure constitutes a modified version of a natural nucleoside, act by incorporating themselves into the HIV DNA, interfering with the reverse transcriptase enzyme, thereby stopping the building process. The resulting HIV DNA is incomplete and unable to create new viral material. All NRTIs cause premature termination of the proviral DNA chain, and require phosphorylation in the host's cells prior to their incorporation into the viral DNA.

In the order of FDA approval, from first to last, NRTIs include zidovudine, which is also known as azidothymidine (Retrovir, AZT); didanosine (Videx, VidexEC); zalcitabine (Hivid); lamivudine (Epivir); stavudine (Zerit); abacavir (Ziagen, ABC); tenofovir (Viread); and fixed-dose combinations such as zidovudine and lamivudine (Combivir), and fixed-dose zidovudine, abacavir, and lamivudine (Trizivir). NRTIs under investigation include emtricitabine (Voviracil, FTC) and amdoxovir (DAPD).

Nucleotide sequences

DNA is composed of nucleotides. Nucleotides are formed from the amino acid bases thymine, cytosine, adenine, and guanine, combined with the sugar deoxyribose linked to a phosphate molecule. The way in which the sugar and phosphate are attached to the carbons in the bases determines the specific nucleotides that are formed. Paired nucleotides form the double-stranded helix of DNA. The exact configuration of nucleotides in a compound is known as a sequence, and all forms of DNA have distinct nucleotide sequences. Mutations occur when specific chemicals in a sequence are altered. DNA sequences found in biological specimens such as blood can be used to identify specific organisms, including organisms that cause STDs.

Nutrition

Nutrition plays an important role in immune system health and consequently one's risk for infectious disease development and treatment response. The immune system depends on nutrient-rich foods for its proper function, whereas certain foods, particularly sugar and saturated fats, injure immune system cells. Highly processed foods often contain chemical preservatives that harm the immune system.

Occupational exposures

Although the risk is small, healthcare workers may be exposed to HIV, hepatitis, and other infectious diseases through "needle sticks," laboratory accidents, and similar injuries. The Health Resources and Services Administration (HRSA) of the U.S Department of Health & Human Services supports a Post-Exposure Prophylaxis hotline for healthcare workers to call for advice after exposure to HIV: 1-888-HIV-4911. HRSA also works with state and local health departments, and hospital and healthcare organizations worldwide to prevent and manage accidental occupational exposures.

Workers with occupational exposures to HIV and hepatitis should receive follow-up counseling and medical evaluation. HIV and hepatitis antibody tests should be performed at baseline and at six weeks, 12 weeks and six months. In some instances, particularly when the needle stick involves source patients with HIV, post-exposure prophylactic treatment may be indicated. It is the employer's responsibility to offer treatment when it is indicated, although the employee has the right to refuse treatment.

For skin exposures, follow-up is indicated if it involves direct contact with body fluids and if there is evidence of compromised skin integrity. This may be difficult to tell, especially when the hands are involved. Therefore, if contact with HIV contaminated blood is prolonged or involves a large area of skin, post-exposure prophylactic therapy may be indicated. Bites that result in blood exposure may also require prophylactic therapy if the source patient is HIV positive. When the source patient is HIV positive, the patient's CD4+ T cell count and viral load should be used in determining the need for other anti-retroviral therapy.

A large national study found that prophylactic treatment with zidovudine (AZT, ZDV) may reduce the risk of HIV infection after a percutaneous exposure by 81 percent. Among the people in the study who still developed HIV, the virus was found to be resistant to AZT in one of the cases. When prophylactic treatment is initiated, it should be started within 1–2 hours after the exposure. The Public Health Services recommends four weeks of treatment with zidovudine. In some instances both zidovudine and lamivudine are used. The addition of a third drug, usually a protease inhibitor such as indinavir or nelfinavir, should be considered for exposures that pose an increased risk of transmission or where resistance to other drugs is known or suspected. The specific prophylactic treatment should be administered with the guidance of an infectious disease specialist.

Individuals who receive post-exposure prophylaxis should be monitored for drug toxicity with blood tests that assess renal and liver function and with a complete blood count. Blood glucose should also be monitored if protease inhibitors are used. If indinavir is used, the urine should be tested for blood and crystals.

The side effects associated with antiretroviral therapy may cause non-compliance. Common side effects include headache, malaise, fatigue, and insomnia. More serious side effects include kidney stones, hepatitis, and low platelet count. Protease inhibitors also have serious drug interactions, so individuals using them must report all other medications that they are using. The effects of antiretroviral therapy on individuals who do not have HIV infection are unknown. The CDC and two pharmaceutical companies have created a registry to determine these effects. Healthcare workers and providers can receive more information by calling 1-888-737-4448. *See also* **Needle sticks**.

Onconase

Onconase is an extract of the Northern leopard frog, *Rana pipies*, with properties similar to those of an RNA enzyme. Onconase is undergoing phase III trials as an anti-cancer drug because of its ability to destroy damaged cells. Researchers are also investigating Onconase because it has also been shown to inhibit HIV-1 replication when used in low concentrations. In mammalian studies, levels of HIV-1 RNA (viral load) declined significantly. Onconase appears to affect viral life cycle directly by degrading viral RNA and indirectly by cleaving reverse transcriptase. Onconase may offer a valuable tool for HIV therapy when combined with other antiretroviral agents, since it affects stages not targeted by antiretroviral drugs.

Saxena, S., et al. "Onconase and Its Therapeutic Potential." *Laboratory Medicine*, May 2003; 5(34): 380-387.

1592U89

1592U89 is the experimental code for a nucleoside analog reverse transcriptase inhibitor (NRTI) drug used in the treatment of AIDS. 1592U89, which is marketed as abacavir (Aiagen) works well with other nucleoside analogs and with the protease inhibitor saquinavir. In addition, AZT-resistant HIV strains remain sensitive to abacavir although there appears to be slight cross-resistance with lamivudine.

Ophthalmia neonatorum

Ophthalmia neonatorum is a condition of conjunctivitis occurring in neonates caused by infection with *C. trachomatis* or *N. gonorrhoeae* during exposure to the cervical canal during vaginal delivery. Infection may be also related to *Moraxella catarrhalis* and other *Neisseria* species that are indistinguishable from N. gonorrhoeae on gram stains.

Infants at increased risk include those who do not receive ophthalmia prophylactic therapy after birth and those whose mothers have had no prenatal care or who have a history of STDs or substance abuse. Ophthalmia prophylactic treatment is required in many states, and includes applications of one percent silver nitrate, 0.5 percent erythromycin, or one percent tetracycline administered as an ophthalmic ointment in a single application into both eyes of newborns as soon as possible after birth. If prophylaxis is delayed, a monitoring system should be established to ensure that all infants receive prophylactic treatment, whether they are delivered by vaginal or cesarean section. Single-use ampules or tubes are preferable to multiple-use tubes. Bacitracin is not considered effective and the use of povidone iodine has not been adequately studied.

In ophthalmia neonatorum caused by chlamydia, numerous inclusion bodies are found in the cytoplasm of affected cells. When related to gonorrhea, a gram stain of exudates shows gram negative diplococci and white blood cells.

Presumptive treatment for gonorrhea may be indicated for newborns who are at increased risk for gonococcal ophthalmia and who have conjunctivitis but do not have gonococci demonstrated in gram stains of conjunctival exudates. Treatment for infection caused by gonorrhea includes ceftriaxone, using 25–50 mg/kg administered IV or IM in a single dose, not to exceed 125 mg. Topical antibiotic therapy used alone is inadequate and is unnecessary when systemic treatment is administered. Simultaneous infection with both *N. gonorrhoeae* and *C. trachomatis* should also be considered. *See also* **Chlamydia** and **Gonorrhea**.

Opportunistic infections

Opportunistic infections refer to infections that develop in patients with suppressed or damaged immune systems, either as a result of diseases such as HIV or HTLV infection, or as a result of immunosuppressant drugs, including drugs used for cancer. A healthy immune system normally prevents these infections from occurring. Therefore they are rarely seen in the normal population. The CDC regards the presence of certain opportunistic infections, such as *Pneumocystis jiroveci* pneumonia (PCP) in people infected with HIV as a sign that they have AIDS.

With the advent of highly active anti-retroviral therapy (HAART), the guidelines for prophylactic treatment of opportunistic infections have changed. The U.S. Public Health Service and the Infectious Diseases Society of America created a compendium of prophylactic treatment guidelines in 2002, which take advances in anti-retroviral therapy into consideration for patients with HIV infection. The guidelines are available at the CDC website and can be directly accessed at http://www.cdc.gov/mmwr/preview/mmwrhtml/rr5108a1.htm.

Before HAART therapy, patients with opportunistic infections were told that lifelong therapy was required to prevent recurrence. Now that HAART therapy can effectively raise levels of CD4+ lymphocytes, lifelong therapy is not always required. HAART is considered the most effective approach to preventing opportunistic infections and should be considered for all HIV-infected persons who qualify for such therapy. Patients who do not qualify for HAART therapy or who have failed HAART therapy require life-long prophylaxis. The new guidelines also include revised recommendations for vaccinating HIV-infected adults and HIV-exposed or infected children, and new information regarding drug interaction, primarily related to rifamycins and anti-retroviral drugs. *See also* AIDS-defining illnesses in entry on **Acquired Immune Deficiency Syndrome**.

Opportunistic organisms

Opportunistic organisms are microorganisms (bacteria, fungi, viruses) known to cause life-threatening infections in people with suppressed immune systems. Opportunistic organisms usually exist in the body without causing problems. For instance, most people have *Pneumocystis jiroveci* in their bodies, but a healthy immune system keeps this fungus in line, preventing infection. When the immune system is deficient in CD4+ lymphocytes, opportunistic organisms are able to freely proliferate and cause infection.

Oral candidiasis (thrush)

Oral candidiasis or thrush, a disease characterized by oral infection with the yeast *Candida albicans*, is one of the more common signs of AIDS, often appearing before AIDS fully develops. Thrush is also seen in individuals who have been on long-term antibiotic therapy. When the normal bacterial flora of the mouth is destroyed by antibiotics, yeast is allowed to proliferate freely.

Several studies have found that infection with thrush in homosexual men is an early sign of immunosuppression and an early marker for future development of AIDS. Thrush is often associated with esophageal candida infection, which may not cause symptoms until infection is severe.

Oral candidiasis is generally treated with the anti-fungal agent nystatin, with 500,000 units used as a mouth rinse that can be swallowed four to six times daily. Clotrimazole lozenges may also be prescribed, using 10 mg five times daily. When the esophagus is affected, 100 mg fluconazole or 400 mg ketoconazole may be used. Another alternative is amphoteracin B. However, patients with recurrent infections may develop resistance to fluconazole or amphoteracin B. This may be caused by a mutation to new strains of candida or because of reinfection with a different candida strain.

Oral hairy leukoplakia

Oral hairy leukoplakia is a proliferative disorder caused by the Epstein-Barr virus (EBV) that affects mucocutaneous epithelial cells within the oral cavity. Oral hairy leukoplakia is seen in up to 25 percent of homosexual men with AIDS and has also been reported in other immunocompromised patients and healthy individuals.

Clinically, the lesion appears as a poorly demarcated area with a grooved or "hairy" surface varying in size from a few millimeters to extensive lingual and oral mucosal involvement. The lesions typically occur on the lateral borders of the tongue and appear as whitish, slightly raised lesions that are often mistaken for thrush. Tissue studies show a thickening of the epithelial cell layer, with characteristic balloon cells with characteristic hair-like projections. An abundance of viral particles can be seen in the outer layers of epithelium indicating active EBV replication. The lesions do not show signs of dysplasia and do not typically become malignant.

Organ transplants

In some instances STDs that are transmissible through blood products can be transmitted through organ transplants. Although human sources of harvested organs are tested for infectious disease before transplantation occurs, if they have been recently infected with hepatitis, HIV, or other blood borne diseases, they will have not yet seroconverted and infectious disease screening tests for antibodies may be negative. With the use of newer techniques such as nucleic acid (DNA) amplification tests, infections can be detected earlier.

Oropharyngeal

Oropharyngeal refers to the division of the pharynx between the soft palate and the epiglottis. The pharynx is a tube that connects the mouth and nasal passages with the esophagus, the connection to the stomach. The epiglottis is a thin, valve-like structure that covers the glottis, the opening of the upper part of the larynx (the part of the throat containing the vocal cords), during swallowing.

Pap smear

The Pap smear or Papanicolaou test was developed by the Greek physician George N. Papanicolaou. In his post-doctoral work, Dr. Papanicolaou hypothesized that cells could be affected by the hormonal environment in which they exist. In 1925, he examined a smear of a female patient known to have cancer of the uterus and found the abnormal cellular changes now known to exist in cervical cancer. After reviewing more cases, in 1928 he published his legendary article, "New Cancer Diagnosis." Initially met with skepticism, Papanicolaou's finding eventually led to the use of the Pap smear as the most well known test used for detecting cervical cancer as well as distinct cellular changes that foreshadow cancer.

The Pap smear is a screening test, not a diagnostic test, and can be used to detect abnormal cell changes in other tissues, including those found in anal lesions, and also urine. As a screening test, the Pap smear can have a certain percentage of false positives and false negatives, although the percentage of false negatives is usually as low as five percent. Cervical cancer screening is based on repeated examinations at appropriate intervals. Abnormal Pap smears are generally followed by colposcopically-directed biopsy, which is considered the diagnostic gold smear.

Currently, the thin-layer Pap smear test is most widely used, and it may be combined with a DNA test for the human papillomavirus (HPV).

Papillomavirus *see* Human papillomavirus (HPV)

Parenteral treatment

Parenteral treatment refers to treatments that do not pass through the stomach. Most parenteral treatments are administered intravenously (IV) or intramuscularly (IM).

Parasites

Parasites are organisms that live on or in other organisms. Some parasites are known to cause STDs, and some parasites occur in patients who are immunosuppressed as a result of STD infections. For instance, the parasite *Strongyloides stercoralis* is often seen in people infected with HTLV-I.

Amebiasis (*Entamoeba histolytica* infection) of the penis, vulva, and cervix have also been reported, indicating that amoeba are likely sexually transmitted among heterosexual couples. Parasitic infections that occur in homosexual men include *Giardia lamblia, Iodamoeba butschlii, Dientamoeba fragilis, Entamoeba histolytica,* and *Enterobius vermicularis.* In addition, mixed infections with a variety of intestinal parasites, including other protozoans and nematodes, have also been described in homosexual men.

Most parasitic infections including amebiasis cause mild diarrhea to rare cases of fulminant bloody dysentery. Infection may be spread to the liver and rarely to the lungs and brain. Amebic proctocolitis causes diffuse inflammation and ulceration of the distal colon. Symptoms may be similar to those of irritable bowel disease, shigellosis, *Campylobacter jejuni* infection, or *Yersinisa* enterocolitis. Symptoms may wax and wane for weeks to months.

Diagnosis is made by examination of stool samples for ova and parasites.

Parent notification programs

Currently, most states have provisions for medical information of minors, generally individuals younger than 18, to be shared with parents and legal guardians. However, under HIPPA laws, even if individuals 18 years old and older are being covered by their parent's insurance policies, medical information cannot be given to their parents without their written consent.

Mandatory parental notification for adolescents to obtain prescribed contraceptives is a controversial issue. As of August 2002, legislation that would prohibit contraceptives without parental involvement had been introduced in 10 states and the U.S. Congress. Researchers at the University of Wisconsin in a study published in the August 14, 2002, *JAMA* reported finding that mandatory parental notification for prescribed contraceptives would impede girls' use of sexual health care services, potentially increasing teen pregnancies and the spread of STDs.

Partner notification programs

Partner notification (PN) programs are a key element in STD/HIV prevention programs. These programs originated in Europe in the 19th century as "contact tracing." Most city and county health departments have formal partner notification programs in which public health officials contact all of the sexual partners of patients with certain STDs, such as syphilis and HIV/AIDS. For most STDs, sex partners within 60 days of the onset of patient symptoms are notified, although for some STDs, such as the tertiary stage of syphilis, sex partners within the past year are notified.

PN programs are designed to link sexual and needle-sharing partners of people infected with HIV and other STDs with a comprehensive set of services intended to limit further spread of infection or a relapse in the infected partner.

However, it is difficult to evaluate the success of these programs because not all patients are willing to name all of their partners. Undoubtedly, some unsuspecting individuals receive diagnosis and treatment that they might not otherwise receive, but the programs encourage some patients to see doctors who guarantee confidentiality, interfering with the essential process of case-reporting.

In a study of adolescents with STDs, which was conducted by researchers at the Indiana University School of Medicine in Indianapolis, Indiana, partner notification was found to be increased among partners with higher levels of self-efficacy and in relationships with stronger affiliative and emotional ties. In this study sex partners were listed at enrollment, and at one month following treatment patients were asked if they had notified partners and when. In this study, 61 percent of women's partners and 52 percent of the men's partners had been notified. The study concluded that self-efficacy and partner communication could be especially amenable to interventions intended to increase patient-initiated partner notification for curable STD infections.

In the United States, PN is a voluntary process that is conducted using two basic approaches. In "provider referral," the infected person's partners are informed of their potential STD/HIV exposure and advised by a health care worker to obtain care. A disease intervention specialist usually provides this service in public clinics. Confidentiality is maintained by not revealing the identity of the original infected patient. In "patient referral," patients are relied on to inform their own partners. In addition, if patients admit that they haven't informed their own partners, health care workers will inform the partners.

Partner notification programs today serve to reduce disease transmission, provide counseling and treatment to persons exposed to STDs, and to increase knowledge about risk factors in different populations. *See also* **Contact tracing** and **Reportable diseases.**

Pediatric AIDS

Pediatric AIDS refers to the condition of AIDS occurring in children younger than 18 years. The first cases of AIDS in children were reported in 1982. Of the 7,296 cases of AIDS in children under 13 years in the U.S. reported to the CDC from 1981 to June 1996, 90 percent occurred in children whose mothers had HIV infection or were at risk of it (perinatally acquired).

Etiology

Almost all HIV-infected children acquire the virus from their mothers before or during childbirth (perinatally) or through breast-feeding. In maternally transmitted pediatric infection, disease progression appears to follow two distinct modes. One subgroup of children progresses rapidly to AIDS at a median age of approximately five months, and the other 20 percent of maternally transmitted pediatric AIDS patients develops AIDS at about 12 months.

Timeframe

In maternally transmitted AIDS, the mean time from birth to a stage of AIDS causing severe symptoms is estimated to be 6.3 to 6.6 years. The time to death is estimated to be approximately 6.3 to 9.4 years from birth. In studies involving 2,148 perinatally infected children (infected around the time of childbirth), the mean durations of the stages of infection were 10 months for the symptom-free internal (stage N of the CDC's 1994 pediatric guidelines), four months for stage A (mild signs or symptoms), 65 months for stage B (moderate signs or symptoms), and 34 months for stage C (severe signs or symptoms). Although children with perinatally transmitted AIDS usually develop moderate symptoms by the second year of life, they may not progress for a long time. In one study, as many as one-third of children with perinatal HIV infection are estimated to remain free of AIDS by 15 years. The rapid progression of HIV in infants compared to adults is thought to be related to the immaturity of the neonatal immune response. Normally, the immune system does not fully mature until about two years of age.

One landmark study (ACTG 076) conducted in 1994 by the Pediatric AIDS Clinical Trials Group (PACTG) found that the anti-retroviral drug AZT, given to HIV-infected women who had very little or no anti-retroviral treatment in the past but had CD4+ T cell counts greater than 200 cells per cubic millimeter of blood, reduced the risk of maternal transmission by two-thirds, from 25 percent to eight percent. In this study, therapy was initiated in the second or third trimester and continued during labor. In addition , infants were treated with AZT for six weeks following birth. AZT produced no serious side effects in the mothers or infants in this study. Ongoing studies have shown the rate of neonatal infection using this protocol to be as low as five percent.

Epidemiology

The U.S. cities that had the four highest rates of pediatric AIDS during 1998 were New York City; Miami, Florida; Newark, New Jersey; and Washington, D.C. The primary maternal risk factors related to pediatric HIV infection include advanced HIV disease, increased levels of HIV in the maternal bloodstream, and decreased numbers of CD4+ T cells in the maternal circulation. Other maternal risk factors include maternal drug use, severe inflammation of fetal membranes, or a prolonged period between membrane rupture and delivery.

Symptoms

Compared to adults, children have a different pattern of primary and secondary HIV-related abnormalities. The most important primary symptoms in children include growth delay or failure to thrive and central nervous system abnormalities, such as microcephaly (abnormally small head) and developmental delay. Other symptoms seen in children include cardiomyopathy (heart disease), kidney disease, swollen parotid glands, a condition of lymphoid interstitial pneumonitis (LIP), enlarged liver, enlarged spleen, and painful swollen lymph nodes. Opportunistic infections seen in children include *Pneumocystis jiroveci* pneumonia and recurrent serious bacterial infections, particularly with *Streptococcus pneumoniae* and *Haemophilus influenzae*, group b. Children with HIV infection also have an increased risk of developing osteoporosis and osteonecrosis. Osteonecrosis of the hip in children is known as Legg-Calve-Perthes disease, or Perthes disease.

CDC Classification of Children under 13 years with HIV infection

• N: NOT SYMPTOMATIC—No signs or symptoms of HIV infection or only one of the conditions in category A. Appropriate HIV tests for HIV protein or HIV culture should be performed in children <18 months; in older children, the HIV antibody tests must be confirmed with the Western blot or a comparable test.

• A: MILDLY SYMPTOMATIC—Two or more signs in category A, but none of the conditions in categories B or C. Category A includes: lymphadenopathy greater than 0.5 cm at more than two sites or bilaterally at one site; enlarged liver; enlarged spleen; dermatitis; swollen parotid glands; recurrent or persistent upper respiratory infection, sinusitis, or otitis media ear infection.

• B: MODERATELY SYMPTOMATIC—Symptoms from Group B which include but are not limited to: anemia (Hgb <8 grams);

neutropenia (<1,000 WBC); or thrombocytopenia (<100,000 platelets/mm^3); bacterial meningitis, pneumonia or sepsis; candidiasis or thrush persisting in children >6 months for more than two months; cardiomyopathy (heart disease); cytomegalovirus infection with onset before one month of age; recurrent or chronic diarrhea or hepatitis; recurrent herpes simplex; herpes simplex bronchitis, pneumonitis, or esophagitis, with onset before one month of age; herpes zoster with two or more episodes; leimyosarcoma, LIP or pulmonary lymphoid hyperplasia (PHL); nocardiosis; persistent fever lasting >1 month; Toxoplasmosis with onset <1 month of age; and varicella (complicated chickenpox).

• C: SEVERELY SYMPTOMATIC—Any condition listed in the 1987 case definition for AIDS with the exception of LIP, including: Two serious bacterial infections within two years, such as sepsis, pneumonia, meningitis, bone or joint infection, abscess of organ or body cavity excluding otitis media, skin or mucosal abscesses, and indwelling catheter infection; candidiasis (esophageal, tracheal, bronchial, or pulmonary); disseminated or extrapulmonary coccidiomycosis; extrapulmonary cryptococcosis; cryptosporidiosis or isosporiasis lasting >1 month; cytomegalovirus disease with onset >1 month affecting other than the liver, spleen, or lymph nodes; encephalopathy not related to infection and impaired brain growth or acquired microcephaly; acquired symmetric motor deficit, including sleep and gait disturbances; histoplasmosis; Kaposi's sarcoma; primary brain lymphoma and non–Hodgkin's lymphoma; mycobacterium infection; pneumocystis jiroveci infection; progressive multifocal leukoencephalopathy; recurrent salmonella infection; and wasting syndrome without other causes. *See also* **Acquired immune deficiency syndrome; lymphoid interstitial pneumonitis;** and **pulmonary lymphoid hyperplasia.**

CDC Classification for Children under 13 years with HIV Infection, 1994.

Havens, Peter. "Pediatric AIDS." Chapter 20 in *Infectious Diseases*. Donald Armstrong, Editor. London: Mosey Imprint of Harcourt, 1999.

Schupbach, Jorg. "Human Immunodeficiency Viruses." Chapter 63 in *Manual of Clinical Microbiology*. 7th edition. Washington, DC: ASM Press, 1999).

Pediatric AIDS Clinical Trials Group (PACTG)

PACTG is a nationwide clinical trials network that evaluates treatments from HIV infected children and adolescents and develops new approaches for the interruption of mother-to-infant transmission. PACTG is jointly sponsored by the National Institute of Allergy and Infectious Disease (NIAID) and the National Institute of Child Health and Human Development (NICHD).

Pediatric STDs

Pediatric STDs can occur as a result of perinatal infections, such as with HIV or syphilis, that have not been previously diagnosed. They most often occur, however, as a result of sexual abuse, and often, more than one STD is present. When an STD is diagnosed in a child, it is important to screen for the presence of other STDs. Management of children who have STDs requires close cooperation among clinicians, laboratorians, and child-protection authorities. Investigations, when indicated, should be initiated promptly. The CDC guidelines state that some diseases, such as gonorrhea, syphilis, and chlamydia, if acquired after the neonatal period, are almost 100 percent indicative of sexual assault. For other diseases, such as HPV and vaginitis, the association with sexual contact is not as clear.

Centers for Disease Control and Prevention. *Sexually Transmitted Diseases Treatment Guidelines 2002.* Atlanta: U.S. Dept. of Health and Human Services, 2002.

Pediculus pubis (Crabs)

Pediculus pubis is the infectious agent responsible for pubic lice, an STD commonly known as crabs. *See also* **Pubic lice**.

Pelvic inflammatory disease (PID)

Pelvic inflammatory disease is a term referring to a spectrum of different upper genital tract inflammatory disorders, including any combination of endometritis, salpingitis, tubo-ovarian abscess, and pelvic peritonitis. PID refers to infections caused by microorganisms that ascend from the cervix or vagina and enter the endometrium, fallopian tubes, or contiguous structures. PID does not include blood-born infections such as tuberculosis, nor does it include infections following delivery or induced abortion.

Etiology

PID is usually caused by *Chlamydia trachomatis* or *Neisseria gonorrhoeae*, although other organisms may be responsible. Ten to 19 percent of women with gonorrhea of the cervix have clinical signs of acute PID. In populations with a high endemic rate of gonorrhea, PID is usually related to gonorrhea. In populations where gonorrhea is rarely seen, the cause is more likely chlamydia.

Epidemiology

The instance of PID varies with different populations. Because PID is not a reportable disease, epidemiological data is limited. Women with children and married women have a lower incidence of PID than women who are single, divorced, or widowed and have not had children. American data indicate a particularly high incidence of PID among young, nonwhite, single, or divorced women from urban areas. In 1993, approximately 313,000 women aged 15–44 were seen in emergency rooms for PID.

Symptoms

PID associated with gonorrhea may cause pain in the first part of the menstrual cycle, although often symptoms are vague or not noticed. Salpingitis, which is an infection of the fallopian tubes, occurs in two-thirds of women with PID. Salpingitis may cause infertility, and one of the goals of early treatment for PID is to prevent salpingitis from developing. Abscess formation is a late manifestation of PID and is rarely caused by gonorrhea or chlamydia infection alone. Abscesses typically result from a combination of aerobic and anaerobic bacteria. A delay in treatment is responsible for scarring, salpingitis, more frequent periods and infertility. Severe cases may even spread to the liver and kidneys, causing dangerous internal bleeding and death.

Diagnosis

PID is usually diagnosed by direct culture of upper genital tract tissue, such as endometrial tissue obtained by cervical biopsy, peritoneal fluid obtained by cul-de-sac puncture, or abscess material from vaginal drainage. Specimens can also be collected from the pelvic cavity during laparoscopy or laparotomy surgical procedures.

Treatment

Treatment depends on the specific organism responsible for PID and is included under the sections for chlamydia and gonorrhea. If the infectious agent is unknown, PID treatment regimens must provide empiric, broad-spectrum coverage of likely pathogens. Antimicrobial coverage should be effective against *N. gonorrhoeae*, *C. trachomatis*, anaerobes, Gram-negative facultative bacteria, and streptococci.

Recommended treatment regimens include cefotetan, using two grams administered IV every 12 hours; or cefoxitin, using two grams IV every six hours; or doxycycline, using 100 mg orally or IV every

12 hours. Because of pain associated with infusion, doxycycline should be administered orally if possible, even if the patient is hospitalized. Parenteral therapy may be discontinued 24 hours after the patient shows clinical improvement and oral therapy with doxycycline should continue until 14 days of therapy are completed.

An alternative regimen includes clindamycin, using 900 mg IV every eight hours plus gentamicin, using a loading dose IV or IM containing 2mg/kg of body weight, followed by a maintenance dose (1.5 mg/kg) every eight hours. Single daily dosing may be substituted.

Another alternative parenteral regimen includes ofloxacin, using 400 mg IV every 12 hours; or levofloxacin, using 500 mg IV once daily with or without the addition of metronidazole, using 500 mg IV every eight hours; or ampicillin/sulbactam, using three grams IV every six hours along with doxycycline, using 100 mg orally or IV every 12 hours.

Patients who do not respond to oral therapy within 72 hours should be reevaluated to confirm the diagnosis and should be administered parenteral therapy on either an outpatient or inpatient basis.

Risk factors

Risk factors include unprotected sex, age, ecological disturbances of the vaginal flora caused by concurrent infection with bacterial vaginosis, HIV, multiple sex partners, smoking, drug and alcohol abuse, and frequent douching. Induced abortion also predisposes to PID, presumably from the introduction of pathogenic cervical or vaginal bacteria into the endometrium.

Precautions

Often, episodes of PID go unrecognized. Although some cases are asymptomatic, others remain undiagnosed because the patient or the health care provider fails to recognize the implications of mild or nonspecific symptoms or signs, such as abnormal bleeding, painful menstruation, and vaginal discharge. Because of the difficulty of diagnosing PID and the potential for damage to the reproductive health of women caused by even mild or atypical PID, health-care providers must make a vigilant effort to diagnose PID, even when symptoms are vague.

Empiric treatment of PID is recommended for sexually active young women and other women at risk for STDs if the following minimum criteria are present and no other cause or causes for the illness can be readily identified: uterine/side tenderness, or cervical motion tenderness. In patients with both pelvic tenderness and signs of lower genital tract inflammation, the diagnosis of PID should be considered.

Additional criteria that can be used to support a diagnosis of PID include oral temperature greater than 101° F; abnormal cervical or vaginal mucopurulent discharge; presence of white blood cells on saline microscopy of vaginal secretions; elevated erythrocyte sedimentation rate (blood test useful in detecting inflammatory processes); elevated C-reactive protein; and laboratory documentation of cervical infection with *N. gonorrhoeae* or *C. trachomatis*.

Male sex partners of women with PID should be examined and treated if they had sexual contact with the patient during the 60 days preceding the patient's onset of symptoms. Evaluation and treatment are essential because of the risk for reinfection of the patient and the strong likelihood of urethral gonococcal or chlamydial infection in the sex partner. Male partners of women who have PID related to chlamydial infection or gonorrhea often do not have symptoms.

Treatment for PID is the same for women with HIV infection. Early observational studies indicate that women with HIV are more likely to require surgical intervention.

Centers for Disease Control and Prevention. *Sexually Transmitted Diseases Treatment Guidelines 2002.* Atlanta: U.S. Dept. of Health and Human Services, 2002.

Penicillin

Alexander Fleming, a Scottish doctor, whose early experiments demonstrated the bactericidal power of the mold *Penicillium notatum*, is credited with discovering penicillin in 1928. In 1939, a team of Oxford researchers managed to purify this substance while preserving its antimicrobial properties. After conclusive experiments on humans in 1941, the United States began producing penicillin to be used as the first antibiotic. In 1943, a team of physicians successfully treated early cases of syphilis with penicillin, and it has remained the mainstay of syphilis treatment since that time. Penicillin was once used as the primary treatment for gonorrhea, but by the 1980s, a number of mutated strains began showing penicillin resistance.

Penicillin desensitization

Penicillin is the recommended treatment regimen for pregnant patients with syphilis and also for patients with syphilis and HIV. Approximately three to 10 percent of the adult population have experienced urticaria (hives), angiodema (welts) or anaphylaxis (upper airway obstruction) after penicillin therapy. Re-administration of penicillin to these patients can cause severe, immediate reactions. Because these reactions can be fatal, every effort should be made to avoid administering penicillin to these patients unless they undergo acute desensitization to eliminate anaphylactic sensitivity.

An estimated 10 percent of people reporting a reaction to penicillin remain allergic. However, with the passage of time after a reaction to penicillin, these people may stop expressing penicillin specific immunoglobulin E, which is released as a first step in the allergic response. These people will not react to skin tests and can be safely administered penicillin after having skin tests with dilute and full-strength skin test reagents.

Patients who have a positive skin test to

one of the penicillin determinants can be desensitized by administering gradually higher amounts of penicillin after starting with a very dilute dose of penicillin. The doses can be administered orally or intravenously (IV) in a hospital setting, because serious allergic reactions can rarely occur. Desensitization can be completed in approximately four hours, after which the first dose of therapeutic penicillin can be safely administered. After desensitization patients must be maintained on penicillin continuously for the duration of the course of therapy.

Penicillinase producing *Neisseria Gonorrhoeae* (PPNG)

PPNG is a term used to describe strains of *Neisseria gonorrhoeae* that produce the enzyme penicillinase, which causes resistance to penicillin antibiotics.

Pentamidine, aerosolized (Nebupent, AP)

Aerosolized pentamidine is a drug inhaled as a fine mist used for the prevention of *Pneumocystis jiroveci* pneumonia (PCP).

Perinatal transmission

Perinatal transmission refers to the transmission of a pathogen, such as HIV, from mother to baby before, during, or after the birth process. Ninety percent of children reported with AIDS acquired HIV infection from their HIV-infected mothers.

Peripheral neuropathy (PN)

Peripheral neuropathy is a condition characterized by damage to the peripheral nerves, which may cause sensory loss, pain, muscle weakness, and wasting of muscle in the hands or legs and feet.

PN occurs at similar rates in men, women, and children. The peripheral nervous system consists of sensory and motor neurons (nervous system cells). Sensory neurons carry impulses of sensation such as touch, pain, vibration, and temperature to the brain. Motor neurons send messages from the brain and spinal cord to the muscles. Neuropathy impairs these signals. About one-third of people with AIDS develop peripheral neuropathy, usually in the late stages of disease.

Symptoms of PN may be mild or severe; PN may progress slowly or rapidly worsen within a few days. Common symptoms include altered sensations known as paresthesias. Paresthesias include numbness, tickling, tingling, prickling, burning, pain, pins and needles sensations, and hypersensitivity. Symptoms are often more severe at night. Severe cases may result in paralysis.

In HIV/AIDS, PN is thought to be related to immune system changes that cause infiltration and compression of peripheral nerves or damage to the protective myelin coating of nerves. PN may also arise as a side effect of certain drugs, especially some of the nucleoside analogs. Other conditions that can cause PN, such as diabetes, hypothyroidism, and nutrient deficiency states, can contribute to PN or worsen symptoms.

Persons with HIV/AIDS may experience several different types of peripheral neuropathy. The most common type is distal sensory polyneuropathy, or DSP (also known as distal symmetrical sensory neuropathy and distal sensory axonal polyneuropathy). Distal refers to nerve damage at the farthest point from the spinal cord, particularly the hands and feet. The longest nerves are affected first, with the first symptoms typically occurring in the toes and soles of the feet. Polyneuropathy means that many nerves are affected, and symmetrical means that symptoms occur equally on both sides of the body. This syndrome is sometimes referred to as "dying back" neuropathy because the damage progresses from the extremities inward toward the spinal cord.

Other types of PN seen in HIV/AIDS include acute or chronic inflammatory demyelinating polyneuropathy (AIDP or CIPD respectively), progressive polyradiculopathy, mononeuropathy (mononeuritis) multiplex, and diffuse infiltrative lymphocytosis syndrome (DILS).

AIDP, which is also known as Guillain-Barré Syndrome, is an autoimmune condition that often develops in people after viral infection or vaccinations. In HIV infection, it usually occurs early in infection. It is a rapidly progressing, potentially fatal condition characterized by myelin inflammation, mild sensory loss, and severe motor loss or paralysis. Polyradiculopathy is an often painful condition of inflammation of the nerve roots adjacent to the spinal cord. Polyradiculopathy may result from cytomegaloviral (CMV) infection in the nerve roots. It can lead to rapidly progressive motor and sensory nerve damage. Mononeuropathy multiplex affects individual peripheral nerves, including facial nerves. DILS is a condition in which immune system cells, typically CD8+ lymphocytes, infiltrate neurons, causing various symptoms of neuropathy.

The various types of PN are often seen at different stages of infection. AIDP and CIDP typically occur in early infection, whereas DSP is more likely to be seen in the middle and late stages as immune system damage progresses. Other forms of PN may occur as a result of opportunistic infections. For example, polyradiculopathy is likely to occur in patients with CMV infection.

PN is also associated with certain NRTI drug therapies, specifically ddl (didanosine), ddC (zalcitabine), d4T (stavudine), and 3TC (lamivudine). The NRTIs AZT and abacavir are associated with absence of PN. PN can also occur in patients using dapsone for *Pneumocystis jiroveci* pneumonia; disulfiram (Antabuse); ethambutol, which is used to treat Mycobacterium avium complex; isoniazid, which is used for tuberculosis; metronidazole, used to treat parasitic and bacterial infections; and several drugs used for the treatment of cancer.

PN is usually diagnosed on the basis of symptoms, and diagnosis can be confirmed with nerve conduction studies. PN related to specific medications is often treated by changing drug therapy. Tricyclic antidepressant, anticonvulsant medications, and narcotic analgesics such as methadone, morphine, and fentanyl are often used to relieve pain.

Complementary medicines for PN include acupuncture, alpha lipoic acid, gamma linolenic acid (GLA), L-acetylcarnitine, and B vitamins.

The NCCAM is conducting clinical trials at the University of California in San Francisco to evaluate the benefits of marijuana on peripheral neuropathy. For more information, contact Hector Vizoso, RN at (415) 476-9554, ext. 21, or email him at hvizoso@php.ucsf.edu.

Lands, Linda. "Neuropathy: nutrient therapies." *AIDS Treatment News*, 1996 July 5: 250.
The Neuropathy Association, http://www.neuropathy.org, (800) 247-6968.
Senneff, J.A. *Numb Toes and Other Woes*. San Antonio: MedPress, 2001.

Persistent generalized lymphadenopathy (PGL)

PGL is characterized by chronic, diffuse, non-cancerous lymph node enlargement. Typically, PGL occurs in persons with persistent bacterial, viral, or fungal infections. PGL in HIV infection is a condition in which lymph nodes are chronically swollen in at least two areas of the body for three months or more with no obvious cause other than the HIV infection.

Phase I trials

Phase I trials involve the initial introduction of an investigational new drug into humans. Phase I trials are closely monitored and may be conducted in patients or in healthy volunteers. The studies are designed to determine the metabolism and pharmacologic actions of the drugs in humans; safety; side effects associated with increasing doses; and if possible, early indications of effectiveness. Usually, about 20 to 80 subjects are involved in Phase I trials.

Phase II trials

Phase II trials include controlled clinical studies of effectiveness of a drug for a particular indication or indications in patients with the disease or condition under study. Phase II studies also determine common, short-term side effects and risks associated with the drug. Phase II studies are typically well controlled, closely monitored, and usually involve no more than several hundred patients.

Phase III trials

Phase III trials include expanded controlled and uncontrolled studies. They are performed after preliminary evidence of drug effectiveness and safety have been obtained. Phase III trials are intended to gather additional information about effectiveness and safety that is needed to evaluate the overall benefit-risk relationship of the drug and to provide an adequate basis for physician labeling. These studies usually include anywhere from several hundred to several thousand subjects.

Phase IV trials

Phase IV trials include post-marketing studies that are carried out after licensure of the drug. Generally, a Phase IV trial is a randomized, controlled trial that is designed to evaluate the long-term safety and efficacy of a drug for a given indication. Phase IV trials are important in evaluating AIDS drugs because many drugs for HIV infection have been given accelerated approval with small amounts of clinical data regarding the drugs' effectiveness.

Phenotype assay

Phenotype or phenotypic assays are laboratory procedures whereby a DNA sample of a patient's HIV is tested against various antiretroviral drugs to see if the virus is susceptible or resistant to these drugs. Phenotype assays also measure the amount of drug needed to suppress the growth of HIV in a laboratory setting. Smaller amounts of drug are needed to stop reproduction of non-resistant HIV, whereas higher amounts of an antiretroviral drug are needed to stop reproduction of resistant strains.

Resistance is usually reported as the level of drug needed to reduce viral replication by 50 percent (inhibitory concentration 50 or IC50), or by 90 percent (IC90). The level of resistance is graded by comparing this value for an individual's HIV with the levels for non-resistant (or wild-type) virus. Low level represents a two to fourfold increase in the amount of drug needed to stop HIV replication; moderate level represents a 4–10-fold increase, and high level represents a 10-fold or greater increase. With most antiretroviral drugs, high-level resistance means that this drug is no longer able to block viral growth in the body. Moderate resistance might be overcome by achieving higher drug levels in the blood or by using novel drug combinations. The protease inhibitor ritonavir, for instance, can increase the blood levels of many other drugs, including other protease inhibitors.

Phenotype assays are more expensive than genotype assays, and these tests are not as widely available as genotype assays.

Phimosis

Phimosis is a condition characterized by tightening and constriction of the foreskin of the penis caused by inflammation, making it impossible to bare the glans. Phimosis may occur as a consequence of STD infection, particularly chancroid infection.

Piercing *see* Body piercing

Pneumocystis jiroveci pneumonia (PCP)

In the early 1980s, reports of *Pneumocystis carinii* (now classified as *Pneumocystis jiroveci*) pneumonia in American homosexuals without previously known immune deficiency heralded the spread of a new epidemic. During the first decade of the AIDS epidemic, PCP remained the most frequent AIDS-defining diagnosis in industrialized countries, at one time affecting 75–90 percent of all HIV infected people.

Etiology

Pneumocystis jiroveci is a fungus that may normally exist in the human body. In people with suppressed immune systems, particularly HIV infected patients with CD4+ T cell counts below 200 cells/mm^3, *Pneumocystis jiroveci* can cause pulmonary infection and pneumonia. Without treatment, up to 85 percent of HIV patients with low CD4+ counts are likely to develop PCP. In the early years of the AIDS epidemic, PCP was the most prevalent opportunistic infection to occur in individuals with HIV/AIDS. Although new antiretroviral therapies have markedly decreased the incidence of PCP, it remains frequent, especially in patients unaware of their HIV status or who have poor access to the health-care system. It is generally thought that PCP infection is due to reactivation of latent infection acquired during childhood or adolescence. The rate of relapse after a first episode is high, approximately 60 percent incidence within one year, when no specific prophylactic treatment is used.

Epidemiology

Since the start of the AIDS pandemic, approximately 20,000 to 60,000 cases of PCP have been reported each year in the United States. Without prophylactic treatment, PCP occurs in 75 to 90 percent of immunosuppressed patients at some time during the course of their illness. With prophylactic treatment and the introduction of effective antiretroviral therapies, the incidence of PCP has declined.

PCP primarily occurs in patients with CD4+ T cell counts less than 200,000 cells/mm^3. However, in five to 15 percent of cases it occurs in patients with higher CD4+ T cell counts. In patients on prophylactic therapy, the lifetime risk of developing PCP in patients with AIDS is 28 percent. Data from the Multicenter AIDS Cohort Study (MACS) found that regardless of CD4+ cell count, the presence of unexplained fevers or oropharyngeal candidiasis is independently associated with an increased risk of developing PCP.

Symptoms

Pneumocystis jiroveci primarily causes a pulmonary infection, although disseminated disease involving the skin, eye, ear, spleen, bone marrow, heart, lymph nodes, and thyroid gland can occur, especially in those receiving aerosolized petamidine prophylactic treatment. Symptoms are often insidious in onset, with fatigue, weight loss, and fever. As the disease progresses, shortness of breath, chest pain, and a nonproductive cough usually occur.

Diagnosis

The chest radiograph shows a diffuse bilateral interstitial pattern (evenly distributed symptoms in both lungs) early in infection. Numerous atypical patterns may be seen, including localized infiltrates, notably of the upper lobes. Parenchymal tissue involvement can be assessed using computed tomography (CT) scans. Small pulmonary cysts with thin walls throughout the lungs are common in AIDS-related PCP.

Diagnosis is generally made by detecting the organisms in either induced-sputum specimens or bronchoalveolar lavage fluid. Laboratory methods using polymerase chain reaction techniques are often used, although their sensitivity is not optimal. Because many other conditions, including Kaposi's sarcoma, can cause lung involvement, it is important to differentiate PCP from these other conditions. The level of serum LDH, and more precisely, its decrease during the first day of treatment, can be used to aid in diagnosis.

Treatment

Trimethoprim-sulfamethoxazole (TMP-SMX) is the first choice for treatment for PCP, even in patients who have moderate to severe adverse reactions to this medication. Pentamidine is equally effective but less convenient because it must be given parenterally, and it is considerably more toxic, potentially causing hypoglycemia, hypotension, renal impairment, and pancreatitis. Other agents commonly used include dapsone-trimethoprim, clindamycin plus primaquine, atrovaquone, and trimetrexate with leucovorin. Dapsone-trimethoprim is thought to be as effective as TMP-SMX but less toxic. Moderate to severe disease, as defined by an increased room air blood gas result (greater than 35 mm Hg, and/ or an arterial PO2 of less than 70 mm Hg) indicates the need for adjunctive corticosteroid treatment in addition to the antibiotics.

TMP-SMX may cause rash, fever, itching, nausea, anemia and leukopenia. Unless severe toxicity occurs, such as Stevens-Johnson reaction, severe hematologic changes, or immediate hypersensitivity, many experts recommend challenging the patient with TMP-SMX.

Prophylactic Treatment

Primary prophylactic treatment is frequently used when the CD4+ T lymphocyte count falls below 200 cells/mm^3 or if the patient develops oral candidiasis or unexplained fever for more than two weeks. Secondary prophylactic treatment is used for all patients with a history of PCP. TMP-XMX is considered the agent of choice for both primary and secondary prophylaxis. Monthly aerosolized pentamidine is also effective although not as effective as TMP-SMX therapy.

Risk Factors

Risk factors include a CD4+ T cell count less than 200/mm^3 or clinical manifestations such as thrush (oral candidiasis), herpes zoster (shingles), unexplained fever or weight loss.

Pol (*pol*)

Pol is an HIV gene that codes for the enzymes protease, reverse transcriptase and integrase.

Polymerase chain reaction (PCR)

PCR is a laboratory process or method that selects a DNA segment from a mixture of DNA chains and rapidly replicates it to create a sample of a piece of DNA. For HIV, this is called RT-PCR, which allows the laboratory to detect and quantify the amount of HIV (viral load) that is present in a person's blood or lymph nodes based on reverse transcriptase levels. PCR is also used for the diagnosis of HIV infection in exposed infants and to detect the presence of chlamydia in genital swabs and urine specimens.

Postexposure prophylaxis

Postexposure prophylaxis refers to treatment which is prescribed after exposure to an infectious agent. For instance, health professionals who receive needle sticks from needles used to inject someone with HIV infection, are given the medicine AZT to help protect them against developing infection.

Pox *see* Syphilis

Pregnancy

Intrauterine (transmitted to the uterus) or perinatally (transmitted around the time of childbirth) transmitted STDs can have severely debilitating effects on pregnant women, their partners, and their fetuses. All pregnant women and their sex partners should be asked about STDs, counseled about the possibility of perinatal infections, and provided access to treatment, if needed.

All pregnant women should be offered voluntary HIV testing and syphilis, chlamydia, gonorrhea, hepatitis C virus (HCV), and hepatitis B virus (HBV) screening at their first prenatal visit. Women who test negative but are at high risk for gonorrhea, syphilis, HIV or HBV infection, should be re-tested for these STDs in the 3rd trimester, preferably before 36 weeks gestation. In addition, women who have not received prenatal counseling should be encouraged to be tested for HIV infection at delivery. Women who have a new or more than one sex partner are at increased risk for chlamydia and should be re-tested in the 3rd trimester for chlamydia infection.

At the first prenatal visit, women should also be evaluated for bacterial vaginosis (BV) if they have a high risk for pre-term labor (due to previous history of preterm delivery). Current evidence does not support routine testing for BV during pregnancy. A Pap smear should be obtained at the first prenatal visit if a Pap test hasn't been performed in the previous year.

Women infected with HBV should be reported to the state so appropriate testing and treatment are available for household members, partners, and for their infants. Treatment is not available for women with HCV, but they should receive appropriate counseling. In the absence of lesions during the 3rd trimester, routine serial cultures for HSV are not indicated for women who have a history of recurrent genital herpes. Prophylactic cesarean section is not indicated for women who do not have active genital lesions at the time of delivery. The presence of genital warts is not an indication for cesarean section. Not enough evidence exists to recommend routine screening for *Trichomonas vaginalis* in pregnant women who do not have symptoms.

Centers for Disease Control and Prevention. *Sexually Transmitted Diseases Treatment Guidelines* 2002. Atlanta: U.S. Dept. of Health and Human Services, 2002.

Presidential Advisory Council on HIV and AIDS (PACHA)

The Presidential Advisory Council on HIV and AIDS was established in 1995 by President Bill Clinton, Vice President Al Gore, and then–Secretary of Health and Human Services Donna Shalala to provide recommendations on the U.S. government's response to the AIDS epidemic. President George W. Bush and his Secretary of Health and Human Services Tommy G. Thompson renewed the council's charter on July 19, 2001. The council may have up to 35 members, including the chair. The council may also include ex-officio members from relevant HHS components as deemed appropriate by the secretary or designee.

Prevention guidelines

The prevention and control of STDs is based on the following five major concepts: education and counseling of persons at risk on ways to adopt safer sexual behavior; identification of asymptomatically infected persons and of symptomatic persons unlikely to seek diagnosis and treatment services; effective diagnosis and treatment of infected persons; evaluation, treatment, and counseling of sex partners; and pre-exposure vaccination of persons at risk for vaccine-preventable STDs.

Centers for Disease Control and Prevention. *Sexually Transmitted diseases Treatment Guidelines 2002.* Atlanta: U.S. Dept. of Health and Human Sources, 2002.

Primary effusion lymphoma (PEL)

Primary effusion lymphoma occasionally develops in patients with HIV/AIDS.

Studies have demonstrated DNA of human herpesvirus-8 (HHV-8) in these lymphomas, which typically form in serous body cavities. Up to 70 percent of primary effusion lymphomas also show evidence of Epstein Barr virus (EBV).

Prisons

The United States has the second highest rate of incarceration in the world. Early reports indicate that 17 percent of people living with HIV/AIDS are reported to have spent time in the U.S. correctional system, where the prevalence rate of AIDS is six times higher than in the general public. However, at the 14th International AIDS Conference in Barcelona, Spain, in July 2002, the CDC presented data showing that of the 2,639 patients questioned 48 percent answered that they had been incarcerated at least once. Twelve percent of the patients in this group were initially diagnosed in a correctional facility.

CDC data from 1996 also show that 46,000–76,000 inmates had syphilis; 43,000 inmates had chlamydia infection; 18,000 inmates had gonorrhea; 36,000 inmates had hepatitis B, and 303,000–332,000 inmates had hepatitis C, a rate nine to 10 times higher than that in the general population.

Certain high-risk behaviors that are prevalent in correction facilities make prisoners more susceptible to HIV/AIDS. The geographic distribution of this risk is reported to be markedly uneven. Some prisons have HIV/AIDS rates as low as one percent and some institutions have HIV/AIDS rates that exceed 20 percent. In New York City, a voluntary test among the incarcerated population showed that 22 percent of female prisoners and nine percent of male prisoners were HIV-positive.

The Center for AIDS Prevention Studies at the University of California, San Francisco, reports that most HIV infected prisoners were HIV positive before entering jails and prisons. However, for those who are not yet HIV-positive, continued intravenous drug use, tattooing, and consensual sexual activity that occurs in prisons increase the risk of contracting HIV. Other high-risk activities, such as rape or coerced sex among inmates, also contribute to HIV transmission. The Federal Bureau of Prisons reports that up to 30 percent of federal inmates engage in homosexual activity while incarcerated. However, only four percent of jails, specifically the urban jail systems of New York, Washington, D.C., San Francisco, and Philadelphia, make condoms available to inmates. Ten percent of prison systems allow condom distribution.

The Office of National Drug Control Policy reports that 60 to 83 percent of inmates have used drugs at some time in their lives. Inmates who continue to inject drugs in prison are most likely to share needles. However, only 20 percent of prisons make bleach kits for sterilizing needles available.

The World Health Organization (WHO) supports the provision of voluntary, not mandatory, HIV testing for incarcerated populations that includes counseling both before and after the test. HIV testing is performed in 47 states if there is an indication of AIDS.

In a January 2003, press release, the CDC reported that 12 to 15 percent of all Americans with chronic hepatitis B virus and 39 percent of those with hepatitis C virus infections were released from a correctional facility during the previous year. The CDC recommendations include that all persons who have not been previously vaccinated receive vaccinations for hepatitis B. The recommendations also include medical evaluation for behavioral risk factor and testing for hepatitis C for inmates with risk factors. Those inmates who test positive for hepatitis C should be evaluated to determine the extent of their liver disease. Inmates with chronic hepatitis C should be evaluated for antiviral treatment, which should be considered based on criteria developed by each jurisdiction and incorporate current treatment guidelines. Substance abuse treatment is recommended for persons with chronic hepatitis B or C infection to limit disease transmission, reinfection and disease progression. The CDC also recommends that education regarding the prevention of viral hepatitis be incorporated into health education programs available for all correctional facility inmates.

Most states have their own regulations regarding HIV testing. Under a Florida bill passed in March 2002, Florida inmates whose HIV status is unknown will be tested for HIV before being released from prison. Positive test results are sent to the county where the inmate plans to reside.

CDC Issues Recommendations Designed to Prevent Hepatitis Infections in Correctional Settings. CDC Press Release, January 23, 2003.
Policy Facts: Incarcerated Populations and HIV/AIDS. AIDS Action: The Body: An AIDS and HIV Information Resource. http://www.thebody.com/aac/brochures/incarcerated.html.

Proctitis

Proctitis is a gastrointestinal syndrome that primarily occurs in persons who participate in anal intercourse. Proctitis is an inflammation limited to the outer 10–12 centimeters of the rectum. It is associated with anorectal pain, spasms, and rectal discharge. Infection is primarily with *Neisseria gonorrhoeae*, *Chlamydia trachomatis*, *Treponema pallidum* and Herpes simplex virus. Patients co-infected with the HSV virus may have particularly severe proctitis. Diagnosis is based on microscopic examination of the rectal discharge and treatment is specific to the particular infectious agent responsible for symptoms.

Proctolitis

Proctolitis is a sexually transmitted gastrointestinal syndrome with symptoms of proctitis plus diarrhea and/or abdominal cramps and inflammation of the colonic mucosa extending to 12 centimeters. Proctolitis occurs predominantly among persons who engage in anal intercourse and whose sexual practices include oral-fecal contact. Fecal examination shows the presence of white blood cells depending on the responsible infectious agent. Pathogenic organisms associated with proctolitis include *Campylobacter* species, *Shigella* species, *Entamoeba histolytica*, and rarely *Chlamydia trachomatis*. Cytomegalovirus or other opportunistic agents may be involved in patients co-infected with HIV who are immunosuppressed. Culture of a rectal swab is used to identify the responsible infectious agent, and treatment is specific to the particular infectious agent responsible for symptoms.

Progressive multifocal leukoencephalopathy (PML)

PML is a rapidly debilitating opportunistic infection caused by the JC virus that infects brain tissue and causes damage to the brain and the spinal cord. Symptoms vary from patient to patient, and include loss of muscle control, paralysis, blindness, problems with speech, and an altered mental state. PML can lead to coma and death.

Prostitution *see* Sex workers

Protease

Proteases are enzymes that trigger the breakdown of proteins into their component peptides. Proteases are naturally occurring chemicals. HIV's protease enzyme breaks apart long strands of viral protein into separate proteins, containing the viral core and the enzyme it contains. HIV protease acts as new virus particles are budding off a cell membrane. *See also* **Retrovirus replication.**

Protease inhibitors

Protease inhibitors are drugs that bind to and block HIV protease from working, interfering with HIV replication and preventing the production of new functional viral particles. Specifically, these drugs block the protease enzyme from breaking apart long strands of viral proteins to make the smaller, active HIV proteins that comprise the virion. If the larger HIV proteins are not broken apart, they cannot assemble themselves into new functional HIV particles. Discovered by Dr. David Ho, protease inhibitors, when used in combination with medications affecting other stages of viral replication, are effective at reducing viral load in patients with AIDS. The earliest protease inhibitors in the order of FDA approval, from first to last, include saquinavir (Invirase, Fortovase); ritonavir (Norvir); indinavir (Crixivan); nelfinavir (Viracept); amprenavir (Agenerase); and Lipinavir/ritonavir in a fixed dose (Kaletra).

Protease-sparing regimen

A protease-sparing regimen is an antiretroviral drug regimen that does not include a protease inhibitor.

Provirus

Provirus refers to viral genetic material, in the form of DNA that has been integrated into the host genome of the infected cell. HIV, when it is dormant in human cells, is in a proviral form.

P24 (p24)

P24 is a bullet-shaped core made of another protein that surrounds the viral RNA within the envelope of HIV. P24 appears in the blood shortly after HIV infection.

P24 antigen test

P24 is an HIV-1 core protein encoded by the *gag* gene. It is expressed shortly after acquisition of HIV-1, and antibody to p24 forms shortly thereafter. The p24 antigen, which may wane one to two weeks after infection, can be detected in serum, plasma, and cerebrospinal fluid using an ELISA technique. The sensitivity of the p24 antigen assay during acute HIV-1 infection is approximately 89 percent, with a specificity of 100 percent. False-positive results have been found in neonates younger than one month, making tests for HIV-1 proviral DNA more useful for diagnosing HIV infection in newborns, an instance in which HIV antibody tests are not useful because of the possibility of the temporary presence of maternal HIV antibodies.

Before the introduction of tests to measure plasma HIV-1 RNA, the p24 antigen test was used as a prognostic tool. Levels of p24 antigen were found to reappear or increase in HIV-1-infected patients shortly before or during the development of AIDS. This test was also useful in measuring the response to anti-retroviral therapy. Although it is not FDA-approved as a diagnostic test, p24 antigen testing has played a role in diagnosing acute HIV infection and HIV infection in infants born to mothers who are HIV-infected. Measurement of serum p24 antigen may be useful during the serologic window period before antibodies to HIV-1 become detectable.

Pubic lice (*Pediculus pubis*)

Pubic lice (pediculosis or crabs) is an infectious disease caused by the parasite *Pediculus pubis*. Pubic lice are not the same as body lice, which commonly infest hair. Pubic lice need blood to survive, but they are capable of living off a human body for up to 24 hours. Pubic lice have three distinct phases: the egg, the nit, and the louse. The louse is the parasite responsible for itching.

Epidemiology

In the United States there are an estimated three million cases of crabs annually.

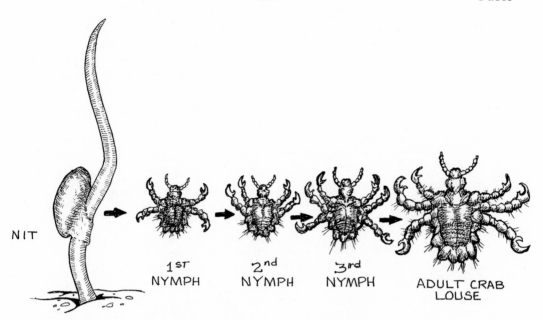

Life cycle of pubic lice (Marvin G. Miller).

Pubic lice are transmitted by skin-to-skin contact with another person. Even in the absence of sexual penetration, public lice can be transmitted. Non-sexual transmission of pubic lice can occur. It is possible to get pubic lice from sleeping in an infested bed, using infested towels, wearing infested clothing, and possibly from an infested toilet seat.

Symptoms

The most common symptom of pubic lice is itching or pruritis in the pubic area. Itching is caused by an allergic reaction to the bites and usually occurs about five days after the initial infestation.

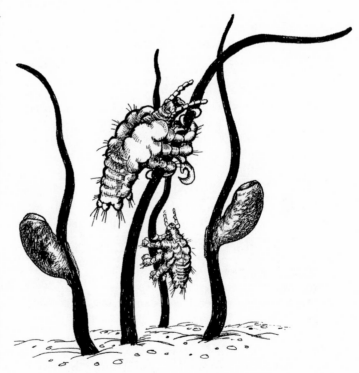

Pubic lice and nits (crabs) (Marvin G. Miller).

Diagnosis

Pubic lice are visible to the naked eye and are seen as small crab-like parasites that may be whitish-gray or rust colored.

Eggs, sometimes called nits, are small and oval-shaped. They become attached to the base of the hair follicle. While the prime target is the pubic area, pubic lice may also be found in armpits, eyelashes, beards, mustaches and rarely in scalp hair. Skin near the infested area may have blue colored spots caused by bites. Patients are usually able to determine if they have pubic lice, but they can see a health care provider if they are uncertain.

Treatment

Pubic lice may be treated with permethrin, which is applied as a cream rinse and left on for 10 minutes and then rinsed. Another option is pyrethrins with piperonyl butoxide, which is also applied to the affected area and left on for 10 minutes. Alternately, lindane (Kwell) may be used, although it cannot be used in pregnancy or on children younger than two years. All clothing and bedding must be washed in hot water to prevent recurrences. Clothes and other items that cannot be washed can be sealed in a plastic bag for two weeks at which time they are considered decontaminated.

Risk Factors

Risk factors include multiple sex partners and having sex with people who have pubic lice. It is important to notify all sexual partners so that they can be treated.

Public policy issues

Public health and public policy go hand in hand. In the 18th century, public health organizations patrolled port cities at the eastern seaboard. Their duties involved quarantining persons suspected of having communicable disease. They also regulated graveyards, tanneries, and slaughterhouses.

In the 19th century more stringent regulations for quarantine were implemented due to the threat of yellow fever and cholera. In 1864, the Council of Public Health and Hygiene was formed to investigate tenement housing congestion, slaughterhouse conditions, sewage drainage, dumps, and slums.

Public officials who studied diseases soon learned the importance of gathering statistics, and the Civil War helped emphasize the importance of containing epidemics when two-thirds of the Union soldiers' deaths resulted from infections. Public policies relating to health were born of necessity rather than as a means to punish those who were ill.

In the great depression, the New Deal and Social Security Act granted old-age benefits, unemployment insurance and public health service. In 1935, the federal government set aside funds for public health education and began awarding grants to be used toward the study and treatment of maternal and child services, venereal diseases, tuberculosis, mental health, industrial hygiene, and dental services. Twenty-five states and territories have general provisions in their public health codes, most passed before 1930 that make it a crime to expose any other person to a communicable or sexually transmitted disease. Twenty of the 25 states define the crime as a misdemeanor. To see which states criminalize STD transmission, see the HIV Criminal Law and Policy Project at http://www.hivcriminallaw.org/laws/std.cfm.

During the 1950s, funds to maintain public health agencies were reduced. Duties of public health officers were limited to well-child care, tuberculosis clinics, STD clinics, and immunization clinics. During the 1960s, the trend changed and public health became more of a focus. The Social Security Act of 1965 established Medicare and Medicaid. During the Reagan Era of the 1980s, federal funding was reduced and block grants were created. These resulted in significant cuts in existing programs. The AIDS epidemic grew and tuberculosis became a serious public health threat.

From the start of the AIDS epidemic, politicians decided that states would provide care and treatment services while the federal government focused on finding a cure and a vaccine. The role of the federal government also includes measures to help with the global relief effort. With the added expenses of war and an unstable economy, Congress holds a tight rein on federal spending.

Despite recommendations by more than 60 AIDS and STD organizations, the federal government spends more than $100 million dollars annually on abstinence-only education, and the Bush administration continues to push for these programs. In February 2002, more than 70 groups, including Human Rights Watch, SIECUS, and Planned Parenthood, signed letters urging President Bush to reconsider his decision to support only abstinence-only sex education programs. For specific information on public policy decisions and proposals that affect STDs and HIV, see http://www.hivdent.org/publicp/pubpolicy.htm, http://www.amfar.org, http://www.kaiser network.org/dailyreports/hiv and http://www.ncsl.org/programs/health/pp/aids mainpg.htm.

Pulmonary lymphoid hyperplasia (PHL)

PHL is a focal pulmonary disorder related to an infiltration of lymphocytes into lung tissue. PHL is often seen with lymphoid interstitial pneumonitis, which causes a similar disease with a more diffuse infiltration of lung tissue (PHL-LIP). PHL initially causes nodular infiltrates that may progress to an illness characterized by chronic cough and a progressive lowering of blood oxygen level (hypoxemia) that entails a typical clubbing of the fingers similar to that seen in the initial ascent to high altitudes. PHL has an association with the Epstein-Barr virus (EBV). Children with PHL frequently show high titers of EBV antigen.

Other symptoms include enlarged lymph nodes and salivary glands. PHL is associated with a higher survival rate in children compared to that caused by *Pneumocystis jiroveci* infection. Conditions of PHL-LIP

are less likely to cause fever. PHL often improves with antiretroviral therapy either as a direct result of EBV eradication or from immune system improvement.

Quantitative RNA (QRNA) test

The presence of viral RNA can be used to detect specific viral diseases. Researchers at Emory University School of Medicine in Atlanta studied 156 HIV-exposed non-breast-fed infants, comparing QRNA testing with DNA testing using PCR or ELISA/ Western blot testing for the diagnosis of HIV infections. Researchers report there was no difference in the sensitivity and specificity of QRNA and DNA results overall. In addition, results were concordant at least 88 percent of the time. Although false positive results may occur, QRNA may be most useful as a confirmatory test in infants who have tested positive with another testing method.

Daily Newsbriefs.
Medical Laboratory Observer, March 12, 2003.

Quinolones

Quinolones represent a class of synthetic broad-spectrum antimicrobial agents, such as ciprofloxacin, which are used for the systemic treatment of infection. The safety of quinolones in pediatric patients, pregnant women, and lactating women has not been established. In animal studies, some quinolone class drugs have been found to cause lesions and erosions of the cartilage of weight-bearing joints.

Rarely, patients may occasionally exhibit potentially fatal hypersensitivity reactions following the first dose of quinolone therapy. Some of these reactions may be accompanied by cardiovascular collapse, loss of consciousness, tingling, pharyngeal or facial edema, dyspnea (shortness of breath), and itching. The condition of pseudo-membranous colitis has been reported with nearly all antibacterial agents, including those of the quinolone class, and is often related to overgrowth of *Clostridium difficile* bacteria. Achilles and other tendon ruptures requiring surgical repair or causing disability have been reported with ciprofloxacin and other antibiotics.

Convulsions, increased intracranial (within the brain) pressure, and toxic psychosis have also been reported in patients receiving quinolones. Other side effects include dizziness, nightmares, nervousness, agitation, insomnia, anxiety, paranoia, tremors, hallucinations, and depression. Quinolones may also cause moderate to severe phototoxicity, which may cause an exaggerated sunburn reaction in patients exposed to direct sunlight during drug therapy. Quinolones should not be simultaneously administered to patients using theophylline or medications containing caffeine.

Racial & ethnic minorities *see* Health Disparities Initiative

Rapid HIV tests

One of the drawbacks to traditional antibody screening tests for HIV is the length of time for the test to be performed. For this reason, a number of rapid HIV-1 and HIV-1/2 antibody tests have been developed that provide results within 20 minutes or less. Rapid results are important in occupational exposures, and in public clinics and emergency rooms where patients may not return for results. The Single Use Diagnostic System (SUDS) test was the first rapid HIV test to be approved for hospital use, although it has since been removed from the market. The rapid tests with FDA approval as of June 2003, include the OraQuick rapid HIV-1 antibody assay and the MedMira Reveal Rapid HIV-1 antibody test.

In April 2003, the Food and Drug Administration categorized the OraQuick rapid HIV-1 antibody assay as waived under CLIA '88 regulations. With this new categorization, all 180,000-plus CLIA-registered test sites, including those with certificates of waiver, will now be able to perform the OraQuick rapid HIV test. Individual state laws will ultimately determine whether small CLIA laboratories associated with clinics and doctors' offices can perform these tests.

Tests for performing HIV testing on urine were also approved in 2003, including Calypte Biomedical's HIV-1 Urine Western Blot test and its HIV-1 urine EIA test. These tests are also approved for use in CLIA laboratories.

Receptors

Receptors are protein molecules located on the surface of a cell that serve as recognition or binding sites for antigens, antibodies, hormones, drugs, or other cellular or immunological components. These agents cause activity by reacting with cell receptors.

Regulatory genes

HIV has three regulatory genes, *tat*, *rev*, and *nef*, and three so-called auxiliary genes, *vif*, *vpr* and *vpu*, that contain essential information for the production of proteins that regulate the ability of HIV to infect a cell, produce new copies of the virus, or cause disease.

Reiki

The National Center for Complementary and Alternative Medicine (NCCAM) is conducting clinical trials to investigate the use of Reiki, an energy-based complementary and alternative medicine intervention, as an approach to improve well being for patients with advanced AIDS. The study, which ended in September 2003, is also evaluating the effects of Reiki on dimensions of well being and quality of life. The study, centered in Philadelphia, consisted of 146 patients with advanced AIDS.

The study compares patients using medical treatment alone to patients using medical treatment and three one-hour Reiki sessions over a period of six weeks. This is one segment of a large NCCAM study designed to evaluate the use of complementary medicine in advanced AIDS.

Reiter's syndrome (Reiter's disease)

Reiter's syndrome or disease is an autoimmune arthritic condition that occurs after exposure to certain infectious organisms that cause urethritis, including several organisms that cause STDs. The pathology in Reiter's syndrome is incompletely understood. Reiter's syndrome usually develops after infection involving a mucosal surface, such as the urethra or mouth, and persists even after the infectious organism has been eradicated. Reiter's syndrome is characterized by a triad of urethritis (nor related to gonorrhea), arthritis, and skin manifestations that consist of keratoderma (skin thickening), balantitis, and oral ulcerations.

Etiology

Infectious organisms that have been implicated in the immunological response that leads to Reiter's syndrome include *Chlamydia trachomatis, Shigella flexneri, Salmonella* species, *Yersinia enterocolitica*, and *Campylobacter* species, and perhaps *Neisseria gonorrhoeae*, the genital mycoplasmas, or other organisms. In several studies, up to 50 percent of men with Reiter's syndrome had documented genital *Chlamydia trachomatis* infections. Antibodies to chlamydia are commonly seen in Reiter's, usually in higher titer than in patients with uncomplicated chlamydial infection. There have also been reports of Reiter's syndrome after successful treatment of gonorrhea.

Epidemiology

Reiter's syndrome typically has an endemic form, usually sexually acquired and a less common epidemic form, most often associated with enteric infection. Reiter's syndrome usually follows sexual contact with a new partner, although sexual transmission of Reiter's syndrome has not been proven. Enteric Reiter's syndrome may occur in children following infectious diarrhea, although it most often occurs in adults. Nonspecific rheumatic complaints haven been seen in women with Reiter's syndrome who had histories of salpingitis, gonorrhea, bacterial urinary-tract infection, and trichomoniasis. In one study of patients hospitalized with acute arthritis, 11 percent were found to have Reiter's syndrome. In the general population, Reiter's disease has a prevalence of 0.04 to 0.06 percent. In HIV positive individuals the prevalence ranges from 0.5 to 10 percent. Up to 30 percent of people with Reiter's syndrome have an underlying active infection.

Reiter's syndrome, like most autoimmune disorders, has a genetic component. Individuals with the HLA-B27 haplotype, which is associated with the arthritic condition ankylosing spondylitis, are more likely to develop Reiter' syndrome. HLA-B27 is found in 70 to 80 percent of white patients with Reiter's syndrome, although HLA-B27 only occurs in about six to eight percent of the white population. Among African-Americans, 15 to 75 percent of persons with Reiter's syndrome have HLA-B27. HLA-B57 is seen in about 12 percent of the African-American population. In one small study of patients with Reiter's syndrome, seven of 10 patients who were HLA-B27 negative had HLA antigens that cross-reacted with B27, such as B7, BW22, and BW42.

Other genes are likely involved, because studies show that only 25 percent of men with nongonococcal urethritis who have HLA-B27 go on to develop Reiter's syndrome. Of those who do, symptoms are generally initially more severe than the symptoms of patients who do not have HLA-B27 antigen.

Symptoms

Although it is often associated with disseminated gonococcal infection (DGI) and the reactive arthritis it causes, Reiter's syndrome is a distinct arthritic disorder and may be accompanied or followed by conjunctivitis or mucocutaneous lesions. Clinically, Reiter's syndrome is associated with acute arthritis, lower-urogenital-tract inflammation, conjunctivitis, and mucocutaneous inflammatory lesions. Most patients eventually develop all four features, especially if they are HLA-B27 positive, although it is rare to see all four of these conditions at initial presentation.

Patients frequently report having recently had sexual intercourse with a new partner, followed by the development of urethritis. Urethritis related to gonorrhea occurs in up to 20 percent of these patients. Urethritis occurs in up to 90 percent of patients with enteric Reiter's syndrome. Urethritis may also occur in children and adults who are not sexually active who develop Reiter's after enteric infection (usually with Yersinia, Shigella, Salmonella, or Campylobacter). Genital inflammation in Reiter's is not necessarily sexually acquired, especially when reactive arthritis follows diarrhea.

Arthritis in Reiter's syndrome typically affects many joints and tendons. This is followed by persistence of signs and symptoms in a few specific joints. Arthritis usually begins in the knees, ankles, and feet. Mucocutaneous lesions are common in sexually acquired Reiter's syndrome and in reactive arthritis following infection with shigella. Lesions known as keratoderma blennorrhagica begin as reddened flat lesions and plaques, sometimes with red halos and central clearing, primarily affecting the feet and palms of the hands. In up to 30 percent of patients, especially those with the sexually acquired form of Reiter's syndrome, shallow, painless ulcers frequently occur on the tongue, lips, roof of the mouth, or throat. The fingernails in Reiter's may become thickened with brown-yellow discoloration. Conjunctivitis occurs in half of the cases that are sexually acquired and up to 90 percent of cases that follow shigella infection.

Acute Reiter's syndrome causes malaise, fever, anorexia, and weight loss. It may cause changes in heart rhythm, myocarditis, pericarditis, and rarely congestive heart failure.

Diagnosis

Diagnosis is made by a combination of laboratory tests. The erythrocyte sedimentation rate (ESR, sed rate) is elevated, exceeding 50 mm/hour in nearly half of patients. The white blood cell count is usually elevated, up to 20,000 leukocytes/mm^3. Anemia may be present; antinuclear antibodies, rheumatoid factor, cryoglobulins, C-reactive protein, or circulating immune complexes are occasionally present.

Treatment

Without treatment, most episodes of Reiter's syndrome resolve completely within two to six months, although in about 35 percent of cases, symptoms

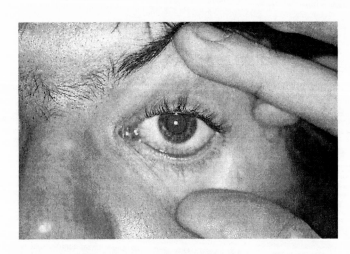

Conjunctivitis in Reiter's syndrome (Joe Miller, CDC).

persist for up to one year. Recurrences may occur. Treatment includes treating any known infectious disease process and ameliorative treatment for symptoms of arthritis.

Rice, Peter, and H. Handsfield. "Arthritis Associated with Sexually Transmitted Diseases." Chapter 68 in *Sexually Transmitted Diseases*. 3rd edition. Edited by King K. Holmes, et al. New York: McGraw-Hill, 1999.

Reportable diseases

All states require that healthcare institutions (laboratories and physicians primarily) report all cases of syphilis, gonorrhea, and HIV/AIDS to state health departments. In some states, healthcare workers report these infections to the county health department, which passes them on to the state office. Some states require reporting of other STDs, such as hepatitis.

The accurate identification and timely reporting of STDs are integral components of disease control efforts. Timely reporting assists in the assessment of morbidity trends, targets areas where resources may be limited, and assists local health authorities in identifying sex partners who may be infected. STD/HIV and AIDS cases should be reported in accordance with local statutory requirements. All reports of STDs remain in strict confidence. In most jurisdictions, these reports are protected by statute from subpoena. Before public health representatives conduct follow-up of a positive STD test result, these persons should consult the patient's primary health-care provider to verify the diagnosis and treatment.

Reproduction

Reproduction is the process in which individuals produce new individuals of the same species. Reproduction can occur as a sexual process (in human beings and other primates) or as an asexual process in bacteria and viruses), which is also called replication.

Reproductive organs

In humans, both males and females have several reproductive organs that serve to produce various hormones and proteins necessary for reproduction and successful pregnancy.

Retrovir *see* Zidovudine

Retrovirus replication

The retroviral life cycle is the key to its ability to survive. Retroviruses contain viral RNA along with several copies of the enzyme reverse transcriptase (DNA polymerase). The following steps show how the HIV virus is replicated.

1. The first step in replication is attachment or entry. Here, the virus attaches to CD4+ surface markers on white blood cells and enters the cell. Infection typically begins when an HIV particle, which contains two copies of the HIV RNA, encounters a cell with a surface molecule called cluster designation 4 (CD4). One or more of the virus's gp120 molecules binds tightly to the CD4 molecules on the host cell's surface. While CD4+ T cells are the main target, other immune system cells such as monocytes and macrophages that have CD4+ surface markers may also be infected. Monocytes and macrophages are long-lived cells that may harbor the HIV virus in a stable, inactive form after they have been infected.

2. After infecting a cell, HIV reverse transcriptase, working within the host cell's cytoplasm, is used to make the initial copies of viral DNA from viral RNA. DNA is the nucleic acid form of the virus in which the cell carries its genes. Once a DNA strand has been synthesized, a complementary strand of viral DNA (cDNA) is produced.

3. These double strand copies of viral DNA are transported into the host cell nucleus.

4. The new DNA is then integrated with the host cell's DNA. The newly made HIV DNA is spliced into the host's DNA with the help of the enzyme HIV integrase. Once incorporated into the cell's genes, HIV DNA is called a "provirus."

5. Through a process of transcription, new copies of the viral RNA are produced from the provirus. Host cell RNA polymerase is used to make this virus-related RNA. These RNA strands serve as templates for making new copies of the viral chromosomal RNA, and they also serve as messenger RNA (mRNA). Messenger RNA is then translated into viral proteins that are used to form the retroviral envelope. New viral particles are then assembled and released from the cell's plasma membrane. Proteins known as cytokines that are released during the immune response may also regulate transcription. The cytokines, tumor necrosis factor (TNF) alpha and interleukin (IL)-6, secreted in elevated levels by the immune system cells of persons with HIV infection, may help to activate HIV proviruses.

6. Viral proteins are then produced. After HIV mRNA is processed in the host cell's nucleus, it is transported to the cytoplasm. HIV proteins encoded by HIV genes are critical to this process. For instance, the gene rev allows HIV structural proteins encoding mRNA to be transferred from the cell nucleus to the cytoplasm. If the rev gene is defective, structural proteins cannot be produced.

7. The virus is then assembled. Components of the virus gather near the cell membrane and combine or form by a "pinching" action of the cell membrane.

8. The newly created virus then buds off from the host cell.

9. The virus matures as long strands of viral RNA and protein are cleaved or split into smaller segments by protease enzymes. *See also* **Assembly and budding.**

Retroviruses

Retroviruses belong to a class of viruses that synthesize viral DNA from an RNA template. When not infecting cells, retroviruses store their genetic information on a single-stranded RNA molecule instead of the usual double-stranded DNA molecule. HIV is an example of a retrovirus. After a retrovirus penetrates a cell, it constructs a DNA version of its genes using a special enzyme, reverse transcriptase. This DNA then becomes part of the infected cell's genetic material. The reverse flow of genetic information that characterizes retroviruses is not unique to this viral class.

Retroviruses are divided into seven distinct genera, and humans have been infected by viruses from several of these genera. The family of retroviruses include the primate lentiviruses, which include HIV-1, HIV-2, HIV-O and SIV; the human T-cell leukemia virus (HTLV-1), which causes adult T-cell leukemia and tropical spastic paraparesis/HTLV-associated myelopathy (HAM); HTLV-2, which is possibly associated with hairy cell leukemia; Rous sarcoma virus (RSV); Genus Gammaretrovirus, which includes mouse mammary tumor virus (MMTV); and murine leukemia virus (MLV).

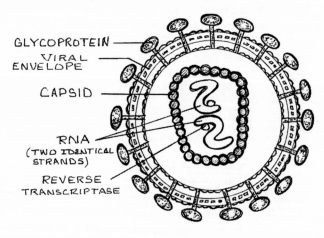

GLYCOPROTEIN

VIRAL ENVELOPE

CAPSID

RNA (TWO IDENTICAL STRANDS)

REVERSE TRANSCRIPTASE

Retrovirus (Marvin G. Miller).

Rev (*rev*)

Rev is a regulatory gene of HIV needed for the virus's ability to infect host cells, replicate and cause disease.

Reverse transcriptase

Reverse transcriptase is a uniquely viral enzyme that constructs DNA from an RNA template. This ability to construct DNA is an essential step in the life cycle of a retrovirus such as HIV, and depends on the presence of reverse transcriptase. The RNA based genes of HIV and other retroviruses must be converted to DNA if they are to integrate into the cellular genome. Some antiviral drugs approved by the FDA for the treatment of HIV infection work by interfering with this stage of the retroviral life cycle. *See also* **Retrovirus replication.**

Reverse transcriptase inhibitors

Reverse transcriptase inhibitors represent a class of anti-retroviral drugs used in the treatment of HIV infection. Reverse transcriptase inhibitors include nucleoside and nucleotide analog reverse transcriptase inhibitors (NRTIs), which act as chain terminators when incorporated into proviral DNA, and nonnucleoside reverse transcriptase inhibitors (NNRTIs), which interfere with enzyme function.

In the order of FDA approval, the early NNRTs include zidovudine (Retrovir); didanosine (Videx); zalcitabine (Hivid); lamivudine (Epivir); stavudine (Zerit); abacavir (Ziagen); tenofovir (Viread); and fixed dose combinations such as zidovudine and lamivudine (Combivir), and fixed dose zidovudine, abacavir, and lamivudine (Trizivir).

In the order of FDA approval, the early NNRTs include nevirapine (Viramune), efavirenz (Sustiva), and delaviridine (Rescriptor).

Ribonucleic acid (RNA)

Ribonucleic acid is a type of messenger protein used in the intermediate steps leading to DNA production. RNA is primarily found in the cell cytoplasm. Retroviruses, such as HIV, carry RNA instead of the more usual genetic material DNA and use the enzyme reverse transcriptase to replicate RNA into DNA. The presence of viral RNA can be used to diagnose infection. For instance, quantitative RNA (QRNA) can be used to diagnose infection in HIV-exposed infants, although false-positive results are possible. *See also* **HIV-1 RNA** and **Viral load.**

Ricord, Phillipe (1799–1889)

A French physician specializing in the treatment of venereal diseases, Ricord established the specificity of gonorrhea and syphilis. Prior to Ricord's discovery, gonorrhea was considered a manifestation of syphilis and not a separate disease. Ricord is also known for differentiating the primary, secondary, and tertiary stages of syphilis infection.

Risk factor

A risk factor is a behavior or characteristic (physical, social, or epidemiological) that places a person at risk for a specific disease. For most STDs, unprotected sex, multiple sex partners, and commercial sex work are risk factors. For HIV and hepatitis, injection drug use is also a risk factor. A complete list of risk factors for specific STDs, such as HIV, is included in the specific STD sections.

Rural areas

To address HIV and related health concerns of rural and underserved communities, the Health Resources and Services Administration's Bureau of Primary Health Care has created community health centers that provide health screening, counseling, and treatment services.

Ryan White *see* White, Ryan

Ryan White Comprehensive AIDS Resources Emergency Act (Ryan White CARE Act or the CARE Act)

The goal of this federal act is to improve the quality and availability of care for individuals and families affected by HIV/AIDS. The act achieves its goal by funding primary health care and support services that enhance access and retention in care. Current legislation related to the CARE law is designed to address the unmet health needs of persons living with HIV diseases (PLWH).

This law was originally enacted in 1990 under Public Law 101-381. It was reauthorized on May 20, 1996, under Public Law 104-146 and again in 2000. This act was named after Ryan Wayne White, a teenager with hemophilia who contracted HIV through a blood transfusion. He died in 1990 at the age of 18 after courageously giving testimony to the needs of people with AIDS and the need for HIV/AIDS public awareness and education.

The CARE act is intended to help communities and states increase the availability of primary health care and support services, increase access to care for underserved populations, and improve the quality of life of those affected by the epidemic. The act also has provisions for the treatment and care of emergency response workers, medical case management, clinical training, and patient outreach.

Title I of the act provides emergency funding to localities disproportionately affected by HIV/AIDS. Title II provides formula funding to each state and eligible territory to improve the quality, availability, and organization of health and support services for people and families living with HIV/AIDS. Title III(b) supports early intervention in clinical settings such as community and migrant health centers, health care for the homeless programs, and Native Hawaiian health programs, including projects to organize and coordinate a broad range of medical, social, and support services for children, youth, women, and families with HIV/AIDS, and provides enhanced access to clinical research. Title IV supports services for women, children, adolescents, and families affected by the HIV epidemic, including the Dental Reimbursement Program.

Part F of the act supports Special Projects of National Significance (SPNC) which advance the knowledge and skills in the delivery of HIV health care and support services, including education and training for health care providers. Each state has a service directory listing funded services and agencies for their communities.

The CARE Act reaches more than 500,000 individuals each year, making it the federal government's largest program specifically for people living with HIV disease. Programs funded by the CARE Act are the payer of last resort, in that they fill gaps in care not covered by other resources. Most likely users of CARE Act services include people with no other source of healthcare and those with Medicaid or private insurance whose care needs are not being met.

CARE Act services are intended to reduce the use of more costly inpatient care, increase access to care for underserved populations, and improve the quality of life for those affected by the epidemic. The CARE Act works toward these goals by funding local and state programs that provide primary medical care and support services, healthcare provider training, and technical assistance to help funded programs address implementation and emerging HIV care issues. The CARE Act also provides for significant local and state control of HIV/AIDS healthcare planning and service delivery. For more information, see http://hab.hrsa.gov/care.html.

Salpingitis

Salpingitis is a condition of infection of the fallopian tubes. Salpingitis is one of the most serious complications of pelvic inflammatory disease (PID), and some doctors refer to salpingitis and PID as if they are the same disorder. However, salpingitis only occurs in about two-thirds of all women with PID.

Several different infectious agents can cause salpingitis, including *Chlamydia trachomatis, Neisseria gonorrhoeae,* and *Mycoplasma hominis.* Studies show that women infected with chlamydia who are between 15 and 19 are 70 percent more likely to develop salpingitis than women between the ages of 20 and 24. Women with gonorrhea who are between 15 and 19 are 20 percent less likely to develop salpingitis than women between the ages of 20 and 24.

At the end of the 19th century, physicians discovered that salpingitis could result in infertility. The surgical procedure of laparoscopy is usually used to diagnose salpingitis accurately.

The organisms responsible for salpingitis are generally transmitted through sexual intercourse, but these bacteria, if present in the genital tract, can be transmitted into the endometrial cavity through various medical procedures, including dilation and curettage, induced abortion, intrauterine device (IUD) insertion, and imaging studies (hysterosalpingography). Changes in levels of sex steroids affect the protective cervical mucus plug. Combination oral contraceptives appear to offer protection against salpingitis because of their influence on estrogen and progesterone levels. Progesterone, in particular, offers protection against ascending infection.

Safe sex

The term safe sex refers to certain precautions that reduce the risk of contracting sexually transmitted diseases.

Limiting the number of sex partners an individual has reduces the risk of STD transmission. A monogamous relationship reduces risk. It is important to avoid sexual contact (both with and without penetration) with anyone whose medical history for STDs is uncertain. Even in individuals who have been tested, there are limitations to most tests, and the results only pertain to the date testing was completed.

Condoms protect against most STDs, but partners may have herpes or HPV in areas that are not covered by condoms. Condoms should be made of latex or polyurethane, and if possible a spermicide containing nonoxynol-9 should also be used to protect against some STDs. Women hesitant to insist on condoms need to be aware that most STDs are more harmful to women than men. Also, females have fewer obvious symptoms and a higher risk of serious health consequences.

Safe sex also includes not touching the genital organs of an individual infected with genital warts, herpes, molluscums, and chancroid. These diseases can be spread by touching, either genital-to-genital or hand/finger to genital. It is important to be aware of certain symptoms such as herpes blisters, warts, and genital ulcers.

Safe sex also includes an avoidance of drugs and alcohol in potentially intimate situations. These drugs can affect one's ability to make serious decisions. *See also* **Condoms** and **Risk factors.**

Salmonella

Salmonella is a family of gram-negative bacteria, found in undercooked poultry or eggs, which is a well known cause of food poisoning. Salmonella can also be transmitted as an enteric infection in anal sex, and it can cause serious disseminated disease in persons infected with HIV.

Salvarsan

In 1909 the Nobel laureate immunologist Paul Ehrlich (1854–1915) announced the discovery of the arsenic compound, Salvarsan, as a chemotherapeutic treatment for syphilis. This discovery was important because it was the first time a compound had been demonstrated to kill a specific organism, in this case, *Treponema pallidum*, the cause of syphilis.

However, Salvarsan was not the "magic bullet" Ehrlich described. Although the compound was effective, it was toxic, difficult to administer, and required a lengthy treatment regimen, sometimes as long as two years. Only about 25 percent of patients were able to complete treatment because of its toxic side effects. New arsenic compounds, the neo-arsphenamines, proved to be more effective. But until 1943 when the efficacy of penicillin was discovered, there were no safe and effective treatments for syphilis.

Sanru III Project

In 2000, the U.S. government began financing the Sanru III Project, which supports the provision of integrated health services in rural areas of the Congo. Phase I activities of the project focused on the distribution of medicines and medical equipment to health zones. Phase II is working to provide extensive training of rural health workers, create community-based polio surveillance programs, and upgrade the notification and supervisory systems in 53 health zones.

Sarcoptes scabiei

Sarcoptes scabiei (itch mite) is a parasite belonging to the class Arachnida. *Sarcoptes scabiei* infection causes the disorder scabies.

Scabies

Scabies in an infectious disease caused

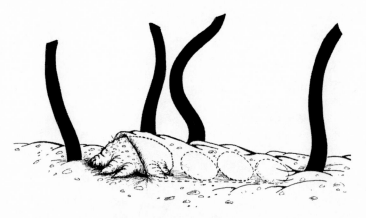

Scabies (Marvin G. Miller).

by infestation with the scabies mite, also known as the itch mite.

Etiology

Scabies is a highly contagious infestation caused by the itch mite *Sarcoptes scabiei*. The itch mite, like spiders, ticks, and chiggers, is most closely related to the dust mite. The scabies mite is a parasite that burrows into and resides and reproduces in human skin. Adult scabies mites have a body structure and short legs that facilitate entry into the skin. They have four pairs of legs and lay chiggers. Mites can move rapidly on the skin when choosing a site to burrow.

Epidemiology

Scabies is transmitted by intimate personal contact, often sexual in nature. Scabies may also be transmitted by casual contact, such as during care provided by health providers, which can result in institutional epidemics. Epidemics of scabies appear to cycle at approximately 10 to 30 year intervals. Scabies can occur in any population, but is least likely to occur in African-Americans. Among young adults, sexual transmission is the most likely method of infection.

Symptoms

Most individuals infested with the scabies mite complain of severe itching that is

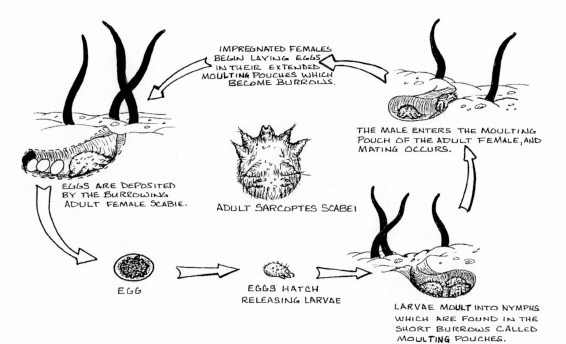

IMPREGNATED FEMALES BEGIN LAYING EGGS IN THEIR EXTENDED MOULTING POUCHES WHICH BECOME BURROWS.

THE MALE ENTERS THE MOULTING POUCH OF THE ADULT FEMALE, AND MATING OCCURS.

EGGS ARE DEPOSITED BY THE BURROWING ADULT FEMALE SCABIE.

ADULT SARCOPTES SCABEI

EGG

EGGS HATCH RELEASING LARVAE

LARVAE MOULT INTO NYMPHS WHICH ARE FOUND IN THE SHORT BURROWS CALLED MOULTING POUCHES.

Scabies life cycle (Marvin G. Miller).

usually more intense at night. Skin lesions occur in the form of reddened papules, burrows, and open sores. Mite burrows concentrate on the hands and wrists, but they can also be found on axillary folds, breasts, the umbilical area, and the penis. Reddened papules and blisters may also develop between the fingers and toes and on abdominal skin, the pelvic girdle, and ankles. Burrows may be clearly visible on the wrist and elbows, whereas lesions on other parts of the body are usually papular, nodular, or crusted.

Patients with HIV/AIDS are at special risk for scabies and generally develop crusted lesions. Although scabies rarely involves the face and scalp in patients without HIV infection, patients with HIV/AIDS frequently develop lesions in these areas.

Secondary infections, generally with *Staphylococcus aureus* bacteria, may develop over the infested area, obscuring the lesions. The skin surrounding lesions may become eczematous, probably as a result of sensitivity to the scabies mite.

Diagnosis

Examination revealing visible burrows on the hands is diagnostic for scabies. Lesions can also be scraped and examined microscopically for the presence of mites, eggs, and fecal pellets.

Treatment

Scabies is generally treated with weekly applications of scabecides, such as lindane or permethrin, using one to several applications. The CDC recommends treatment with five percent permethrin cream applied topically. The cream should be massaged in the skin from head to feet using approximately 30 gm for an adult, and it should be washed off after 8–14 hours. Patients may experience burning of the skin and increased itching after application. Patients should be advised that itching may persist for days or weeks after successful treatment. This may be a result of hypersensitivity to fecal pellets, and may require treatment with an antihistamine.

Alternatively, lindane cream (one percent) using one ounce of lotion of 30 grams of cream can be applied in a thin layer to all areas of the body from the neck down and thoroughly washed off after eight hours. Lindane can be toxic, especially when applied repeatedly to children or old persons, and should not be used in persons with extensive dermatitis or in pregnant or lactating women or children younger than two years old. Lindane applied after bathing may cause high blood levels and should not be used immediately after a bath or shower.

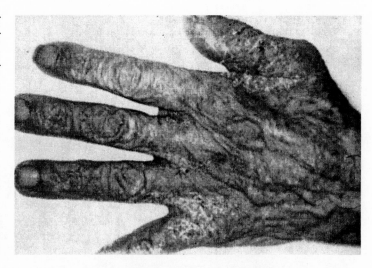

Hand with scabies eczema (Navy Environmental Health Center Training and Health Communication Branch).

Alternatively, the anti-parasitic agent ivermectin, using 200ug/kg orally, can be used once and repeated in two weeks. One study reported increased mortality among elderly, debilitated persons receiving ivermectin, but this observation has not been repeated in subsequent reports. In studies of AIDS patients with scabies, oral ivermectin was shown to be effective.

Weekly application of lindane over six weeks may be required for the crusted scabies seen in AIDS patients. When permethrin is used externally, concomitant use of a keratinolytic agent such as six percent salicylic acid is often recommended.

All sexual partners should also be treated. Although the scabies mite only survives for a short time outside the body, it can live briefly in bedding and clothing. Scabies mites are killed by washing in hot water.

Precautions

Patients with persistent symptoms may be inclined to extend or repeat treatment. This carries a risk of sensitization and contact eczema, that may be confused with scabies infestation.

Crusted scabies (Norwegian scabies) is an aggressive infestation that usually occurs in immunodeficient, debilitated, or malnourished persons. Persons who are receiving systemic or potent topical glucocorticoids, organ transplant recipients, HIV-infected persons, HTLV-1 infected persons, and persons with various malignancies are at risk for developing crusted scabies. Crusted scabies is associated with greater transmissibility than scabies. Lindane should be avoided because of risks of neurotoxicity with heavy applications and denuded skin.

Centers for Disease Control and Prevention. *Sexually Transmitted Diseases Treatment Guidelines 2002.* Atlanta: U.S. Dept. of Health and Human Services, 2002.

Platts-Mills, Thomas A.E., and Michael F. Rein. "Scabies." Chapter 47 in *Sexually Transmitted Diseases.* 3rd edition. Edited by King K. Holmes, et al. New York: McGraw-Hill, 1999.

Schaudinn, Fritz (1871–1906)

The protozoologist Fritz Schaudinn, along with Erich Hoffman, isolated *Treponema pallidum* as the infectious agent of syphilis in 1905.

Seroconversion

Seroconversion refers to the development of detectable antibodies to infectious agents, such as hepatitis and HIV, as a result of infection. It normally takes several weeks to several months for antibodies to the virus to develop after HIV transmission. When antibodies to HIV appear in the blood a person will test positive using the standard ELISA test for HIV.

Seroconversion window

Seroconversion window refers to the time between one's exposure to an infectious agent and the time in which one becomes seropositive (antibodies develop). During this seroconversion window, individuals can be infectious although their blood tests are negative. In some infectious diseases, including HIV, there is also a post-conversion window, in which patients no longer have detectable antibodies.

Serology

Serology refers to the study of serum, the liquid portion of blood. Serology tests are used to detect antibodies, proteins, and other specific disease markers.

Seropositive

Individuals with antibodies to specific infectious organisms are said to be seropositive. For instance, when individuals exposed to HIV develop antibodies to HIV, demonstrated by a positive HIV antibody test, these individuals are said to be seropositive for HIV. This shows that they have been previously exposed to the infectious agent. As a consequence, their immune systems produced antibodies, which are present in the blood.

However, antibodies are not immediately detectable, so a window exists in which individuals may have been exposed to an infectious agent but are not yet seropositive. During this window, the individual who has been exposed to an infectious agent but has not yet developed measurable antibodies can infect others. Since 1999, when blood tests for HIV became highly sensitive, there have been two instances in which individuals contracted HIV after receiving blood from donors who had been exposed to HIV but were not yet seropositive. On future blood donations, these donors tested positive. *See also* **Antibody-positive** and **Seroconversion window**.

Sex education

The World Health Organization (WHO) has conducted comprehensive reviews of the scientific literature on sex and AIDS education. In 1993, WHO reported that there was no of evidence of sex education leading to earlier or increased sexual activity in the young people who were exposed to it. In fact, six studies showed that sex education led to either a delay in the onset of sexual activity or to a decrease in overall sexual activity. Ten studies showed that education programs increased safer sex practices among young people who were already sexually active.

In 1995, the Office of Technology Assessment (OTA), at the request of the 103rd Congress, examined the effectiveness of prevention programs and found no scientific evidence that curricula focusing only on abstinence delay the onset of sexual intercourse. The report concluded that discussions of abstinence and contraception in combination with other topics such as resistance skills, do not lead to earlier initiation of sex, and in fact, result in lowered incidence of sexual intercourse in some cases.

Sex workers

Sex workers are individuals (women, men, or children) who exchange sexual services for an immediate cash or in-kind return such as drugs. Sex work takes many different forms in different societies and nations, and includes highly paid call girls, slum prostitutes, and Japanese geishas. Sex work may be viewed in some cultures as the only means for a family's economic survival. Despite their differences, all sex workers, or prostitutes, along with their clients form a group of individuals whose members are at highest risk of acquiring and transmitting sexually transmitted diseases.

Until the beginning of the 20th century, STDs were generally considered to spread almost exclusively through prostitution. Restrictions to control prostitution served the purpose of controlling STDs. The high level of condom use and medical examinations among sex workers in developed countries is directly related to a lower level of HIV infection when compared to sex workers of low socioeconomic status in developing countries. Prostitutes in Africa have an extremely high incidence of HIV infection. The annual HIV incidence among female sex workers is also very high, ranging from 24 to 29 percent. Genital inflammation and genital tract infections are also thought to increase HIV shedding, making sex workers with HIV more infectious to sexual partners.

The use of preventive antibiotics among sex workers has contributed to the development of strains of *Neisseria gonorrhoeae* resistant to antimicrobial agents, particularly penicillin.

Programs designed to reduce STD transmission by regulating sex work must be made on an individual basis, taking the economic and sociological reasons for sex work of the particular community into consideration. Effective STD control programs also focus on preventive measures and prompt detection and treatment for those infected with STDs.

Researchers at the Department of Sociology and Human Geography at the University of Oslo in Norway conducted a study of adolescents reported to sell sexual favors. The study found that three times

as many adolescent boys or girls sold sex, and most were under the age of 16. The researchers concluded that adolescents who take part in these activities are often heavily involved in delinquent behaviors and abuse drugs and that they are at risk for STDs as well as delinquent and criminal development.

Pedersen, W., and K. Hegna. "Children and adolescents who sell sex: a community study." *Social Science and Medicine*, Jan. 2003; 56(1):135–147.

Sexual assault

Survivors of sexual assault should be examined by an experienced clinician. Samples of hair, blood, urine, and scrapings can be used to test for STDs and DNA. These reports are then available if charges are filed. Laws in all 50 states strictly limit the evidentiary use of a survivor's prior sexual history, including evidence of previously acquired STDs. Patients should also be offered counseling in a way that minimizes further trauma. Results of tests that can be performed immediately can help the clinician decide what, if any, prophylactic treatment is needed.

The CDC reports that trichomoniasis, bacterial vaginosis, gonorrhea, and chlamydial infection are the most frequently diagnosed infections among women who have been sexually assaulted. Because the prevalence of these infections is high among sexually active women, their presence after an assault does not necessarily signify that these conditions resulted from the assault. Initial examinations should include cultures for *N. gonorrhoeae* and *C. trachomatis*, and NAT testing for these organisms. Blood should be tested for HIV, hepatitis B, and syphilis, and genital swabs should be collected for Trichomonas.

Patients should have follow-up visits in which they are advised of test results and given prophylactic treatment if indicated. The risk for acquiring HIV through assault is low, but patients should still be advised to have follow-up tests for HIV antibodies.

In certain circumstances, the potential of HIV transmission has been reduced by postexposure prophylaxis with antiretroviral agents. Postexposure prophylaxis with AZT has been associated with a reduced risk of infection.

Sexually transmitted diseases (STDs)

Sexually transmitted diseases include more than 30 infectious diseases that are primarily transmitted through anal, oral, or vaginal intercourse, although some STDs may be transmitted through other means. The modes of transmission are described in the specific disease entries. Various infectious agents, including bacteria, viruses, fungi, and parasites, cause sexually transmitted diseases. Most, but not all, STDs can be prevented with the proper use of condoms.

STDs caused by bacteria include gonorrhea, chlamydia, mycoplasma, syphilis, donovanosis, epididymitis, genital ulcer disease, bacterial vaginosis, chancroid, proctitis, proctocolitis, Reiter's syndrome, shigellosis, urethritis, cervicitis, salpingitis, and pelvic inflammatory disease.

STDs caused by viruses include HIV types 1 and 2 disease, AIDS, human papillomavirus (HPV), condyloma acuminata, genital warts, Kaposi's sarcoma, genital molluscum contagiosum, genital ulcer disease, cytomegalovirus, laryngeal papillomatosis, herpes simplex, hepatitis A, hepatitis B, hepatitis C, tropical spastic paraparesis, and Human T cell leukemia.

STDs caused by fungi include candidiasis and thrush. STDs caused by parasites include pubic lice infestation, scabies, trichomoniasis, and giardiasis.

Shigellosis

Shigellosis refers to infection with the enteric pathogens, *Shigella sonnei* and *Shigella flexneri*. Epidemiologic studies suggest that Shigella may be sexually transmitted, causing enteritis and proctocolitis in homosexual men. Shigellosis is also more common in AIDS patients than in similar patients without AIDS. In AIDS patients, shigellosis also tends to be more severe and is associated with more frequent recurrences, more frequent bacteremia, and more antibiotic resistance than in patients without AIDS.

The sexual transmission of Shigella was first recognized in 1972, when reports from San Francisco and later from Seattle and New York documented that 30 to 70 percent of patients with Shigella were homosexual men. Contact tracing demonstrated recovery of the identical Shigella strain from sexual partners, although no contaminated food or water source could be demonstrated as a common source of infection.

Shigelloisis causes an abrupt onset of diarrhea, fever, nausea, and cramps. The diarrhea is usually thin and watery, but may contain mucus or blood. Infection may be complicated by the development of toxic megacolon. Sigmoidoscopy usually reveals an inflamed mucosa with friability not limited to the distal rectum. Tissue studies show inflammation and bacterial infiltrates. Treatment is usually supportive, and antibiotics are used after culture and sensitivity studies demonstrate the effectiveness of specific antibiotics. Ciprofloxacin using 500 mg orally twice daily for seven days is usually effective.

Shilts, Randy

Randy Shilts, a reporter from the *San Francisco Chronicle*, documented the early years of the AIDS epidemic in his book *And The Band Played On*, which was later made into a movie. Shilts, who later died of AIDS, is credited with moving the AIDS epidemic to the public policy arena by his accurate portrayal of hindrances caused by the National Cancer Institute's internal conflicts and the country's homophobia.

SHIV

SHIV is a recombinant hybrid virus with an HIV envelope and an SIV core.

Silver nitrate

Silver nitrate is used as a prophylactic treatment in newborns to prevent eye infection related to STD infection. Used as a one percent solution in the form of an ointment, silver nitrate is administered into both eyes as soon as possible after delivery.

Simian immunodeficiency virus (SIV)

SIV is a lentivirus that affects the simian population and is similar to HIV, a lentivirus that affects humans. Studies of SIV have been helpful in studying HIV. As in humans, SIV infection of Rhesus macaques results in CD4+ lymphocyte depletion, immunosuppression, secondary malignancies, direct organ damage related to viral infection, and opportunistic infections. Many infections found in simians with SIV, such as those caused by *Toxoplasma gondii* and *Pneumocystis jiroveci*, are also found in humans with HIV.

Similarities between HIV-2 and SIV strongly suggest that the presence of HIV-2 in humans represents an interspecies transfer of SIV to humans caused by multiple introduction of SIV to humans. The case for HIV-1 having crossed species with monkeys is not as clear as the case for HIV-2, which is more commonly seen in Africa, but HIV-1 and chimpanzee SIV share many characteristics.

Social Security Disability for HIV/AIDS

People with HIV/AIDS may qualify for Social Security Administration (SSA) benefits, including Social Security Disability Insurance (SSDI) and Supplemental Security Income (SSI). SSI provides financial support for people with disabilities and low incomes. SSDI provides insurance for people with disabilities. Medical requirements are the same for SSI and SSDI, and the same process determines disability. Disability is based on the client's inability to work because of a medical condition. Qualifications include: U.S. citizenship, a Social Security number, medical disability, unemployment, and inability to earn gainfully more than $500/month. Also, to qualify individuals must have worked at least five of the past 10 years. The amount one receives in SSDI benefits depends on one's individual earnings history.

Certain criteria are also used to determine disability in AIDS. For instance, conditions of pulmonary tuberculosis resistant to treatment, Kaposi's sarcoma, pneumocystis jiroveci infection, herpes simplex, HIV wasting syndrome, and candidiasis are all considered disabling in people infected with HIV. In HIV, presumptive benefits may be paid for six months before a final decision is made on a claim. For more information and publications, call the SSA at (800) 772-1213 or visit http://www.ssa.gov.

Socioeconomic differences *see* Health Disparities Initiative

Special Projects of National Significance (SPNS)

The SPNS program is the research and demonstration program of the Ryan White CARE Act. The program's mission is to advance knowledge and skills in health and support services for persons with HIV/AIDS. The authorizing legislation specifies three objectives for this program: 1) to assess the effectiveness of particular models of care; 2) to support innovative program design, and 3) to promote replication of effective models.

Spermicides

Recent evidence suggests that vaginal spermicides containing nonoxynol-9 (N-9), the most frequently used spermicide in the United States, are not effective in preventing cervical gonorrhea, chlamydia, or HIV infection. Therefore, the Centers for Disease Control and Prevention (CDC) do not recommend using spermicide alone for STD/HIV prevention. Furthermore, frequent use of spermicides containing N-9 has been associated with genital lesions, which may cause an increased risk of HIV transmission. Spermicide use has also been associated with an increased risk of bacterial urinary tract infection in women.

Condoms containing N-9 are no more effective than other lubricated condoms in protecting against the transmission of HIV and other STDs. Condoms with N-9 are not recommended because they have a shorter shelf life than regular condoms (they have a shorter expiration date), and they are more expensive. Condoms containing N-9 have also been associated with an increased rate of urinary tract infection in women.

Recent studies indicate than N-9 may increase the risk for HIV because N-9 may cause genital lesions in women. Studies of rectal N-9 use have not been conducted, but it is likely that N-9 could also increase the risk of HIV infection in men when used as a rectal spermicide. Studies show that N-9 can damage the cells lining the rectum, thus providing a portal of entry for HIV and other sexually transmissible agents. The CDC recommends that N-9 should not be used as a microbicide or lubricant during anal intercourse.

Spirochete

Spirochetes are slender undulating bacteria. The most well known spirochete is *Treponema pallidum*, the infectious agent in syphilis.

Sponges

Vaginal sponges are sometimes used as contraceptives. The vaginal contraceptive sponge appears to protect against cervical gonorrhea and chlamydia, but its use increases the risk for candidiasis. Vaginal sponges cannot be relied on as protection against HIV infection because the use of sponges has not been evaluated for this purpose.

Squamous intraepithelial lesions (SILs)

Squamous intraepithelial lesions are abnormal cellular changes indicative of malignancy that are often associated with the human papillomavirus (HPV). Squamous cell lesions of the anal and genital tract are generally divided into invasive cancer and non-invasive lesions. The term invasive refers to tumors in which the malignant cells have penetrated the underlying basement membrane and have invaded into the stromal layer of tissue. Invasive squamous cancers are graded as well, moderately, or poorly differentiated.

Grade 1 tumors have a well defined margin and resemble normal squamous epithelium, with many keratinizing cells and keratin pearls present. Grade 2, or moderately differentiated cancer, shows less keratin formation and greater nuclear changes. Grade 3, or poorly differentiated squamous cell cancer, is composed of cells with a high nuclear/cytoplasmic ratio and many mitotic figures but no keratin formation. Invasive cervical cancers are further classified as being either frankly invasive or microinvasive.

Statistics

Statistics are used to monitor changes in the rates of infectious diseases and to determine what factors contribute to a low or high risk for specific STDs. Surveillance programs rely on statistics to develop preventive measures and to establish effective treatment guidelines for STDs.

Stavudine (d4T)

Stavudine (Zerit) is a nucleoside reverse transcriptase inhibitor (NRTI) used as an antiretroviral agent in the treatment of HIV infection.

STD history

The oldest illustration of a condom was found in Egypt and dates back more than 3,000 years. However, the oldest condoms discovered were found in the foundations of Dudley Castle near Birmingham, England, and date to 1640, during the European syphilis epidemic. These condoms were made of fish and animal skin.

Between the dates involved in these reports from Egypt and England, there are reports of *chlamydia trachomatis* infection, gonorrhea (which was often confused with syphilis), and chancroid. Syphilis dates back to the 15th century, and gonorrhea was recognized as early as the 13th century. Up until 1786, gonorrhea, syphilis, and chancroid were all referred to loosely as "venereal disease" because the symptoms were similar and there were no tests to differentiate one from the other.

In England, Lock hospital was the name given to institutions treating venereal diseases. The original lock hospital was built in the Southwark region of London during the 12th century, and specialized in treating leprosy. By the 18th century, however, it specialized in venereal diseases.

In North America

Reports from Mexico show that venereal diseases occurred in men and women during the Pre-Conquest Period from 1325 to 1521. When infected women experienced "fetid secretions" from their genitals or any type of genital lesion, they were segregated or forced to live outside of the town until cured.

An increase in venereal disease occurred from 1529 on during the Colonial Period. Problems with venereal diseases intensified in the 17th century because of the arrival of a large number of immigrants who were highly promiscuous and did not practice good hygiene. Reports which describe the venereal problems in Mexico show that they were similar to those existing in Europe at this time.

In the 19th and 20th centuries, ideas for reducing venereal diseases in Mexico included the simple inspection of women involved in prostitution. Records show that there were 563 commercial sex workers at the start of the 20th century, and 60 percent were between 14 and 20 years of age. A third of the women were isolated at some time because of an unspecified urogenital infection.

With the introduction of the Wasserman test and penicillin, the first anti-venereal dispensary was established in Mexico City in 1921. Other clinics opened later, and the Department of Public Hygiene intensified its campaign against venereal disease.

In the United States, the American Social Hygiene Association (ASHA) was founded in 1914 by a group of public health reformers committed to attacking the undesirable social condition of venereal disease. The moral crusade during World War I focused on preventing the spread of venereal disease and protecting the future of the American family. ASHA prepared posters, handbills, pamphlets, and exhibits instructing servicemen of the importance of avoiding venereal disease if they were to win the war. ASHA also fought hard to prohibit condom use for these soldiers.

The American Expeditionary Forces, as the U.S. Army was called, were the only armed forces in Europe during the war that were denied the use of condoms. It is not surprising that U.S. troops had the highest rates of sexually transmitted infections of all. About 70 percent of these soldiers were apparently unable to "just say no." The secretary of the Navy was only one of the many military leaders who did not believe that condom use was immoral or "un–Christian." It was this Navy officer, Franklin Delano Roosevelt, who, when his boss was away from the office, ordered the distribution of condoms to sailors. Around this time, in 1935, Connecticut became the first state to require blood tests for syphilis before marriage.

By World War II, military leaders had a more realistic attitude about condoms. Concerned that soldiers could bring home diseases and infect their wives, military officials aggressively promoted the use of condoms. Government training films urged soldiers "Don't forget — put it on before you put it in." In 1942, condoms were issued to soldiers during the landing on Dunkirk. They were used to cover and protect rifle barrels from being damaged by salt water as the soldiers waded ashore.

Modern Times

Casual attitudes toward sex and reduced fears of pregnancy following the introduction of IUDs and birth control pills caused a reduction in condom use in the 1960s. Fewer men needed to turn to commercial sex workers, and the most common STDs, syphilis and gonorrhea, were easily treated.

Various STD epidemics surfaced in various parts of the country, and were often associated with escalating drug use. The thought of STDs aroused little fear in the hearts of young people until AIDS emerged in 1983, a time when "safe sex" began to mean something. With this change, rates of most STDs fell, for nearly a decade. But one by one, the rates of various STDs have resumed climbing.

By 2001, epidemiological studies showed a high incidence of both chlamydia and HPV in young adults. By 2002, reports showed an increased incidence of syphilis and a rise in reported cases of HIV in some areas. Reports of reduced mortality with HAART may have caused people to relax their guard. What many of these people may not have heard of is the high failure rates that can occur with HAART, the grueling dietary restrictions and side effects that prevent the use of antiretroviral agents, and the increased incidence of neoplasms and dementia in people who survive AIDS long-term.

With the introduction of new minority initiatives and a wide-ranging preventive program implemented in April 2003, STD and HIV rates should once again begin to decline.

Stevens-Johnson Syndrome

Stevens-Johnson syndrome is a severe and sometimes fatal form of erythema multiforme that is characterized by severe skin manifestations; conjunctivitis, which often results in blindness; Vincent's angina (trench mouth); and ulceration of the genitals and anus.

Streptococcal vaginitis

Streptococcal infections are common because certain strains of streptococcus are normally present in the vagina. When overgrowth of these organisms occurs, often because of antibiotic use, streptococcal infections develop.

Etiology

Three kinds of streptococci, group A, group B, and group D can all cause vaginal symptoms. One common cause of group D streptococcal vaginitis is the use of clindamycin to treat bacterial vaginosis.

Group B *Streptococcus agalactiae* (GBS) poses a serious problem in pregnancy. GBS is the leading cause of life-threatening perinatal infections (sepsis and meningitis) in newborns in the United States. GBS is also a major cause of maternal peripartum infections, resulting in over 1,300 deaths per year in the United States. Group A streptococcal infections may cause vulvovaginitis and toxic shock syndrome. GBS is responsible for sepsis and pneumonia in neonates, urinary tract infection, chorioamnionitis (amniotic fluid infection), post-partum endometritis, and bacteremia in pregnant women, and bacteremia and soft tissue infection in nonpregnant adults.

Epidemiology

In clinical trials evaluating pregnant women, the overall incidence of group B streptococcal infection in the United States is 18.6 percent.

Symptoms

Symptoms include vulvovaginal irritation and discharge.

Diagnosis

An examination of vaginal secretions shows an elevated pH, many white blood cells, and an absence of lactobacilli. On gram stains, streptococcus appears as small cocci occurring in pairs and chains. A culture will identify large numbers of streptococcus belonging to group A, B, or D. To identify group B streptococcal infection, both vaginal and rectal swabs are collected and cultured. Group B streptococcus is routinely tested during pregnancy between 35 and 37 weeks gestation to prevent neonatal transmission. Earlier specimen collection is not advised as it is not predictive. Rapid latex tests, DNA tests with polymerase chain reaction (PCR) methodology (IDID Strep B Assay approved in 2002), and culture techniques with LIM broth enrichment are available for diagnosis. In neonatal infections, Group B streptococcal infection is identified by antigen detection, using blood, urine, spinal fluid, or tracheal aspirates.

Treatment

Antibiotics are used to treat streptococcus vaginitis. Often, anti-fungal creams are prescribed to prevent overgrowth of yeast. Standard treatment is amoxicillin, using 500 mg orally three times daily for 10 days. Over-the-counter anti-fungal creams, such as Diflucan, are used simultaneously. Studies show that nine percent of women infected with GBS change their colonization status between ante- and intrapartum periods when retested at 35 to 37 weeks gestation. Therefore, testing and treatment for GBS in early pregnancy before 35 weeks gestation is not recommended.

Stress

Stress, especially chronic stress, is known to injure immune system cells, weakening the immune system's protective abilities. A weakened immune system causes susceptibility to infection and disease. One large study concluded that persistent stressors and high levels of anxiety predicted genital herpes recurrence, whereas transient mood states, short-term stressors, and life change events did not.

NCCAM is conducting a study at Virginia Commonwealth University, which ends in May 2005, to evaluate the effects of stress management intervention in persons with various stages of HIV disease. The study will determine if these interventions along with booster strategies will, as expected, improve and sustain improvements in psychosocial functioning, quality of life, and somatic health.

Alternative Stress Management Approaches in HIV Disease, sponsored by NCCAM; for more information, contact Nancy McCain, RN, DSN, principal investigator, at 8040828-5930 or nmccain@hsc.vcu.edu.

Cohen, Frances, et. al. "Persistent Stress as a Predictor of Genital Herpes Recurrence." *Archives of Internal Medicine*, Nov. 8, 1999; 159: 2430–2436.

Structured intermittent therapy (SIT)

SIT refers to carefully planned periods or regimens of intermittent therapy that might sustain viral control while reducing costs of HIV treatment.

Structured treatment interruption (STI)

STI refers to the planned interruption of treatment by discontinuation of all antiretroviral drugs. There are four reasons to consider STI: 1) to provide a "drug holiday" to patients to relieve them of the inconvenience and toxicity of unsuccessful antiretroviral therapy and to improve the response to salvage therapy by allowing the emergence of wild-type virus; 2) to "re-immunize" the patient to HIV in the hopes of regaining immunologic control through a regenerated HIV-specific immune response; 3) to decrease the cumulative exposure to antiretroviral agents, reducing toxicity and cost and improving quality of life; and 4) to discontinue antiretroviral drugs during the first trimester of pregnancy.

Subunit HIV vaccine

The subunit HIV vaccine is a genetically engineered vaccine that is based on only part of the HIV molecule.

SUDS test

The Single Use Diagnostic System (SUDS test) manufactured by Abbott Laboratories was the first FDA-approved rapid test kit for HIV. The SUDS test offered a preliminary screening result requiring confirmation with EIA or Western Blot techniques on plasma samples using rapid ELISA or latex agglutination techniques. Providing results within 10 minutes, the SUDS test was primarily used to screen emergency and other healthcare workers who may have been exposed to HIV in the course of their employment. Because of low specificity and sensitivity compared to other test methods, the test was removed from use in June 2003.

Superantigen

Investigators have proposed that a molecule known as a superantigen, made by either HIV or an unrelated agent, may stimulate massive quantities of CD4+ T cells at once, rendering them highly susceptible to HIV infection and subsequent

cell death. For this reason, neutralizing antibodies produced against HIV have little effect.

Symptoms

Symptoms are physical changes or disturbances, such as rash, that can be directly observed by patients. Symptoms typically occur as manifestations of disease, and all STDs are associated with characteristic symptoms.

Some symptoms, such as genital discharge, are common to a number of different STDs. A doctor should be seen if any of the following symptoms occur: any type of discharge from the vagina, penis, or rectum; pain or a burning sensation during urination or sexual intercourse; lower abdominal pain; pain in the genital or anal area; blisters, open sores, warts, rash or swelling in the anogenital area or mouth; flu-like symptoms, including fever and malaise; or swollen glands. Specific STD symptoms are included in the specific STD entries.

Synctia (giant cells)

Synctia are dysfunctional multicellular clumps formed by cell-to-cell fusion. Cells infected with HIV may also fuse with nearby uninfected cells, forming balloon-like giant cells called synctia. In test tube experiments, these giant cells have been associated with the death of uninfected cells. The presence of so-called synctia-inducing variants of HIV has been correlated with rapid disease progression in HIV-infected individuals.

Syphilis (the pox)

Syphilis, a systemic STD once widely known as the pox, was first reported in Europe at the end of the 15th century. The speed with which this first syphilis epidemic spread through Europe led to exclusion measures and accusatory writings in which those afflicted with pox were publicly derided. The history of syphilis, which follows this entry, closely parallels the history of AIDS.

Etiology

The infectious agent in syphilis is the spirochete bacterium *Treponema pallidum*. Nearly all cases of syphilis are acquired by direct sexual contact with lesions of an individual who has active primary or secondary syphilis. Transmission of syphilis occurs in approximately one-half of these contacts. Syphilis can also be transmitted congenitally from mother to child by transplacental passage of the spirochetes to the fetus. Less common modes of syphilis transmission include blood-borne (due to blood transfusions or sharing contaminated needles), nonsexual personal contact, and accidental direct inoculation.

Epidemiology

In the United States, the number of people with syphilis peaked during World War II, then fell dramatically until about 1960, when rates began increasing again. During this period, the incidence of syphilis began to rise in homosexual men. The rate of

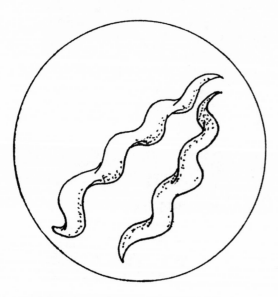

Treponema pallidum (syphilis) (Marvin G. Miller).

syphilis infection remained relatively stable until the mid–1980s. With the emergence of AIDS and education regarding safe sex, the incidence of syphilis among homosexual men fell. This reduction was followed, however, by a rapid increase in new cases of syphilis among crack cocaine users, primarily among women and their newborns.

In October 1999, a year when only 35,600 new cases of syphilis were reported in the United States, the CDC, in collaboration with other federal partners, initiated the National Plan to Eliminate Syphilis in the United States. In the late 1990s the incidence of syphilis fell, only to rise again in certain large cities by early 2001, primarily in homosexual men and presumably due to disregard for preventive measures. The incidence of syphilis, however, continued to decline among women and among non–Hispanic blacks. The highest rates of syphilis are seen in African-Americans, and the rate appears to be increasing among Latino men.

By region, the South has the highest syphilis rate, accounting for 56.2 percent of cases occurring in 2001, and 62.0 percent in 2000. During 2000–2001, although the South still led the country in reported cases of syphilis, the rates decreased in the South and Midwest, but increased 40 percent in the West and 57.1 percent in the Northeast.

Symptoms

As a systemic disease, syphilis can affect all of the body's organs and systems. Specific symptoms are associated with the various disease stages. Syphilis has three distinct stages: the primary, secondary, and tertiary stages. An additional latent stage generally precedes the tertiary stage of syphilis, although latent periods can occur and interrupt any periods of active disease. Infection may persist for many years and can lead to bone and joint damage, heart damage, brain damage, and death.

• PRIMARY STAGE— In the first or primary

stage, symptoms generally occur one to 13 weeks after the initial infection, with most symptoms occurring after 3–4 weeks. Small, round, red, raised, painless sores known as chancres may appear on the penis, vulva, vagina, anus, rectum, lips, tongue, fingers, cervix, mouth, or rarely on other parts of the body. The sores do not bleed, but they frequently form open sores or ulcerations, and when rubbed, they may leak a clear fluid that is highly infectious. Nearby lymph nodes usually become enlarged, but they are painless.

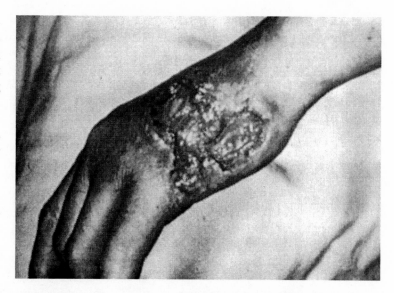

Late syphilis, ulcerating gumma (Navy Environmental Health Center Training and Health Communication Branch, CDC).

Because the primary sores cause few symptoms, they are often ignored. About half of infected women and a third of the infected men are unaware of their sores although some may seek treatment. Syphilitic chancres generally disappear without treatment within three to 12 weeks without any apparent residual side effects. Syphilis is usually transmitted through direct contact with these sores, but transmission may occur even when sores aren't visible.

• SECONDARY STAGE— Secondary syphilis represents the disseminated disease stage that results from the multiplication and dissemination of treponemal spirochetes throughout the body. In this stage, which typically occurs six to 12 weeks after the initial infection, a rash, which is usually reddish, appears. Alternately, the rash may appear as brown spots. This rash occurs on the palms, soles, or other parts of the body, and is highly contagious. About 25 percent of people in this stage still have one or more primary healing sores. Other symptoms include fever, swollen lymph glands, hair loss, headaches, extreme tiredness, and muscle loss. The rash usually clears up spontaneously, but new rashes may appear weeks or months later.

In the secondary stage of syphilis, mouth sores are common and affect more than 80 percent of patients. About 50 percent of patients have enlarged lymph nodes throughout the body, and about 10 percent have eye inflammation, although there are no other eye symptoms at this time. About 10 percent of patients have inflamed bones and aching joints. Kidney inflammation may cause protein to leak into the urine, and liver inflammation may lead to jaundice. A small number of people develop an inflammation of the lining of the brain known as acute syphilitic meningitis. This condition causes headaches, neck stiffness, and sometimes deafness.

Raised pustules known as condylomata lata may develop where the skin adjoins mucous membranes, for instance, at the inner edges of the lips and vulva, and in moist areas of the skin. Hair may fall out in patches, leaving the scalp with a moth-eaten appearance. Other symptoms include a feeling of illness or malaise, loss of appetite, nausea, fatigue, fever, and anemia.

• TERTIARY STAGE—The tertiary or late stage of syphilis occurs in approximately one-third of untreated patients. The third disease stage can occur soon after the second stage although it may occur many years later following a benign latent stage. During the tertiary stage, the disease is not transmitted to others, although the disease process can be particularly destructive, affecting the eyes, skin, cartilage of the nose, and also bone. In the tertiary stage, syphilis can also damage nerve cells in the brain and spinal cord and cause cardiovascular problems, paralysis, blindness, insanity, and death.

Cardiovascular syphilis usually appears 10 to 25 years after the initial infection. Patients with cardiovascular syphilis are prone to aneurysm, a weakening and dilation of the aorta (the main artery leading from the heart) and leakage of the aortic valve. This condition may lead to chest pain, heart failure, and death.

Some patients may develop a benign form of tertiary syphilis, although this form is rarely seen today. In the benign stage, lumps called gummas appear in various organs, where they grow slowly, heal gradually, and leave scars. Gummas may occur in almost any part of the body, but they are most common on the leg, just below the knee, and on the upper trunk, face and scalp. The bones may also be affected, causing a deep, penetrating pain that is usually worse at night.

• LATENT STAGE—The latent stage of syphilis generally follows the secondary stage. Latent syphilis is defined as syphilis characterized by sero-reactivity (positive serology tests) without other evidence of disease. Latent syphilis acquired within the preceding year and documented with serology tests is referred to as early latent syphilis; all other cases of latent syphilis are classified as either late latent syphilis or latent syphilis of unknown duration. During the latent stage, patients generally remain free of symptoms. However, in the early part of the latent stage, infectious sores occasionally occur.

Early latent syphilis cannot be reliably distinguished from late latent syphilis solely on the basis of nontreponemal test (RPR or VDRL) titers. All patients with latent syphilis should have careful examination of all accessible mucosal surfaces, such as the oral cavity, the perineum in women, and underneath the foreskin in uncircumcised men, to evaluate for internal mucosal lesions.

Neurosyphilis

Syphilis affects the nervous system in about five percent of all untreated people. Overall, about 75 percent of infected people are unable to clear the infection from their nervous system. Among those who do not clear infection from their nervous system, a small number of patients will go on to develop neurosyphilis. Patients with serum RPR titers greater than or equal to 1:32 have an increased risk of developing neurosyphilis. Among patients co-infected with HIV, those with peripheral CD4 cell counts less than or equal to 350 cells/uL are significantly more likely to develop neurosyphilis. The three major types of neurosyphilis are meningovascular neurosyphilis, paretic neurosyphilis, and tabetic neurosyphilis, each with its own cluster of symptoms.

Meningovascular neurosyphilis is a chronic form of meningitis that occurs in people with syphilis. The specific symptoms depend on whether the brain is primarily affected or whether both the brain and spinal cord are affected. When the brain is primarily affected, symptoms include headache, dizziness, poor concentration, tiredness and lack of energy, difficulty sleeping, stiff neck, blurred vision, mental confusion, seizures, swelling of the optic nerve (papilledema), abnormalities of the pupils, difficulty speaking (aphasia), and paralysis of a limb or of half the body.

When both the brain and spinal cord are affected, symptoms include increasing difficulty in chewing, swallowing, and talking, weakness and wasting of shoulder and arm muscles, a slowly progressive paralysis with muscle spasms known as spastic paralysis, an inability to empty the bladder, and spinal cord inflammation causing a loss of bladder control (incontinence) and sudden paralysis while the muscles remain relaxed (flaccid paralysis).

Paretic neurosyphilis, which was once referred to as general paralysis of the insane, begins gradually with behavioral changes occurring in the middle-aged, which gradually progress to dementia. Symptoms may include convulsions, difficulty in speaking, temporary paralysis affecting half of the body, irritability, difficulty in concentrating, memory loss, defective judgment, headaches, insomnia, fatigue, lethargy, deterioration in personal hygiene and grooming habits, mood swings, loss of strength and energy, depression, delusions of grandeur, and lack of insight.

Tabetic neurosyphilis, which is also known as tabes dorsalis, is a progressive disease of the spinal cord that emerges gradually. Typically, the first symptom is an intense, intermittent stabbing pain affecting both legs. The person becomes unsteady while walking, especially in poor lighting. Gait changes include walking with the feet kept wide apart, and stamping the feet. Because the sensations signaling a full bladder are impaired, incontinence and urinary tract infections are common, and impotence is a frequent occurrence. Patients with tabetic neurosyphilis may also experience tremors of the mouth, tongue, and hands, and the entire body may tremble. Handwriting often becomes shaky and illegible.

Most people with tabetic neurosyphilis are thin and appear sad. They can experience spasms of pain in various organs, especially the stomach, and stomach spasms may cause vomiting. Similar painful spasms may affect the rectum, bladder, and larynx. Because the feet lose the sensation of feeling and pain, open sores may develop on the soles, and these sores may reach the underlying bone and joints.

Diagnosis

Today, syphilis is usually presumptively diagnosed by a blood test known as the rapid plasma regain (RPR) test. The RPR may be negative in the early weeks of infection and should be repeated after several weeks in people with symptoms characteristic of syphilis. Because latex polymers in the test can react with other proteins, false-positive test results may occasionally occur, especially in people with rheumatoid arthritis.

Before the introduction of the RPR test, laboratories relied on a test known as the venereal disease research laboratory (VDRL) test. Today the VDRL test is primarily used to test for syphilis in spinal fluid specimens. Before the VDRL test was introduced, variations of the Wasserman test were used to diagnose syphilis. The RPR and VDRL tests are nontreponemal tests.

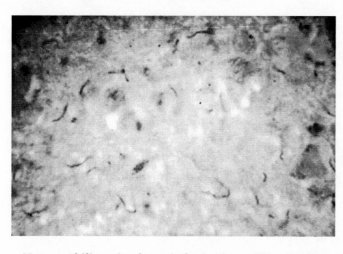

Neurosyphilis; spirochetes in brain tissue (Navy Environmental Health Center Training and Health Communication Branch, CDC).

For this reason, positive tests are usually repeated with a second test employing a treponemal methodology, such as the fluorescent treponemal antibody absorption (FTA-ABS) test, which is more specific and detects antibodies to *Treponema pallidum* or the T. pallidum particle agglutination (TP-PA) test. In the latent and tertiary stages the RPR blood test is used for presumptive diagnosis and confirmed with a treponemal test method. Nontreponemal test antibody titers usually correlate with disease activity.

Nontreponemal tests usually become non-reactive with time after treatment, although nontreponemal antibodies can persist at a low titer for a long time, sometimes for life (this response is referred to as the serofast reaction). Most patients with reactive treponemal tests have reactive tests for the remainder of their lives, regardless of treatment or disease activity. However, 15 to 25 percent of patients who receive treatment during the primary disease stage revert, becoming serologically non-reactive after two to three years.

Syphilis can also be definitively diagnosed in the primary or secondary stages with a darkfield exam of lesion exudates from skin or mouth sores that demonstrates the characteristic undulating *Treponema* spirochetes.

No test alone can be used to diagnose neurosyphilis. The VDRL test performed on cerebrospinal fluid (CSF) is highly specific, but it is insensitive. Most other tests are both insensitive and nonspecific and must be interpreted in relation to other test results and the clinical assessment. Therefore, diagnosis of neurosyphilis usually depends on various combinations of reactive serologic test results, and abnormalities in CSF assays, such as elevated protein or white blood cells. Some specialists also perform the FTA-ABS test on spinal fluid. Because this test is very sensitive but not as specific, a negative test can be used to rule out neurosyphilis.

Treatment

In the early years of the epidemic, mercury and potassium iodide were used to treat syphilis, and by 1848 arsenic compounds emerged as the treatment of choice. It is not surprising that many patients found it difficult to complete their courses of treatment. In 1943, a team of doctors successfully used the newly discovered antibiotic penicillin to successfully treat syphilis. Since then, penicillin has remained the primary treatment for syphilis.

Penicillin is used for all stages of syphilis and is administered parenterally (by injection). Researchers theorize that treatment for both late latent syphilis and tertiary syphilis may require a longer duration of therapy because organisms are dividing more slowly. The specific preparation (i.e., benzathine, aqueous procaine, or aqueous crystalline), its dosage, and length of treatment depends on the stage and clinical manifestations of disease. However, neither combinations of benzathine penicillin and procaine penicillin nor oral penicillin preparations are considered appropriate for the treatment of syphilis. Parenteral penicillin G is the only therapy with documented efficacy for syphilis during pregnancy. Pregnant women with allergy to penicillin should be desensitized and then treated with penicillin.

More than half of the people with early stage syphilis, especially secondary syphilis, develop an acute febrile reaction (the Jarisch-Herxheimer reaction) within two to 24 hours after the first treatment. Patients should be warned of this reaction for which aspirin can be used to help relieve symptoms. This reaction is thought to result from the sudden death of bacteria. Symptoms include fever, headache, sweating, shaking, chills, and a temporary worsening of syphilitic sores. Rarely, people with neurosyphilis may experience seizures or paralysis. In pregnant women, this reaction can induce early labor or cause fetal distress, although it should not prevent or delay therapy.

• PRIMARY AND SECONDARY SYPHILIS TREATMENT— The recommended regimen for adults is Benzathine penicillin G, using 2.4 million units IM in a single dose. The recommended regimen for children is Benzathine penicillin G, using 50,000 units/kg IM, up to the adult dose of 2.4 million units in a single dose.

• LATENT SYPHILIS TREATMENT— Treatment of latent syphilis usually does not affect transmission and is intended to prevent occurrence or progression of late complications. The recommended regimen for adults with early late syphilis is Benzathine penicillin G, using 2.4 million units, IM in a single dose. For late latent syphilis or latent syphilis of unknown duration, Benzathine penicillin G, using 2.4 million units should be administered IM in three consecutive weekly injections for a total of 7.2 million units.

For children with early late syphilis, Benzathine penicillin G, using 50,000 units/kg administered IM, up to the adult dose of 2.4 million units in a single dose, is recommended. For late latent syphilis or latent syphilis of unknown duration in children, Benzathine penicillin G should be administered IM, using 50,000 units/kg, up to 2.4 million units repeated for three consecutive weeks, up to the adult total dose of 7.2 million units.

Non-pregnant patients with late latent syphilis who have penicillin allergy can be treated with doxycycline, using 100 mg twice daily or tetracycline, using 500 mg orally four times daily for 28 days. These therapies should be used in conjunction with close follow-up and evaluation for symptoms.

• TERTIARY SYPHILIS TREATMENT— Patients who are not allergic to penicillin and have no evidence of neurosyphilis should be treated with Benzathine penicillin G, administered as three doses of 2.4 million units IM each at one week intervals for a total of 7.2 million units. Patients with

penicillin allergy should follow treatment guidelines for late latent syphilis.

• NEUROSYPHILIS TREATMENT— The recommended regimen for neurosyphilis is Aqueous crystalline penicillin G, using 18–24 million units daily, administered as 3–4 million units every four hours, or continuous infusion for 10–14 days. If compliance with therapy can be ensured, patients can be treated with Procaine penicillin, using 2.4 million units IM once daily along with Probencid, using 500 mg orally four times a day, both for 10–14 days. Patients with penicillin allergy can be treated with ceftriaxone, using two grams daily administered IM or IV for 10–14 days.

Treatment Management and Follow-up

All patients with syphilis should be tested for HIV infection. In geographical areas where the incidence of HIV infection is high, patients who test negative for HIV should be retested after three months. Patients with symptoms of neurologic or ophthalmic disease should have an evaluation that includes CSF analysis and an ocular slit-lamp examination.

All patients with latent syphilis should be evaluated for evidence of tertiary disease, such as aortitis, gumma, and iritis (inflammation of the iris). Patients with neurologic or ophthalmic signs or symptoms, evidence of active tertiary syphilis, treatment failure, or HIV infection with latent syphilis should have a prompt CSF examination. Patients with latent syphilis should have serological tests repeated at 6, 12, and 24 months.

Patients with primary or secondary syphilis should not be routinely retested after treatment because serologic tests generally remain reactive for some time. However, patients who have signs or symptoms that persist or recur should be tested with nontreponemal serological tests, such as the RPR. Patients with a sustained fourfold increase in titer probably failed treatment or have become rein-fected. When patients are retreated, most STD specialists recommend administering weekly injections of Benzathine penicillin G, using 2.4 million units IM for three weeks unless a CSF examination shows that neurosyphilis is present.

Precautions

Sexual transmission of *T. pallidum* only occurs when mucocutaneous syphilitic lesions are present. Because people with primary and secondary stage syphilis are infectious, they must avoid sexual intercourse until they and their sex partners have completed treatment.

However, persons exposed sexually to a patient with any stage of syphilis should be evaluated clinically and serologically according to the following CDC recommendations: 1) Persons exposed within the 90 days preceding a partner's diagnosis of primary, secondary, or early latent syphilis might be infected even if serology tests are non-reactive. Therefore, such persons should be treated presumptively. 2) Persons exposed more than 90 days before the diagnosis of primary, secondary, or early latent syphilis in a sex partner should be treated presumptively if serologic test results are not immediately available and the opportunity for follow-up is uncertain. 3) For purposes of partner notification and presumptive treatment of exposed sex partners, patients with syphilis of unknown duration who have nontreponemal test titers equal to or greater than 1:32 can be assumed to have early syphilis. However, serologic titers should not be used to differentiate early from late latent syphilis for the purpose of determining treatment. 4) Long-term sex partners of patients with latent syphilis should be evaluated clinically and serologically for syphilis and treated on the basis of the evaluation findings.

Pregnancy

Syphilis infection during pregnancy, including latent infection, can cause neona-tal growth retardation and it can cause serious, permanent disabilities such as blindness or damage to the heart, brain, or skeleton as well as death. Parenteral penicillin G is used for treatment, and patients allergic to penicillin should be desensitized and then treated with penicillin. Penicillin is administered according to the appropriate regimen for the mother's stage of syphilis.

Congenital Syphilis

Syphilis can be transmitted during delivery, but the vast majority of congenital syphilis cases are believed to arise from infections occurring in utero (while in the uterus). *Treponema pallidum* may infect the placenta and umbilical cord and it may also gain access to the fetal circulation by crossing the fetal membranes and infecting the amniotic fluid. The risk of congenital syphilis is directly related to the stage of maternal syphilis during pregnancy. The risk is extremely high during the first four years after infection when spirochetes are readily found in the blood, and the risk declines during late syphilis. During the high risk period, the risk of having a stillborn child is high.

Babies with syphilis often have a characteristic appearance, causing them to look aged. Congenital syphilis can involve almost every fetal organ, with liver, kidneys, bone, pancreas, spleen, lungs, heart, and brain being the most frequently affected. Studies of the nervous system show gross meningeal involvement, especially around the brainstem. Fibrosis during healing may result in obstructive hydrocephalus and entrapment of cranial nerves. Teeth, when they emerge, show abnormalities of form, structure and size, with apical notching, defective enamel, and an irregular amilo-dentinal junction. The first molars (six year) and central incisors of the permanent teeth are most affected. Fibrosis and gummas are frequently found in congenitally infected tissues.

Congenital syphilis can be divided into

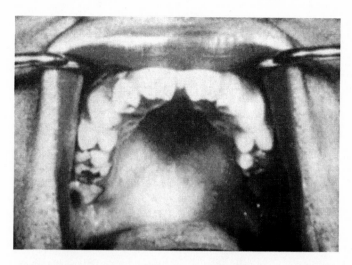

Congenital syphilis, Hutchinson's teeth (Navy Environmental Health Center Training and Health Communication Branch, CDC).

early and late disease. Those features that typically appear within the first two years of life represent congenital syphilis while symptoms that occur after age two represent late congenital syphilis. Severity of early congenital infections varies, ranging from life-threatening involvement of multiple organs and body systems to laboratory abnormalities in an otherwise normal appearing infant.

Nasal discharge is the earliest sign of congenital syphilis, and occurs one to two weeks before the rash. The nasal discharge is initially watery but later becomes progressively thicker and purulent and then blood-tinged. The nasal discharge interferes with feeding and causes necrosis and eventually septal perforation or the characteristic saddle-nose deformity of late congenital syphilis.

As in adults, infants develop many skin lesions, with the most common lesion forming a large round pink macule that fades to a dusky or coppery hue after one to three months, leaving a residual pigmentation. The lesions are typically distributed over the back, perineum, extremities, palms, and soles. Clusters of lesions may form around a large central plaque, and blisters may erupt. When the blisters

rupture, they leave a dusky red surface that dries and crusts. These lesions typically occur on the face, perineum, and between fingers and toes, and may become infected.

Blood changes are common in congenital syphilis, with anemia, low platelet counts, and abnormally low or high white blood cell counts frequently seen. Neurologic symptoms are common and similar to those seen in meningitis. Three distinct ocular lesions are associated with early congenital syphilis: chorioretinitis, glaucoma, and uveitis.

Late congenital syphilis can be prevented by prompt treatment of early congenital syphilis. Late congenital syphilis causes craniofacial malformations, such as frontal bossing, which can cause the forehead to appear mis-shapen, and the face may appear flattened. As mentioned, a saddle-nose deformity also frequently develops. The teeth are also usually misshapen, and the lower incisors may have parallel sides and lack a notch, and the upper incisors are sometimes pointed rather than notched. The tibia may be thickened due to bone changes, causing a condition of saber shin. Interstitial keratitis, which may lead to blindness, typically develops between ages five and 16.

All infants born to mothers with reactive syphilis serology tests should be evaluated with a quantitative RPR or VDRL performed on infant serum. Cord blood specimens cannot be used because they can be contaminated with maternal blood. These infants should also be examined thoroughly for evidence of congenital syphilis, such as nonimmune hydrops, jaundice, enlarged spleen, rhinitis, skin rash, and pseudoparalysis of an extremity. Darkfield exam can be performed on any skin lesions and on nasal secretions. For infants with reactive serological tests and symptoms, treatment regimens involve the use of Aqueous crystalline penicillin G or Procaine penicillin with doses determined by the presenting symptoms and serologic test results.

Risk Factors

Risk factors for syphilis include unprotected sex, sexual or direct contact with syphilitic lesions, drug abuse, and commercial sex work.

Syphilis and other STDs that produce genital lesions or evoke an inflammatory response are important risk factors for the acquisition and transmission of HIV. This may be because ulcerations allow direct entry of infectious agents or because the cells and chemicals released during the immune response in syphilis may facilitate HIV replication.

Complications

Complications related to syphilis include coronary artery disease, aortic valve disease, aortic aneurysm, nasal cartilage destruction, arthritis, bone and joint inflammation, eye disease, and arthritis.

Reporting Syphilis

Private healthcare providers, healthcare institutions, and laboratories are required to report positive syphilis tests to city-county health departments. Health departments then forward this information to the CDC, obtain information about sex partners, and notify sexual partners if this is their policy. Information may also be obtained regarding drug use and venues for meeting sex partners to help in identifying high-risk behaviors.

For identification and notification of at-risk partners, the time periods before treatment are a) three months plus duration of symptoms for primary syphilis; b) six months plus duration of symptoms for secondary syphilis; and c) one year for early latent syphilis. *See also* **Genital ulcer disease; National Plan to Eliminate Syphilis in the United States; Penicillin;** **Penicillin desensitization; Syphilis, history of;** and **Tuskegee syphilis experiment.**

Centers for Disease Control and Prevention. *Sexually Transmitted Diseases Treatment Guidelines 2002.* Atlanta: U.S. Dept. of Health and Human Services, 2002.

Syphilis, history of

Syphilis dates back to 15th century Europe, where reports of a disease worse than leprosy and the plague first originated. The reports began circulating shortly after the king of France, Charles VIII, entered Italy at the head of a mercenary army consisting of Flemish, Gascons, Swiss, and even Italians and Spaniards. In the course of their travels the French army had picked up a disease they called "the Neapolitan sickness," and which the Italians called "the French sickness."

By the 16th century, the disease was known as the "great pox," because of the unfortunate lesions that it caused. Besides the lesions, sufferers often lost their eyes, hands, noses, or feet. During autopsy, physicians noted bones that were tumorous and hollow to the marrow. Sufferers complained of violent pain that intensified toward evening, and commented that their bones felt broken and distended. The disfiguring pustules also were said to cause great pain and suffering.

A European Epidemic

Preventive measures involved identifying high-risk groups, such as prostitutes, and advising young men to avoid them. Early treatments consisted of the formidable panacea mercury and gaiac, which were first used separately and then together. On the other side of the Rhine, the epidemic spread throughout Germany. The Germans called it Bosen Blattern or malignant smallpox, which they blamed on France and Italy. Northern and central Europe were affected a little later, and syphilis first swept through Denmark in about 1495.

Here, syphilis was called "the French sca-bies." Later, the Mucovites called it "the Polish sickness," and the Poles called it "the German sickness." The Portuguese called it the "the Castilian sickness," and the Japanese called it "the Portuguese sick-ness." Only the Spanish declined to call it anything.

In 1496, a young scholar from Augsburg, Josephus Grunpeck, reproduced the poems and illustrations of Sebastian Brant, a pro-fessor of civil and canon law. Grunpeck's text is important because it is the oldest printed work to describe syphilis. Several years later, Grunpeck contracted syphilis and wrote one of the finest and most ter-rifying accounts of this illness.

It has long been suspected that Christo-pher Columbus brought syphilis back to Europe after his expeditions. The remains of a medieval woman found in England in 2001, which show syphilitic bone lesions, prove that syphilis already existed at the time of the woman's death, which dates to a period between 1296 and 1445. This is considered proof that Columbus did not bring syphilis to Europe in 1492. Skeletons found in the United States had previously shown that syphilis was in existence in North America before 1492.

The Evolution of Treatment

As early as the 1300s, ore cinnabar, a form of mercury, had been used for lep-rosy. When syphilis emerged, mercury was also used as a treatment in the form of ointments, oral administration, and vapor baths. By the 17th century, a time when as many people were injured by mercury as by syphilis, a moralizing approach was adopted, and people were advised to shun the temptations of the flesh. In Paris, pox-sufferers were sent to the Hotel-Dieu much like lepers. During the 18th century, med-icine again prevailed over morality and new treatments emerged. Mercury reigned supreme at the time although charlatans sold many home-brewed potions offering little in the form of a cure.

By the 19th century, "the pox" was being called syphilis, and it was determined that syphilis and gonorrhea were two separate diseases. Potassium iodide was used as a treatment for syphilis in 1840 and was sometimes combined with mercury. With this poor arsenal of chemicals still the only hope for a cure, condoms came into use, with evidence of the first condoms found in England.

In the 20th century, progress was finally made when, in 1905, Schaudinn and Hoff-man described the pathogenic agent of syphilis, the pale-colored spirochete named Treponema. By 1910, Ehrlich developed Salvarsan (606), a preparation composed of arsenic derivatives known as ar-sphenamines. Ehrlich used the term "silver bullet" to describe the effect he predicted Salvarsan would have on syphilis. This "silver bullet" didn't offer the cure that had been predicted, but it inspired other re-searchers to continue the search. About this time, critics claimed that finding a cure for syphilis only opened the doors to immorality. Importance was placed on sex-ual virtues. While men prepared for World War I, the American Social Health Associ-ation worked to prevent the distribution of condoms. Consequently, Americans were reported as having the highest STD rate of the soldiers in World War I, and condoms were dispensed to American sol-diers fighting in the Second World War.

After the Second World War, the liber-alization of moral codes and the emergence of new high-risk groups (homosexuals, commercial travelers, university students, etc.) led to the abandonment of all dis-criminatory prophylactic measures and an increase in syphilis. In response, morality joined with medicine, and a vigorous cam-paign was initiated on all fronts, with posters, radio, theatre, and the cinema used to frighten people. In addition, newly developed serological tests showed that even with a supposed cure from Salvarsan, Treponema remained dormant within the blood. Frenzy and fear were replaced with relief and a loosening of morals with the discovery of penicillin and its ability to cure syphilis. This same lack of concern led to the upsurge of syphilis in the 1960s, the 1980s, and in late 2002. Scholars find many similarities in the history of syphilis and AIDS, both in public perceptions and in certain symptoms. Both diseases cause depression and a similar type of dementia.

Explanations

Similar to the debates over the origins of HIV, ideas and explanations were given for the emergence of syphilis. Some people proposed that it was the result of the intercourse of a leprous knight and a courtesan, or the coupling of men with monkeys, or of the vengeful Spaniards mixing lepers' blood with Greek wine. God's alleged anger was also mentioned as a cause. The Moors, who were driven out of Spain in 1492, were accused of causing the plague. The Beggars, a mystic-erotic sect that had roamed Europe since the time of the Black Death, were also sometimes accused. The astrological explanation was the most popular. It explained that the positions of certain stars and the conjunction of different planets could work together to cause an epidemic. Of course, the astrologers also predicted the syphilis epidemic would last for seven years.

Quetel, Claude. *History of Syphilis.* Translated by Judith Braddock and Brian Pike. First published as *Le Mal de Naples; histoire de la syphilis.* Paris, 1986; Baltimore, MD: Johns Hopkins University Press, 1992.

Syringe exchange programs

Syringe exchange programs are state or local programs that replace or supply syringes and needles intended for intravenous drug use. The CDC reports that more than 36 percent of all HIV infection and more than 60 percent of all hepatitis C infection can be related to intravenous drug use. In addition, the CDC reports that 50 to 80 percent of intravenous drug users are reported to be infected with hepatitis C

within six to 12 months of initial injection. Studies suggest that drug treatment and syringe exchange programs are effective in reducing transmission of hepatitis and HIV.

Despite these statistics, under the Alcohol, Drug Abuse, and Mental Health Administration (ADAMHA) Reorganization Act of 1992, federal funds cannot be used to carry out any needle exchange program unless the surgeon general determines that they are effective in reducing the spread of HIV and the use of illegal drugs. However, the U.S. Department of Health & Human Services does have the authority to conduct demonstration and research projects that could involve the provision of needles.

In 1991, the National Commission of Substance Use and HIV reported that legal barriers such as drug paraphernalia laws encouraged sharing of injection equipment. In this report the commission cited the value of needle exchange in reducing the risk of HIV infection among those who continue to inject drugs.

In 1993, the GAO prepared a report on needle exchange programs in response to the questions regarding the efficacy of these programs in reducing HIV infections. The report concluded that syringe exchange programs directly reduce unsafe injection practices, reduce the spread of HIV, acquaint drug abusers with treatment programs, and increase proper disposal of used syringes.

The GAO report emphasized the need for exchange programs to protect the health of children. In September 1992, the CDC reported that among children younger than 13, 40 percent of those with AIDS were born to women who contracted HIV through injection drug use and 17 percent were born to women who contracted HIV through sex with an injection drug user.

Women, minorities, urban dwellers, and persons with lower socioeconomic backgrounds are disproportionately affected by the spread of HIV because of their link with intravenous drug use. Studies in high prevalence areas have shown that the rate of newly acquired HIV infections among intravenous drug users may be as high as four percent annually.

Despite the success of these programs, the federal government has banned the use of federal funds for syringe exchange programs. Some states have also denied state funding. Many cities in the United States, including Washington, DC; New York City; New Haven, CT; Portland, OR; and Boulder, CO, have nevertheless maintained successful syringe exchange programs. These programs understand the economic and legal concerns of intravenous drug users. The purchase or rental of injection paraphernalia in shooting galleries is often expensive, and the possession of injection equipment may lead to arrest and incarceration.

Public policymakers and private individuals who oppose exchange programs state that the programs send a wrong message to young people, suggest that the government approves of illegal drug use, undermine the force and efficacy of laws intended to punish drug use, and promote illegal drug use. Despite these arguments against syringe exchange programs, initial results of the program have consistently demonstrated the reduction of newly acquired HIV infection and do not result in increased crime, drug use, or violence within the affected communities.

Results of pilot programs conducted in New Haven, CT, and other cities show that syringe exchange programs decrease illegal drug use as a result of more addicts in treatment, increases less risky methods of drug use, decrease HIV seroprevalence among drug injecting persons in the community, and reduce the number of needles discarded in public by as much as 50 percent in some locations.

Needle Exchange Programs: Research Suggests Promise as an AIDS Prevention Strategy. GAO Report to the Chairman, Select Committee on Narcotics Abuse and Control, House of Representatives, GAO/HRD-93-60, March 1993.

TAT (*tat*)

Tat is one of the regulatory genes of HIV. Tat plays a role in the ability of HIV to infect cells, replicate, and cause disease.

T4 lymphocytes *see* CD4+ T lymphocytes

T8 lymphocytes *see* CD8+ T lymphocytes

3TC *see* Lamivudine

Thrombotic thrombocytopenic purpura

Thrombotic thrombocytopenic purpura is a form of idiopathic thrombocytopenic purpura that causes blood clots or thromboses. *See also* Immune (idiopathic) thrombocytopenic purpura.

Thrush *see* Oral candidiasis

TMP-SMX

TMP-SMX is a first line treatment for *Pneumocystis jiroveci* pneumonia (PCP), which often occurs in patients with AIDS.

Toxoplasmosis

Toxoplasmosis is an opportunistic infection and AIDS-defining illness that is caused by the protozoan parasite *Toxoplasma gondii*.

Etiology

The etiologic agent is the protozoan parasite *Toxoplasma gondii*. This parasite is carried by cats, birds, and other animals, and is found in soil contaminated by cat feces and in meat, particularly pork, and can be contracted by ingestion of oocyst excreted by felines. *T. gondii* is an infection that has crossed species (zoonosis), with felines as the definitive host.

Epidemiology

Toxoplasmosis is a common opportunistic infection in patients with AIDS. It has a prevalence ranging from 10–40 percent in Europe, the Caribbean, and Africa, and a prevalence of 5–10 percent in the United States. Since the widespread use of prophylactic therapies was introduced in 1988, the incidence of this infection has declined in patients with HIV. The underlying immune cellular defect in HIV infection is still the major cause of the reactivation of latent *T. gondii* infection that has persisted in the central nervous system or extraneural tissues after an earlier acute infection. Toxoplasmosis usually occurs late in HIV disease, when the CD4+ lymphocyte count is less than 100 cells/mm^3.

Symptoms

Toxoplasmosis typically causes encephalitis, retinitis, or pneumonitis. Toxoplasmic encephalitis occurs as single or multiple intracerebral abscesses, with focal neurologic signs and constitutional symptoms that progress over a few days or weeks. Fever and headaches are present in 40–70 percent of cases. Neurologic dysfunction, including confusion and lethargy, are seen in 40 percent of cases. Focal central nervous system deficits occur in 50–60 percent of cases, and seizures (the typical presenting symptom) occur in 30–40 percent of cases. The combination of fever, headaches, mild neurologic deficit, or any unexplained neurologic symptoms in persons with HIV infection suggest the possibility of toxoplasmic encephalitis.

Toxoplasmic retinitis represents the third most common opportunistic infection of the retina in AIDS. Symptoms include decreased visual acuity, defects in visual field, "floaters" and loss of peripheral vision. Unlike retinitis caused by cyto-megalovirus, in toxoplasmic retinitis, there is usually little or no hemorrhage.

Toxoplasmic pneumonitis occurs generally in a context of disseminated disease and presents as a bilateral interstitial pneumonia. Symptoms are non-specific and include fever, cough, shortness of breath, and interstitial radiologic abnormalities.

Diagnosis

Because toxoplasmosis typically occurs in AIDS as a reactivation of a latent, pre-existing condition, a diagnosis of toxoplasmic disease should be suspected in patients with a low CD4+ cell count, usually below 100 cells/mm^3, patients with specific antibodies to toxoplasmosis indicating past infection, and in patients receiving no specific prophylactic therapy for toxoplasmosis.

CT scanning or MRI studies of the central nervous system are useful in diagnosing toxoplasmic encephalitis. Toxoplasmic abscesses are typically contrast-enhancing lesions surrounded by edema. MRI may also reveal hemorrhages, which are highly suggestive of toxoplasmic necrosis. A mass effect may also be seen, with displacement of the ventricles.

Diagnosis of toxoplasmic retinitis relies on funduscopic examination, which typically shows a thick, dense, opaque appearance of retinal lesions with very distinct borders, and an intense inflammation of the vitreous eye fluid. The identification of *T. gondii* in tissues or body fluid gives a definitive diagnosis of toxoplasmosis.

Treatment

Treatment consists of initial acute therapy over a period of 3–6 weeks followed by life-long maintenance therapy unless CD4+ T cell counts show significant improvement. The combination of pyrimethamine (50–75 mg daily) administered orally, and sulfadiazine, using 4–6 grams daily, should be the first-line acute therapy. These drugs work together to block the folic acid pathway of the trophozoites, but have no effect on the cyst forms of the parasite. Folinic acid, using 25 mg daily, should be also administered to prevent toxicity. This drug combination should evoke clinical improvement in 5–10 days, although adverse effects such as fever and rash may occur.

Alternately, the combination of pyrimetamine and clindamycin can be used in cases of intolerance to sulfa antibiotics, which is reported to occur in up to 40 percent of patients infected with HIV. Another alternative treatment is atovaquone used with pyrimethamine and clarithromycin.

Risk factors

Risk factors include avoiding contact with raw meat, cooking meat properly, and washing vegetables. High-risk individuals are defined as those with CD4+ T cell counts less than 200 cells/mm³ and positive test results for toxoplasmosis antibodies.

Trachoma

Trachoma is a condition of contagious conjunctivitis (inflammation of the conjunctiva, the inner rim of the eye) marked by inflammatory granulations on the conjunctival surfaces. Caused by infection with the bacterial organism *Chlamydia trachomatis*, trachoma may lead to blindness if left untreated. Infants of mothers with untreated cervical chlamydia infection have a 40 percent chance of developing trachoma. Prophylaxis of the ocular surface with povidone-iodine 2.5 percent solution is the most efficacious and least toxic agent. Silver nitrate solution, tetracycline, and erythromycin ointments are also effective in preventing neonatal conjunctivitis. Infection is treated with erythromycin, administered orally for 14 days.

Child-to-child transmission is the most common method of chlamydial transmission in trachoma endemic areas, usually developing countries. Several hundred million people are known to be afflicted with trachoma, and millions of people have been blinded by it. In some endemic areas, most children are infected by age two. Poor hygiene and unsanitary conditions contribute to trachoma prevalence. Usually, barring complications, the active disease wanes when the children are six to 10 years old. Most of these children have few lingering symptoms with no permanent effect on vision. Children with moderate to severe trachoma often develop severely scarred conjunctivae, which can distort the upper eyelid, eventually abrading the eyelashes and affecting the cells that make up the cornea. This process may take 30 years to evolve, and blindness generally occurs in adults over age 40 years as a result of childhood trachoma.

Trachoma begins as an acute conjunctivitis with pus and may be complicated by a co-existing bacterial infection. *See also* **Chlamydia**.

Transmission modes

Transmission modes refer to the routes that specific infectious agents can use to gain entry to the body. For instance, in most STDs, sexual intercourse is the primary mode of transmission.

Treatment

Treatment in STDs is primarily used to eradicate infectious organisms and to reduce symptoms associated with the specific infection. Patients with the same STD will not necessarily be given the same treatment. This is because different strains of the same organism can have different susceptibilities to antibiotic or antiviral therapies. The specific STD entries in this book describe treatment guidelines recommended by the Centers for Disease Control and Prevention or the U.S. Department of Health & Human Services. Treatment is always prescribed on an individual basis and may vary based on the patient's body weight, specific symptoms or complications, newer treatment guidelines, or the physician's own experience.

Trichomonas vaginalis

Trichomonas vaginalis is a parasitic protozoa and the etiologic agent responsible for the STD trichomoniasis.

Trichomoniasis

Trichomoniasis is the most common curable STD in the United States, with an estimated five million Americans infected annually. Trichomonas was first reported in France in 1836 as a cause of vaginitis.

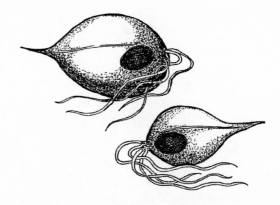

Trichomonas vaginalis (Marvin G. Miller).

cells and causes a reddened appearance in the vaginal tissue.

Etiology

Trichomoniasis is caused by the parasitic protozoa *Trichomonas vaginalis*, a single-celled organism known as a trichomonad or flagellate because it has whip-like tails or flagella. Trichomonads are slightly larger than white blood cells and move rapidly with the help of its five flagella. The vigorous motion of trichomonads damages

Epidemiology

Trichomonas vaginalis is transmitted through sexual intercourse and primarily affects 16 to 35-year-old women, although men may also be infected. In the United States, it is estimated that two million women become infected each year. Trichomonas cannot be transmitted through casual contact.

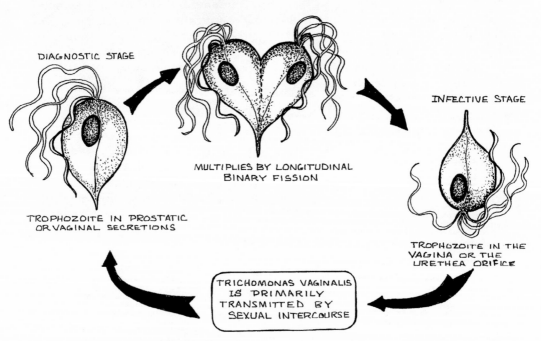

DIAGNOSTIC STAGE

MULTIPLIES BY LONGITUDINAL BINARY FISSION

INFECTIVE STAGE

TROPHOZOITE IN PROSTATIC OR VAGINAL SECRETIONS

TROPHOZOITE IN THE VAGINA OR THE URETHEA ORIFICE

TRICHOMONAS VAGINALIS IS PRIMARILY TRANSMITTED BY SEXUAL INTERCOURSE

Trichomonas life cycle (Marvin G. Miller).

Symptoms

Symptoms generally develop within six months of initial infection. Most men with trichomoniasis do not have symptoms, but some may experience an unusual discharge from the penis or pain during urination or ejaculation. Men may also experience a burning sensation with urination and an urge to urinate. In women, symptoms vary, and may include a yellow-green, malodorous, frothy discharge from the vagina, pain during urination or sexual intercourse, reddened vaginal tissue, itching, and abdominal pain. Occasionally the urinary tract may become infected. Other symptoms include painful sexual intercourse, lower abdominal discomfort, and the urge to urinate.

Diagnosis

Diagnosis in women is made by a wet mount or wet prep test; in this procedure a specimen taken from the vagina with a swab is examined microscopically for the presence of Trichomonas. In men, specimens are collected from the urethra. Direct wet mount testing is positive in about 70 percent of infected patients. The specimen may also be cultured and examined for Trichomonas growth. The culture test is positive in about 90 percent of infected patients. The vaginal pH may also be measured to help in diagnosing Trichomonas. In infections, it is generally elevated to 6.0 or 7.0.

Treatment

Antibiotics, especially metronidazole, are highly effective in treating trichomoniasis. Treatment is recommended for men even if their symptoms have resolved spontaneously to make sure the infection is cleared and cannot be passed on to others. It is also important for sex partners to be treated to prevent recurrence. Clotrimazole (Gyne-Lotrimin) and the spermicide nonoxynol-9 may help relieve symptoms, but they do not eliminate infection and are not FDA approved as a treatment. The usual treatment is metronidazole (Flagyl) using a single oral dose of two grams. Alternately, it may be given for 5–7 days using 250 mg three times daily.

Pregnancy

Pregnant patients with trichomoniasis may experience premature labor. Trichomonas infection can also be spread to the baby, but this is rare. Babies born to infected mothers may contract infection during delivery, causing symptoms of fever in the discharge. Female infants may also have a vaginal discharge. Because trichomoniasis is frequently accompanied by bacterial vaginosis, affected patients should be examined and treated for both disorders. The CDC recommends a single two gram dose of metronidazole, which is safe and effective in all trimesters.

Risk Factors

Latex condoms used properly offer protection against infection with *Trichomonas vaginalis*. Unprotected sex and multiple sex partners are risk factors.

Complications

Trichomonas vaginalis can invade the Bartholin's glands and other small glands near the urethra. For this reason, topical metronidazole gel is not an appropriate treatment. Trichomonads also generate hydrogen molecules that remove oxygen from the vaginal environment. This may promote the growth of anaerobic bacteria and explains why many women with trichomonas also develop bacterial vaginosis (BV). A unique feature of trichomonas is its ability to live on in the vagina for years if not treated. This also explains why trichomonas is sometimes seen in women of advanced age who have not been sexually active for a long time.

Precautions

The anticonvulsant medications Phenobarbital and phenytoin (Dilantin) can interfere with the action of metronidazole, making it less effective. A follow-up treatment with two grams metronidazole daily for five days is often recommended for patients on interfering medications.

Centers for Disease Control and Prevention. *Sexually Transmitted Diseases Treatment Guidelines 2002.* Atlanta: U.S. Dept. of Health and Human Services, 2002.

Tropical spastic paraparesis/HTLV-1 associated myelopathy (TSP/HAM)

TSP/HAM is a chronic neurological disease caused by the HTLV-I retrovirus. This syndrome results from demyelination of the long motor neurons (central nervous system cells) of the spinal cord, causing a variety of symptoms, which can vary in severity.

Etiology

The infectious agent is the HTLV-I retrovirus, which was first isolated in 1979 from an African-American patient with adult T cell lymphoma.

Epidemiology

Females are more likely to develop TSP/HAM, a condition that is more prevalent in Africa, Japan, the Caribbean, the West Indies, and among Australian aborigines than in the United States. HTLV-I, which also causes Adult T Cell Lymphoma (ATL), can be transmitted through sexual intercourse and through blood-to-blood contact. Blood donors in the United States are screened for HTLV-I and HTLV-II, effectively reducing transmission through blood products. Approximately 15 percent of all HTLV-1 infections are transmitted via mother-to-child transmission, particularly through breastfeeding. The majority of cases of TSP/HAM occur in individuals between 30 and 50 years old, although children as young as three years may be infected. It is suspected that TSP/HAM may be immune mediated because it is more likely to occur in patients with specific HLA markers, which control the immune response.

Symptoms

Symptoms include stiff gait, spasticity, lower extremity weakness, back pain, urinary incontinence, impotence, and rarely, ataxia. In some cases, lesions of the central nervous system can be detected.

Diagnosis

Diagnosis is made with serologic tests for HTLV-I antibodies. Viral antibody titers are markedly elevated, indicating a loss of immunological control.

Treatment

Glucocorticoid steroids are used to reduce symptoms in rapidly progressive cases. Treatment with danazol, an androgenic steroid, causes improvement in urinary and fecal continence but not in neurological symptoms. There are clinical results of improvement with high doses of vitamin C.

Risk Factors

Risk factors include commercial sex work, unprotected sex, and past infection with *Chlamydia trachomatis*. In countries where blood donors are not screened for HTLV-I, transfusion with blood products causes a higher risk of HTLV-I infection. Among patients receiving one unit of contaminated blood, 50 percent will show serological evidence (positive blood tests for HTLV-1 antibodies) of HTLV-1 infection. Intravenous drug use is also a significant method for HTLV-1 transmission, although most transmission associated with intravenous drug use involves HTLV-II.

Cleghorn, Farley, and William Blattner. "Human T-cell Lymphotropic Virus and HTLV Infection." Chapter 19 in *Sexually Transmitted Diseases*. 3rd edition. Edited by King K. Holmes, et al. New York: McGraw-Hill, 1999.

Tuberculosis (*Mycobacterium tuberculosis*)

Although it is not a sexually transmitted disease, the infectious disease tuberculosis (TB) is on the rise among individuals infected with HIV/AIDS.

Etiology

Tuberculosis is caused by *Mycobacterium tuberculosis*. The severity of infection depends largely on the host's immune system. The disease, which primarily affects the lungs, is highly contagious and is spread by airborne droplets expelled from the lungs when a person with active TB coughs, sneezes, or speaks. Exposure to these droplets can lead to infection in the air sacs of the lungs.

Epidemiology

According to a study commissioned by the Justice Department, of the 34,000 Americans diagnosed with tuberculosis in 1996, up to 35 percent were recently released inmates. If the body's immune system is impaired due to HIV infection, aging, malnutrition, drugs, or other factors, the TB bacterium may begin to spread more widely in the lungs or to other tissues. TB is seen with increasing frequency among HIV-infected persons. In HIV, the annual risk of developing TB is 10 percent, compared with a lifetime risk of 10 percent in healthy individuals.

Symptoms

Most cases of TB occur in the lungs, although infection may occur in extrapulmonary sites such as the larynx, lymph nodes, brain, kidneys, or bones. Virtually every organ system can be affected, and tuberculosis may present with swollen lymph nodes, bloody sputum, skin lesions, and symptoms of meningitis. Extrapulmonary (other than lung) infections are more commonly seen in patients with HIV.

Diagnosis

Standard PPD skin tests are used to diagnose TB. Skin reactions greater than 5mm to a standard PPD test are considered positive in individuals with HIV. A negative test is not useful for ruling out TB in patients with HIV due to the frequency of anergy, especially in patients with low CD4+ T cell counts. Active tuberculosis may occur at any level of immunosuppression, and may be the first indication of HIV infection. All persons with active TB should be tested for HIV infection.

Definitive diagnosis is based on identifying the acid-fast bacillus (AFB) in any clinical specimen, such as sputum, bronchoalveolar lavage washings, blood, bone marrow, cerebrospinal fluid, urine or biopsy specimens, using stain or culture techniques. Individuals infected with HIV and TB are more likely to have negative sputum stains. Culture takes as long as 10–21 days to identify the organisms. Nucleic acid amplification tests are also available and can detect *M. tuberculosis* with a high degree of sensitivity and specificity within several hours.

Treatment

Treatment relies on a standard regimen of isoniazid, rifampin, and pyrazinamide, with ethambutol commonly added if there is suspicion of possible drug resistance in the community or in the individual patient. If culture and sensitivity do not show resistance to the standard regimen, ethambutol is not necessary. The standard regimen is continued for three months, followed by a two-drug regimen for nine months or at least two months longer than needed to induce a negative AFB stain. Because tuberculosis is very contagious, respiratory isolation is recommended for patients with active tuberculosis.

In November 2002, the CDC reported that isoniazid remains the treatment of choice for latent infection, and that fatal and severe liver injury has been associated with treatment of latent tuberculosis infection with the drug combination rifampin and pyrazinamide. The CDC reports that this combination should be used with caution in latent infection and that blood tests to monitor liver function should be performed at baseline, two, four, and six weeks of treatment. *See also My-cobacterium avium* complex.

Tumor Necrosis Factor (TNF)

TNF is a cytokine produced by macrophages, which helps activate T cells. TNF is also suspected of stimulating HIV activity. TNF levels are high in persons with HIV infection, and TNF is suspected of contributing to HIV-related wasting, neuropathy, and dementia. TNF triggers a biochemical pathway that leads to the programmed form of cell suicide known as apoptosis, and it activates a key molecule that can block this pathway.

The Tuskegee syphilis experiment

From 1932 to 1972, the U.S. Public Health Service, in trying to learn more about syphilis and justify treatment programs for blacks, withheld adequate treatment from a group of poor black men who had the disease, causing needless pain and suffering for the men and their loved ones.

The Public Health Service, working with the Tuskegee Institute, began the study in Macon County, Alabama, to discover how syphilis affected blacks as opposed to whites— with the theory being that whites experienced more neurological complications from syphilis, whereas blacks were more susceptible to cardiovascular damage. It was called the "Tuskegee Study of Untreated Syphilis in the Negro Male."

The study involved 600 black men, generally poor, illiterate sharecroppers. Of these men, 399 had syphilis and 201 did not. Those who were infected were not told what disease they were suffering from or of its dangers. Rather, they were informed that they were being treated for "bad blood." The Public Health Service did not provide treatment for the disease, with the intention of collecting data from the autopsies of the men. Thus they were left to degenerate under the ravages of tertiary syphilis— which can include tumors, heart disease, paralysis, blindness, insanity, and death. In exchange for taking part in the study, the men were provided free medical exams, free meals, and burial insurance. Although originally projected to last six months, the study was conducted for 40 years.

During the years that the study took place, several nationwide campaigns to eradicate venereal disease came to Macon County. However, those involved in the Public Health Service program were prevented from participating. Even when penicillin became the drug of choice for syphilis in 1947, it was not provided to the subjects. Moreover, during World War II, 250 of the men registered for the draft and were consequently ordered to get treatment for syphilis, but the Public Health Services exempted them from treatment.

In addition, the experiment continued in spite of the Henderson Act of 1943, a public health law requiring testing and treatment for venereal disease, and in spite of the World Health Organization's Declaration of Helsinki in 1964, which specified that "informed consent" was needed for experimentation involving human beings.

The story of the experiment broke in the *Washington Star* on July 25, 1972, in an article by Jean Heller of the Associated Press. The source of her information was Peter Buxton, a former Public Health Service venereal disease interviewer, along with officials from the Centers for Disease Control. In response, the Public Health Service remained unrepentant, claiming that the men had been "volunteers" and were "always happy to see the doctors." The story caused a public outcry that lead the assistant secretary for Health and Scientific Affairs to appoint an ad hoc advisory panel to review the study. The panel had nine members from the fields of medicine, law, religion, labor, education, health administration, and public affairs.

The panel found that the men had agreed to be examined and treated. However, there was no evidence that researchers had informed them of the study or its real purpose. Rather, the men had been misled, and not given all the facts required to provide informed consent. The advisory panel concluded that the Tuskegee Study was "ethically unjustified," and in October 1972, advised stopping the study at once. The study was officially ended one month later. By this time, 28 of the men had died directly of syphilis, 100 were dead of related complications, 40 of their wives had been infected, and 19 of their children had been born with congenital syphilis.

A $1.8 billion lawsuit was filed on behalf of the survivors and their families by civil rights attorney Fred Gray. The lawsuit was settled for $10 million. As a part of the settlement, the U.S. government promised to provide free medical and burial services to all living participants. The Tuskegee Health Benefit Program was established to provide these services. It also provided health services for wives, widows, and children who had been infected because of the study. The Centers for Disease Control and Prevention was given responsibility for the program, where it remains today in the National Center for HIV, STD, and TB Prevention.

None of the physician-researchers who ran the study was ever prosecuted. Institutional review boards (IRBS) that must examine most protocols that involve human subjects before research studies begin now exist, in part, because of the revulsions against what happened at Tuskegee. In addition, in 1997, 25 years after the study was exposed, President Bill Clinton issued an official apology to the remaining eight survivors, their families, and the nation's African-American citizens.

The Tuskegee Study raises questions about racism in medical research. It is often paired with the Nazi doctors' experiments on Holocaust victims that were detailed at the war trials at Nuremberg. The Public Health Service rejected such comparisons, claiming that it was just carrying out orders and was exempt from personal responsibility.

In 1990, a survey found that 10 percent of African-Americans believed that the U.S. government created AIDS as a plot to exterminate blacks, and another 20 percent could not rule out the possibility that this might be true. The AIDS epidemic has exposed the Tuskegee Study as an historical marker for the legitimate discontent of African-Americans with the public health system.

In the absence of a cure for AIDS, education and dialogue can contribute to a better understanding of how to develop and implement HIV education programs that are scientifically sound, culturally sensitive, and ethically acceptable.

Jones, James H. *Bad Blood: The Tuskegee Syphilis Experiment.* Expanded edition. New York: Free Press, 1993.

Reverby, Susan M., editor. *Tuskegee's Truths; Rethinking the Tuskegee Syphilis Study.* Chapel Hill, NC: University of North Carolina Press, 2000.

The Tuskegee Syphilis Experiment. http://www.infoplease.com/ipa/A0762136.html.

The Tuskegee Syphilis Study: A Hard Lesson Learned. http:www.cdc.gov/nchstp/od/tuskegee/time.htm.

Ulcers

Ulcers are breaks in the skin or mucous membranes with loss of surface tissue, disintegration, and necrosis (tissue destruction or death) of the upper skin or membrane surface that may exude pus. *See also* **Genital ulcer disease.**

UNAIDS

UNAIDS is a joint program that includes the Joint United Nations Programme on

HIV/AIDS and the World Health Organization (WHO). From 1986, WHO had the lead responsibility on AIDS in the United Nations, helping countries to set up much-needed national AIDS programs. But by the mid–1990s, it became clear that the relentless spread of HIV, and the epidemic's devastating impact on all aspects of human lives and on social and economic development, were creating an emergency that would require a greatly expanded United Nations effort. It was also clear that no single United Nations organization could provide the coordinated level of assistance needed to address the many factors driving the HIV epidemic, or help countries deal with the impact of HIV/AIDS on household, communities, and local economies.

Addressing these challenges head-on, in 1996 the United Nations drew six organizations together in a joint and co-sponsored program: the joint United Nations Programme on HIV/AIDS (UNAIDS), which included the United Nations Children's Fund (UNICEF); the United Nations Development Programme (UNDP); the United Nations Population Fund (UNFPA); the United Nations Educational, Scientific and Cultural Organization (UNESCO); the World Health Organization (WHO); and the World Bank. The United Nations International Drug Control Programme (UNDP) was included in April 1999, and the International Labour Organization (ILO) joined in October 2001.

The goal of UNAIDS is to catalyze, strengthen, and orchestrate the unique expertise, resources, and networks of influence that each of these organizations offers. Working together through UNAIDS, the co-sponsors expand their outreach through strategic alliances with other United Nations agencies, national governments, corporations, media, community-based groups, and networks of people living with HIV/AIDS.

UNAIDS has an annual budget equivalent to $95 million and a staff of 139 professionals based in Geneva, Switzerland. In 2002, UNAIDS received more than $92 million in contributions from 28 donor countries. The largest donors were the U.S. government, which donated $18 million, followed by the governments of the Netherlands, Norway, Sweden, Finland, and Japan. As the main advocate for global action on HIV/AIDS, UNAIDS leads, strengthens, and supports an expanded response aimed at preventing the transmission of HIV, providing care and support, reducing the vulnerability of individuals and communities to HIV/AIDS, and alleviating the impact of the epidemic. For more information see, http://www.unaids.org.

United States Department of Health and Human Services (DHHS or HHS)

The U.S. Department of Health and Human Services supports a vigorous, broad-based public health response to HIV/AIDS that includes extensive research, prevention initiatives, and efforts to expand access to quality health care and services for persons in need. HHS is also working to address the disproportionate impact of HIV/AIDS among ethnic minority populations in the United States. Of the $16 billion budgeted by United States to address HIV/AIDS at home and abroad, HHS is estimated to receive $12.9 billion.

HHS programs, including those of the National Institutes of Health (NIH) and Centers for Disease Prevention and Control (CDC), include vaccine development, prevention research and strategies, clinical trials, safety in the blood supply, a national AIDS hotline, healthcare worker initiatives, the Ryan White CARE Act Program, Medicaid and Medicare Programs, Services for American Indians and Alaska Natives, Global AIDS initiatives, and the Health Disparities Initiative (http://www.hhs.gov/).

United States Department of Justice (DOJ)

The United States Department of Justice serves to enforce the law and defend the interests of the nation according to law. In relation to STDs, the DOJ regulates diagnostic testing and treatment policies of inmates suspected of having or known to have STDs. In this aspect it conducts research and works with other agencies such as the CDC that are involved in STD prevention and treatment.

Universal Precautions

Universal precautions are standard clinical methods used to reduce the risk of blood-borne infection. Universal precautions include the use of latex gloves, protective clothing, safety glasses, and masks, depending on the risk of exposure in specific patient populations. Universal precautions also include proper disposal of biological waste, used needles, and other medical equipment. Universal precautions are routinely used in specific settings, where all patients are considered potentially infectious. Specific recommendations are related to the amount of direct contact and exposure to blood and blood products.

Unprotected sex

Unprotected sex refers to any act of oral, anal, or vaginal intercourse in which barrier protection (condoms or dental dams) is not used.

Ureaplasma urealyticum

Ureaplasma urealyticum is a mycoplasma-like bacterium that occasionally causes urethritis in men. Ureaplasmal infections are usually treated with tetracycline or doxycycline taken orally for at least seven days or with a single one gram dose of azithromycin.

Urethritis

Urethritis is a condition of inflammation of the urethra, the canal that carries off the urine from the bladder and in the male serves also as a genital duct.

Etiology

The clinically significant organisms that cause urethritis in males primarily include *Neisseria gonorrhoeae* and *Chlamydia trachomatis*. Urethritis may also be caused by *Ureaplasma urealyticum, Mycoplasma genitalium, Trichomonas vaginalis* and herpes simplex virus.

Symptoms

Urethritis in male patients is caused by an infection characterized by urethral discharge of mucopurulent (mucus and pus) or purulent (characterized by pus) material, and sometimes by dysuria (difficult or painful discharge of urine) or urethral pruritis (localized itching due to irritation of sensitive nerve endings). Patients may also be free of symptoms.

Diagnosis

Urethritis can be documented on the basis of any of the following signs: mucopurulent or purulent discharge, Gram stain of urethral secretions demonstrating more than five white blood cells for each oil immersion field, positive leukocyte esterase test on first void urine, or microscopic examination of urine showing more than 10 white blood cells for each high power field.

Testing for gonorrhea and chlamydial infection is important to avoid possible complications. In most states these infections must be reported to state health departments, and partners from within the last 60 days are contacted so that they can be treated. If testing methods are not available, men presenting with these symptoms are generally treated for both types of infection. Patients are also instructed to abstain from intercourse until seven days after treatment is started.

Nucleic acid amplification tests performed on urine or urethral swabs enable detection of gonorrhea and chlamydia. These tests are more sensitive than traditional culture techniques for *C. trachomatis* and are the preferred method for the detection of this organism.

Nongonococcal urethritis (NGU) is diagnosed if Gram negative intracellular diplococci are not identified on urethral smears. Complications of NGU among men infected with chlamydia include epididymitis and Reiter's syndrome.

Treatment

The recommended treatment is azithromycin, using one gram orally in a single dose, or doxycycline using 100 mg orally twice a day for seven days. Alternative regimens include erythromycin base, using 500 mg orally four times daily for seven days; or erythromycin ethylsuccinate, using 800 mg orally four times daily for seven days; or ofloxacin, using 300 mg twice a day for seven days; or levofloxacin, using 500 mg once daily for seven days.

Patients should be instructed to return for evaluation if symptoms persist or recur after completion of therapy. Patients should be instructed to abstain from sexual intercourse until seven days after therapy is initiated. Patients should refer all sex partners they have had within the 60 days prior to development of symptoms for evaluation and treatment.

Precautions

Patients may have recurrent and persistent urethritis following therapy. Objective signs of urethritis should be present before initiation of therapy. Some cases of recurrent urethritis following doxycycline treatment may be caused by tetracycline resistant *Ureaplasma urealyticum*. If re-exposure is not likely, patients should be treated with metronidazole, using two grams orally in a single dose, along with erythromycin base, using 500 mg orally; or erythromycin ethylsuccinate, using 800 mg four times daily for seven days. Most forms of urethritis may facilitate HIV infection. *See also* **Chlamydia**; **Gonorrhea**; and *Ureaplasma urealyticum.*

Urine tests

Urine specimens can be tested for infection, evidenced by the presence of white blood cells and bacteria. Yeast and trichomonas may also be found in routine urinalysis testing. Urine can also be used in NAT tests used to detect *Neisseria gonorrhoeae* and *Chlamydia trachomatis,* and in 2003, tests for detecting HIV antibodies in urine were FDA approved.

Urogenital infections

Urogenital infections refer to infections occurring in the organs that are related to or that affect excretion and reproduction. The most common urogenital infections are those caused by the bacteria *Chlamydia trachomatis* and *Neisseria gonorrhoeae.*

USAID-Congo

USAID-Congo is a health program administered by the U.S. for residents of the Congo that addresses key health problems, with an emphasis on the redevelopment of structures for public health care and citizen participation. The rationale for working in child survival, HIV/AIDS/STD prevention, and infectious diseases in the Congo has not changed since the introduction of USAID in 1997. If anything, the health situation has worsened due to ongoing conflict in the region. Reliable health statistics are unavailable, although the maternal and child mortality rates are high. The U.S. Congress permits USAID to work directly with the Congo government to save children's lives, particularly in halting the spread of infectious diseases, and to stop the spread of HIV/AIDS.

USAID-Congo helps with STD prevention by social marketing of condoms, informational and educational campaigns, improving systems for treating STDs, operational research, and materials development. For more information see http://www.usaid.gov/cg/health.html.

Vaccines

Vaccines are substances that contain treated antigenic components from an infectious microorganism. Vaccines stimulate the immune system to produce antibodies directed against the specific microorganism. This offers protection if the person is later exposed to the infectious agents. Vaccines are currently available for hepatitis A and hepatitis B. Clinical trials are currently underway for vaccines to prevent against Chlamydia, Herpes, HPV, and HIV infection.

In clinical trial reports from November 2002, the HPV-16 vaccine was shown to have 100 percent efficacy in protecting women not previously exposed to this virus. HPV-16 is the leading HPV strain associated with cervical cancer. Vaccines against another associated strain HPV-18 are also being tested.

A vaccine against HSV-2 is currently being tested and has been shown to have efficacy against HSV-2 in women who are negative for both HSV-1 and HSV-2. Both vaccines are most effective when they target young women before they have been exposed to the virus.

Barclay, Laurie. "Vaccines May Protect Women from STDs, Cervical Cancer." *Medscape Medical News*, Nov. 20, 2002.

Vaginal infections

Vaginal infections are usually characterized by a vaginal discharge or vulvar itching and irritation, and a vaginal odor may be present. The three diseases most frequently associated with vaginal discharge are trichomoniasis (caused by *Trichomonas vaginalis*), bacterial vaginosis (caused by a replacement of the normal vaginal flora by an overgrowth of anaerobic microorganisms, mycoplasmas, and *Gardnerella vaginalis*), and candidiasis (caused by *Candida albicans*).

Vaginal infection can be diagnosed by a test of vaginal secretions for pH and by a microscopic examination of the discharge.

The pH may be elevated to 4.5 or higher in bacterial vaginosis and trichomoniasis. Microscopic examination (wet prep) is used to detect trichomonas, yeast, and clue cells. The presence of objective signs of external vulvar inflammation in the absence of vaginal pathogens, along with a minimal amount of discharge, suggests the possibility of mechanical, chemical, allergic, or other non-infectious irritation of the vulva. *See also* **Bacterial vaginosis**; **Candidiasis**; and **Trichomoniasis**.

Vaginitis

Vaginitis is a generic term used to describe vaginal itching and discharge. Most cases of vaginitis are caused by yeast infections, bacterial vaginosis, and trichomonas infections. Other causes include mobiluncus and streptococcal infections. Vaginitis may also be caused by a loss of estrogen leading to atrophy (breakdown of tissue). Atrophic vaginitis may also occur in women in the postpartum period and during breastfeeding.

Some medications may also cause symptoms of atrophic vaginitis, including luprolide (Lupron) and danocrine (Danazol), because they interfere with estrogen production.

Vaginosis

Vaginosis is a vaginal condition causing symptoms similar to infection, which is caused by an imbalance of bacterial flora. Vaginosis is not characterized by infection or inflammation. *See also* **Bacterial vaginosis**.

Valacyclovir

Valacyclovir (Valtrex GlaxoSmithKline) is an antiviral medication used for the treatment of herpes simplex virus. Studies show that valacyclovir is also highly effective in preventing HSV transmission to uninfected partners and is safe and well-tolerated. The active metabolite of valacyclovir is acyclovir.

Venereal disease (VD)

Venereal disease is an older term used to describe diseases caused by or associated with genital contact. Venereal disease is derived from the word "venery," which refers to the pursuit of Venus, the goddess of love.

Viral burden

Viral burden refers to the amount of virus, such as HIV, present in the circulating blood. Monitoring a person's viral burden is important because of the apparent correlation between the amount of virus in the blood and disease severity. Sicker patients generally have more virus than those with less advanced disease. The HIV viral load test is effective for monitoring the HIV viral burden.

Viral core

Typically, a virus contains an RNA or DNA core of genetic material surrounded by a protein coat. HIV contains an envelope that contains a bullet-shaped core of another protein, p24, that surrounds the viral RNA. Each strand of HIV RNA contains the virus's nine genes. The structural genes *gag, pol,* and *env* contain the information necessary to make structural proteins.

Viral envelope

Some viruses, such as HIV, contain outer coats or envelopes. The envelope of HIV is composed of two layers of fat-like molecules called lipids, taken from the membranes of human cells. Embedded in the envelope are numerous cellular proteins, as well as mushroom-shaped HIV proteins that protrude from the surface. Each mushroom is thought to consist of four gp41 molecules embedded in the envelope. HIV uses these proteins to attach to and infect host cells.

Viral load

Viral load refers to the quantity of virus present in one's blood; in HIV infections, the quantity of HIV RNA is measured. Viral load is used as a predictor of disease progression, and provides a measure of treatment response. Viral load test results are expressed as the number or copies of RNA per ml of blood plasma.

Plasma viral load has also been shown to predict the rate of decline of CD4+ lymphocytes, progression to AIDS, and death. The higher the HIV RNA value, the faster the CD4+ lymphocyte population declines. This, in turn, leads to a greater chance of developing AIDS or progressing to death. Combined with a CD4+ count, the viral load test has excellent prognostic value.

The typical course of HIV RNA in an infected individual has been well documented. Within weeks of infection the virus rapidly disseminates throughout the body. Before host immune responses are mounted, an explosion of viral replication occurs, with plasma HIV increasing to very high levels for one to two months. CD4+ counts fall at this time. As the immune response is activated, HIV levels fall rapidly and the CD4+ count increases toward pre-infection levels.

Within 6–9 months after the initial exposure, a dynamic equilibrium among cell infection, viral replication, and CD4+ lymphocyte maintenance occurs. The viral load levels off or reaches a plateau, which is referred to as a setpoint. The viral load may remain at this level or gradually increase over time. The higher this setpoint level is, the greater the chance of disease progression. The nadir is the lowest level to which viral load falls after starting antiretroviral treatment. Studies have shown that the nadir of the viral load is the best predictor of long-term viral suppression.

Viral load testing can be used to decide when to start therapy, to assess and monitor the effectiveness of antiretroviral therapy, and to help make ongoing treatment decisions. Because viral load and CD4+ counts do not necessarily correlate as expected, it is important to use both tests in making treatment decisions. Roche Molecular Systems offers a national patient assistance program to help uninsured patients who need viral load testing. Call 1-888-TEST-PCR for more information.

Viremia

Viremia refers to the presence of virus in the blood or its liquid portion, plasma. Plasma viremia is a quantitative measurement of HIV levels similar to viral load but is accomplished by seeing how much of a patient's plasma is required to spark an HIV infection in a laboratory cell culture.

Virions

Virions are complete infectious viral particles that consist of the RNA or DNA viral core with a protein coat and occa-

sionally external envelopes. Virions are the extracellular infective form of viruses.

Viruses

Viruses are any of a large group of submicroscopic infective agents that are regarded either as extremely simple microorganisms or as extremely complex molecules. Viruses are composed mainly of nucleic acid within a protein coat that surrounds an RNA or DNA core of genetic material, but they do not contain a semipermeable membrane. When viruses enter a living plant, animal, or bacterial cell, they use the host cell's chemical energy, protein, and nucleic acid-synthesizing ability to replicate themselves. Viruses are only capable of growth and multiplication when they inhabit living cells.

After the infected host cell makes viral components and virus particles are released, the host cell is often dissolved. Some viruses do not kill cells but transform them into a cancerous state. Some

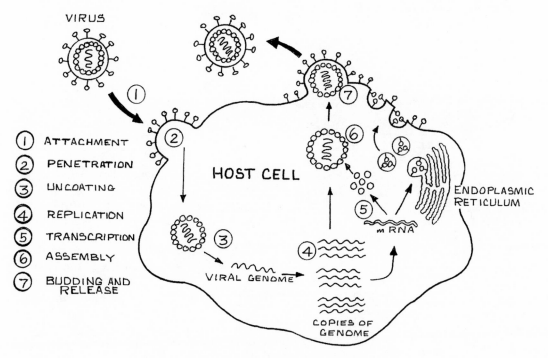

Viral replication (Marvin G. Miller).

viruses cause illness and then seem to disappear, while remaining latent and later causing another, sometimes much more severe, form of disease.

V3 loop

The V3 loop is a section of gp120 protein on the surface of HIV that appears to be important in stimulating neutralizing antibodies.

Warts *see* Condyloma acuminata; Genital warts; Human papillomavirus

Wasserman, August (1866–1925)

The scientist August Wasserman and his colleague Albert Neisser developed the first diagnostic test used for the detection of syphilis, the Wasserman test. The resulting blood test was able to detect syphilis even in patients without symptoms. Beginning in 1935, most states mandated premarital syphilis screening with the Wasserman test as a requisite for a marriage license.

Wasserman test

The first blood test used for the detection of syphilis, the Wasserman test applied the complement fixation technique to detect the presence of the *Treponema pallidum* spirochete.

Wasting syndrome

Wasting syndrome, a complication of HIV infection, refers to a weight loss >10 percent of body weight accompanied by fever or diarrhea for more than 30 days. In the U.S., wasting syndrome occurs in approximately 25 percent of patients who have AIDS at some time during their illness. The incidence of wasting syndrome is expected to rise as mortality from other AIDS-related conditions declines. In some African countries, wasting syndrome is such a common feature of AIDS that the name "slim disease" is often used as a synonym for AIDS.

Wasting syndrome is associated with the increased basal metabolic rate seen in all stages of HIV infection. Other contributing factors include malabsorption of nutrients, gastrointestinal pathogens, and diarrhea. However, the most significant cause of wasting is lowered food (energy), which may be related to nausea, vomiting, chronic gastrointestinal disease, depression, and dementia.

Body mass index (BMI) calculations are usually used to

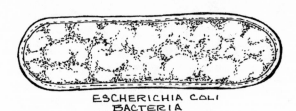

ESCHERICHIA COLI BACTERIA

RETROVIRUS

CHLAMYDIA

CYTOMEGALOVIRUS

HERPES SIMPLEX VIRUS

PAPILLOMAVIRUS

HEPATITIS B VIRUS

Relative sizes of bacteria and viruses (Marvin G. Miller).

determine the severity of wasting with BMI <18.5 as grade I, BMI <17 as grade II, and BMI <16 as grade III. Grade III malnutrition is regarded as life threatening. Complications of malnutrition include bedsores, hypothermia, susceptibility to infection, and absence of menstrual periods in women. Death may occur as a result of wasting even when other specific complications are not present. Laboratory tests are used to measure the complete blood count (CBC) to help determine if anemia or infection is present, and biochemical tests are used to determine if electrolyte (sodium, potassium, chloride) or mineral deficiencies or imbalances are present.

Treatment consists of nutritional and pharmacologic therapies. Nutritional therapies include high-energy oral supplements, nasogastric feeding, percutaneous endoscopic feeding tubes, and total parenteral nutrition. Pharmacologic therapies include growth hormone, testosterone, thalidomide, megestrol acetate, and the synthetic cannabinoid Dronabinol.

Western blot test

The Western blot test is a laboratory method for detecting specific antibodies, such as antibodies to hepatitis B or HIV, in a person's blood. The Western blot test is often used to verify positive enzyme immunoassay (EIA) tests. The Western blot test is more reliable than the EIA method, although it is more difficult and costly to perform. With NAT testing approved for confirmatory hepatitis testing, Western blot is primarily used today for HIV confirmatory testing. EIA and ELISA screening tests may be false positive as a result of technical error, cross-reacting antibodies, and numerous medical conditions.

In the Western blot assay, individual HIV proteins are separated according to size by gel electrophoresis and transferred (blotted) onto nitrocellulose paper. After addition of the patient's serum, the reactivity of antibodies to specific viral pro-

teins can be determined. Interpretation of the Western blot is based on the spectrum of bands that is visualized. The CDC defines a positive Western blot as the presence of any two of the following bands: p24, gp41, or gp120–gp160. If no bands are present the test is considered negative. If one band is present the test is considered indeterminate. In most cases, the sensitivity and specificity of the Western blot for HIV range from 96–100 percent. If the rare group O type of HIV is present, the Western blot could be falsely negative. False-positive HIV-1 Western blot tests have been reported in patients with high levels of bilirubin; HLA antibodies; other human retroviruses including HIV-2; and connective tissue disorders.

Up to 10–20 percent of Western blot tests yield indeterminate results. This may be caused by a false positive result or true HIV-1 infection that has not completely seroconverted. For this reason, it is recommended that indeterminate Western blot tests be repeated in six months. If the test is still indeterminate in the absence of known risk factors or clinical symptoms, the test may be considered negative.

Wet prep test

In the wet prep test, a specimen of vaginal or cervical secretions is collected and placed in 0.5 ml of saline. The specimen is examined microscopically for the presence of white blood cells, bacteria, clue cells, yeast, and trichomonas. *See also* **Clue cells** and **KOH prep.**

Whiff test

In the whiff test, a drop or two of specimen collected from a vaginal discharge is mixed with the chemical potassium hydroxide. The mixture is then smelled (whiffed) by a physician to determine if strong-smelling proteins are present. A positive whiff test is indicated by the presence of a fishy odor released by vaginal bacteria and suggests that the patient has bacterial vaginosis. The whiff test is also positive in patients with trichomonas.

White blood cell (WBC)

White blood cells are immune system cells involved in cellular immunity. The white blood cell population can be divided into two major subtypes, lymphocytes and larger cells known as phagocytes. Derived from the myeloid cell line, phagocytes include monocytes, macrophages, and neutrophils (segmented granulocytes), along with smaller numbers of eosinophils and basophils. Phagocytes engulf and destroy other infected cells and infectious particles. Lymphocytes are derived from the lymphoid cell line. The two major classes of lymphocytes are T cells and B cells. Lymphocytes are the immune system's key players. T cells, which control cellular immunity, are responsible for protecting people from toxic and infectious agents. B cells, which control humoral immunity, are responsible for antibody production.

White, Ryan (1971–1990)

A history of the HIV/AIDS epidemic in the United States would not be complete without an introduction to Ryan Wayne White and a description of his 1987 testimony before the President's Commission on AIDS.

Born on December 6, 1971, in Kokomo, Indiana, three days later Ryan White was diagnosed as having the clotting disorder hemophilia. Hemophilia is a congenital disorder caused by a deficiency of the clotting factor known as Factor VIII. Ryan's condition required him to receive biweekly injections of Factor VIII, which was then primarily derived from human blood donors. Each injection was obtained from a lot or batch of the product containing Factor VIII from thousands of different blood donors.

AIDS emerged in the United States in June 1981. With little knowledge of the cause of AIDS, confusion about the disease was commonplace. During this time, an AIDS panic emerged largely due to the news media. Rather than publicizing factual information to the public, the media published stories, some of which were total lies, about the personal lives of HIV positive people. The media also fostered the notion that AIDS was only seen in the gay community and that heterosexuals were not at risk. Because of the many confusing and conflicting news reports, the general public shunned AIDS patients in a manner bordering on hysteria.

On December 17, 1984, Ryan had surgery on his lungs to repair damage related to pneumonia. During this hospitalization, doctors discovered that Ryan had contracted the HIV virus from a tainted lot of Factor VIII. At this time it was generally known that AIDS was contracted through blood and blood products, but tests to screen blood products for HIV were not yet available. However, there were still people who were frightened and speculated that HIV could be contracted by direct contact. Consequently, the local school board, Ryan's teacher and principal voted to ban Ryan from the classroom. In addition, his home was shot at, and the community ostracized Ryan and his family.

While Ryan attended classes via telephone for nine months, his family became involved in a series of court battles revolving around his right to attend school. Ryan's family eventually won its battle with the school board. After nine months away from the classroom, Ryan was allowed to attend school, provided he used a separate restroom, did not participate in gym, and used a separate drinking fountain as well as disposable eating utensils and trays. Many parents kept their children from school, and parents of 20 students started their own school to keep their children from being exposed to Ryan White.

The news media caught wind of the conflict, and soon Ryan was being publicly labeled as the AIDS Boy. The attention caused Ryan to receive thousands of letters of support from people around the world, including celebrities such as Elton John, Alyssa Milano, and Charlie Sheen. Mayor Ed Koch of New York City was the first public official to support publicly Ryan's right to attend school.

Ryan's social life improved when his family moved to Cicero, Indiana, in 1987. Cicero and the neighboring communities welcomed Ryan and his family with open arms. The school directors there arranged for each student to attend a two-hour seminar on AIDS, and teachers sent informative AIDS material home for parents to read. When a movie of Ryan's life, the *Ryan White Story*, was made, many Americans heard the truth about HIV/AIDS for the first time. Ryan White had a tremendous influence on the initiation of AIDS awareness programs. In addition, Ryan's story affected the media so that a visible shift from information that incited panic to factual, educational information emerged after his story was broadcast.

In his testimony to the presidential Commission on AIDS in 1987, Ryan described the early reaction to his having AIDS. He testified that he had been the target of Ryan White jokes and vicious rumors that said he bit people, spit on vegetables and cookies, and urinated on bathroom walls. His school locker was vandalized and his folders were marked with the words "fag" as well as other obscenities. Ryan's mother was labeled as a troublemaker and an unfit mother. At church, while he lived in Kokomo, people would not shake his hand. Ryan's purpose in testifying was to gain basic human rights for those suffering from HIV/AIDS. Ryan attended Hamilton Heights High School in Cicero, where he made the honor roll and planned to graduate in 1991. However, Ryan White died at the age of 18 on April 8, 1990. As many as 1,500 people, including First Lady Barbara Bush, attended Ryan's funeral.

Even after his death, Ryan's courageous battle with AIDS continues to contribute to AIDS awareness. Ryan White's plight opened doors leading to acceptance of AIDS as a disease that has no social barriers. Ryan White also symbolized to Americans the needs of better AIDS treatment and education. The Ryan White CARE act was first enacted by Congress in 1990. Its provisions have been expanded and the act was reauthorized in 1996 and 2000. Numerous agencies and planning councils for AIDS patients throughout the United States are named after Ryan White. *See also* **Ryan White Comprehensive AIDS Resources Emergency Act.**

Kinsella, James. *Covering the Plague: AIDS and the American Media.* New Brunswick, NJ: Rutgers University Press, 1989.

WHO *see* World Health Organization

Wild type virus

Wild type virus refers to a virus that has not been exposed to antiviral drugs and therefore has not accumulated mutations capable of conferring drug resistance. Wild-type viruses are the prevalent type of virus in the host population before genetic manipulation or mutation occurs. Wild-type viruses also refer to viruses that are isolated from a host as opposed to viruses grown in a laboratory culture.

Women who have sex with women (WSW)

The Centers for Disease Control reports that through December 1998, 109,311 women were reported with AIDS. Of these, 2,220 were reported to have had sex with women. Of the women who reported only having had sex with women, 98 percent had other risk factors, primarily injection drug use. As of December 1998, investigations of these women showed no confirmed cases of female-to-female HIV transmission, although investigators could not prove that the infections were not sexually transmitted. Female sexual contact should be considered a possible means of HIV transmission.

The CDC recommends that these women be aware that exposure of a mucous membrane, such as the mouth, to vaginal secretions and menstrual blood is potentially infectious, particularly during early and late-stage HIV infection when viral load levels are highest. Also, condoms should be used consistently and correctly and for every sexual contact with men or when using sex toys. Sex toys should not be shared. No barrier methods for use during oral sex have been FDA approved, although dental dams, cut-open condoms, or plastic wrap can be used to help protect against contact with body fluids during oral sex.

Women's Interagency HIV Study (WIHS)

WIHS is a multicenter, prospective study that was established in August 1993, to carry out comprehensive investigations of the impact of HIV infection in women. The rationale for establishing the WIHS was to investigate the clinical, laboratory, and psychosocial aspects of HIV infection in women.

World AIDS Day

World AIDS Day, which began in 1998, occurs on December 1 of each year and is a WHO initiative that serves as an international reminder that all must work together to bring an end to the AIDS epidemic. World AIDS Day is commemorated throughout the world with a variety of different educational events and programs designed to promote awareness of AIDS.

World Health Organization (WHO)

The World Health Organization was established on April 7, 1948, as the United Nations' specialized agency for health. Health as defined by WHO is a state of complete physical, mental, and social well-being and not merely the absence of disease or infirmity. WHO is governed by 192 member states through the World Health Assembly, which is composed of representatives from WHO's member states.

Yeast infections

Yeast infections are common causes of vaginitis. However, symptoms of yeast infection are similar to those of bacterial vaginosis and chlamydia, conditions that require different treatment. For this reason, it is best to see a doctor to confirm that yeast infection is present before using antifungal creams.

Yeast occurs in the vagina primarily as a cross-contaminant from the anal area, or it may be transmitted during oral sex. Normally, vaginal yeast is kept in check by the immune system and does not cause problems. Yeast exists in two forms, spores and hyphae, elongated stems with spores inside or budding on the ends. Yeast exist in both acid and alkaline environments, making treatments based on changing pH ineffective. Yeast also proliferates freely in the presence of estrogen. This causes an increase in yeast infections from day 14 to 23 of the menstrual cycle when estrogen levels are highest.

Yeast infections occur when yeast proliferates freely causing overgrowth. About 85 to 90 percent of yeast infections are caused by *Candida albicans*, the infectious agent seen in candidiasis. Most other yeast infections are caused by *Candida glabrata*, which does not respond well to antifungal creams.

Symptoms

Yeast infections cause intense itching and they may cause a cottage-cheese-like white discharge, although the discharge may be watery or uniformly thick. In women, the labia and vulva may be red and swollen, often with small red pimples occurring separately from the central redness.

Diagnosis

Diagnosis is made by examination of vaginal or penile discharge for the presence of yeast or fungal elements. Either the KOH prep or wet prep test can be used, or the specimen can be cultured.

Treatment

Early treatments included Nystatin used orally, but antifungal creams with ingredients from the azole family have proven effective and are now widely available without a prescription. Over-the-counter antifungal creams such as Monistat are effective if the patient has a yeast infection. Unfortunately, many women with lichen sclerosis, vulvodynamia, pre-cancerous skin changes, and chlamydia mistakenly think they have yeast infections and waste time and money using these products inappropriately. Boric acid is also an effective antifungal treatments particularly in the treatment of *C. glabrata*, using 600 mg capsules which are inserted vaginally one or two times daily for 14 days. The capsules are available with a prescription. Boric acid capsules are not recommended as a treatment during pregnancy.

In difficult and severe cases immunotherapy can be used, with patients prescribed yeast-allergy shots weekly for one year.

Risk Factors

Extended periods of antibiotic therapy, especially tetracyclines, tight restrictive clothing, a diet high in sugar, unprotected sex. *See also* **Candidiasis** and **Oral candidiasis (thrush)**.

Zalcitabine (ddC)

Zalcitabine (Hivid) is a nucleoside reverse transcriptase inhibitor (NRTI) used as an antiretroviral agent in the treatment of HIV infection.

Zidovudine (ZDV, AZT, Azidothymidine, Retrovir)

Zidovudine is a nucleoside (thymidine) analog reverse transcriptase inhibitor (NRTI) drug that suppresses the replication of HIV by terminating DNA synthesis. AZT was the first drug approved by the Food and Drug Administration (FDA) for the treatment of HIV infection. Current practice favors the use of AZT in combination with other antiretroviral drugs. AZT crosses the blood-brain barrier and may be effective against AIDS dementia complex.

Adverse side effects include nausea, myopathy, and bone marrow suppression. When initially administered, AZT frequently causes headaches, rash, and nausea. Long-term side effects include anemia and myositis (inflammatory muscle disease). Anemia is reported to occur in 5–10 percent of patients using AZT, and may occur after years of treatment. Like all NRTIs, AZT can cause pancreatitis, alone or in conjunction with elevations of lactic acid (lactic acidosis), although this side effect is most likely to occur with the drug stavudine.

Of greater concern, patients on antiretroviral therapy are likely to develop metabolic abnormalities, including insulin resistance, elevated lipid levels, and a redistribution of body fat known as lipodystrophy. *See also* **Lipodystrophy**; **Nucleoside/Nucleotide analog reverse transcriptase inhibitors**; and the Treatment section of **Acquired immune deficiency syndrome**.

Zinc Finger Inhibitors

Zinc finger inhibitors are a class of experimental anti–HIV drugs which prevents the nucleocapsid part of the gag protein of HIV (which contains the zinc finger amino acid structures) from capturing and packaging new HIV genetic material into newly budding virions.

Zinc Fingers

Zinc fingers are chains of amino acids found in cellular proteins that bind to DNA or messenger RNA, and play important roles in a cell's life cycle. These molecules are called zinc fingers because they capture a zinc ion, which contributes to the array's binding to RNA or DNA. There are two zinc fingers in HIV's nucelocapsid. Zinc fingers are involved in binding and packaging viral RNA into new virions budding from an infected host cell. The nucleocapsid protein and the zinc fingers also play a role during the process of reverse transcription. *See also* **Retrovirus replication.**

Zoonism

Zoonism refers to the process of animal diseases moving into the human population. Zoonotic diseases, including AIDS, which crossed from the simian population, represent one of the leading causes of illness and death from infectious disease. The Institute of Medicine reports that worldwide, zoonotic diseases have a negative impact on commerce, travel, and economies. This was typified by the recent severe acute respiratory syndrome (SARS) epidemic caused by a coronavirus that crossed species.

Resources

Books and Articles

Armstrong, Donald, and Jonathan Cohen, editors. *Infectious Diseases.* London: Mosby, Imprint of Harcourt, 1999.

Bagasri, Omar. *HIV and Molecular Immunity: Prospects for the AIDS Vaccine.* Natuck, MA: Biotechnology Books, 1999.

Centers for Disease Control and Prevention. *1998 Sexually Transmitted Diseases Treatment Guidelines.* 2002 Rev. Atlanta: U.S. Dept. of Health and Human Services, 1997. Also available: http://www.cdc.gov/mmwr/.

_____. *Recommendations for the Prevention and Management of Chlamydia Trachomatis Infections, 1993.* Atlanta: U.S. Dept. of Health and Human Services, 1993. Also available: http://www.cdc.gov/mmwr/.

_____. *Sexually Transmitted Diseases Guidelines 2002.* Atlanta: U.S. Dept. of Health and Human Services, 2002. Also available: http://www.cdc.gov/mmwr/.

Curtis, Tom. "The Origin of AIDS." *Rolling Stone,* March 19, 1992, p. 54.

Dalgleish, Angus, and Robin Weiss, editors. *HIV and the New Viruses.* New York: Academic Press, 1999.

Grmek, Mirko, M.D. *History of AIDS.* Princeton, NJ: Princeton University Press, 1990.

Hooper, Edward. *The River: A Journey Back to the Source of HIV & AIDS.* New York: Penguin, 1999.

Hsiung, G. D., Caroline Fong, and Marie Landry. *Hsiung's Diagnostic Virology.* 4th edition. New Haven, CT: Yale University Press, 1994.

Irwin, Alexander, J. Millen, et al. *Global AIDS: Myths & Facts.* Cambridge, MA: South End Press, 2003.

Martin, Brian. "Polio Vaccines and the Origin of AIDS." *Townsend Letter for Doctors,* No. 26 (Jan. 1994): 97–100.

Matthews, Dawn D., editor. *Sexually Transmitted Diseases Sourcebook.* 2nd edition. Detroit: Omnigraphics, 2001.

Mondoa, Emil, M.D. *Sugars That Heal.* New York: Ballantine, 2001.

"1999 USPHS/IDSA Guidelines for the Prevention of Opportunistic Infections in Persons Infected with Human Immunodeficiency Virus." *Annals of Internal Medicine* 131 (Dec. 7, 1999): 873–908.

Quetel, Claude. *History of Syphilis.* Baltimore: Johns Hopkins University Press, 1990.

Stamm, W.E. In: K. Holmes, P. Mardh, P. Sparline, et al., editors. *Sexually Transmitted Diseases.* 3rd edition. New York: McGraw-Hill, 1999.

Stoto, Michael A., et al. *Reducing the Odds: Preventing Perinatal Transmission of HIV in the United States.* Washington, D.C.: National Academy Press, 1999.

Journals, Reports, and Web Sites

Afraidtoask.com
This site includes in-depth information, graphic photographs, online community based message boards, and a fee-based service allowing users to ask questions of board-certified physicians.
http://www.afraidtoask.com/

AIDScience
http://www.aidscience.org

The Body
Library resource updated daily with excellent STD/AIDS resources with information regarding policies, research, conferences, and quality of life issues.
http://www.thebody.com/

Bulletin of Experimental Treatments for AIDS
http://www.aegis.com/pubs/beta/

HIV Fact Sheets. *Frequently Asked Questions About HIV and AIDS*. Centers for Disease Control and Prevention.
http://www.cdc.gov/HIV/Pubs/Faqs.htm

Healthcare Information Resources
This Canadian site provides information on STDs and links to specialized services.
http://www-hsl.mcmaster.ca/tomflem/intro.html

Horowitz, Leonard G., among others.
Articles on the Origin of AIDS
http://www.originofaids.com/articles/early.htm

JAMA: The Journal of the American Medical Association
http://www.ama-assn.org

Kaiser Daily HIV/AIDS Report
http://www.kaisernetwork.org/dailyreports/hiv
http://www.AIDSinfo.nih.gov
(800) 448-0440

Keske, Tom. *Statistical Analysis Linking U.S. AIDS Outbreak to Hepatitis Experiments.*
http://www.whale.to/v/keske11.html

Medscape
Medscape provides current STD information on reports from clinical journals and conference and educational programs, and it contains material created expressly for Medscape. Visitors must register (free registration) for a category similar to categories on Webmedlit, although they are free to use the search engines in other categories.
http://www.medscape.com

MMWR: Morbidity and Mortality Weekly Report.
"Revised Recommendations for HIV Screening of Pregnant Women." 50 no. RR-19, Nov. 9, 2001. Also available: http://www.cdc.gov/mmwr

New England Journal of Medicine
http://www.nejm.org

New Theory on AIDS Origin Explains Chimpanzee Connection.
Dr. Len Horowitz, LightStream Productions.
http://www.lightstreamers.com/Streaming_05-p2.htm

NIAID Daily News
Subscribe at the NIAID web site for a daily update of infectious disease news, including current research and treatment recommendations.
http://www.niaid.nih.gov

ProMED
The Program for Monitoring Emerging Diseases provides a useful searchable archive and a daily electronic newsletter concerning emerging diseases.
http://www.fas.org/promed/

PubMed
PubMed is a service of the National Library of Medicine that provides access to more than 12 million medical citations, from current citations back to the mid–1960s. PubMed also provides citations to additional life science journals. PubMed includes links to many sites providing full-text articles and other related resources.
http://www.ncbi.nlm.nih.gov/entrez/query.fcgi

STI Online
Sexually Transmitted Infections
Stanford University's High Wire Press
http://sti.bmjjournals.com

U.S. Department of Health and Human Services Reports (all reports available at http://www.aidsinfo.nih.gov/)
Public Health Service Task Force Recommendations for the Use of Antiretroviral Drugs in Pregnant HIV-1 Infected Women for Maternal Health and Interventions to Reduce Perinatal HIV-1 Transmission in the United States. February 4, 2002.
Guidelines for the Use of Antiretroviral Agents in Pediatric HIV Infection. August 8, 2001.

Webmedlit
This site provides access to 22 medical journals including the *New England Journal of Medicine*, *JAMA*, *Cancer*, and the *British Medical Journal*. Categories include AIDS/virology, cardiology, cancer/oncology, dermatology, Diabetes/Endocrinology, Gastroenterology, Immunology, Medical Economics, neurology, and women's health.
http://www.webmedlit.com

Organizations

Alan Guttmacher Institute
This organization provides articles, brochures, and information on sexual behavior, contraception and STDs.

120 Wall Street, 21st Floor
New York, NY 10005
(212) 248-1111
http://www.agi-usa.org/

American College of Physicians
Updated articles and information on internal medicine and subspecialties, including infectious diseases.
http://www.acponline.org

American Herpes Foundation
http://www.herpes-foundation.org/

American Medical Women's Association (AMWA)
801 North Fairfax Street, Suite 400
Alexandria, VA 22314
(703) 838-0500
http://www.amwa-doc.org

American Public Health Association
APHA site that lists its many efforts to prevent disease and promote health in legislative affairs & advocacy, science, public health resources, and other areas.
http://www.apha.org

American Social Health Association
P.O. Box 13827
Research Triangle Park, NC 27709
(800) 783-9877
www.ashastd.org

American Society for Microbiology
The ASM lists archives, ASM news, meetings and workshops, and links to other sites.
http://www.asm.org

Association of Reproductive Health Professionals
Email: arhp@aol.com
http://www.arhp.org

Atlanta Reproductive Healthcare Center for Women
Provides links to information from planned parenthood to STDs; provides women with information on contraception and STDs.
http://www.ivf.com/contrac.html

Family Health International
P.O. 13950
Research Triangle Park, MD 27709
FHI is a very good site for monitoring the status and trends of the HIV/AIDS epidemics and provides information, including STD-related articles, projects and programs.
(919) 544-7040
http://www.fhi.org/

Infectious Diseases Society of America
IDSA site has information on STDs, emerging infectious diseases; links to journal articles and conference information.
http://www.idsociety.org

Institute of Medicine
Site of this nonprofit agency that works for the interest of Public Health and evaluates the efforts of the federal government in this area.
http://www.iom.edu

International Union against Sexually Transmitted Infections (IUSTI)
Founded in 1923 for international cooperation in STD control.
http://www.iusti.org/

Planned Parenthood Federation of America
810 Seventh Ave
New York, NY 10019
(800) 829-7732
http://www.plannedparenthood.org

Alternative Medicine Resources

Alternative Medicine Information Source
http://www.alternative-medicine-info.com

Herbal Medicine Resource
http://www.herbalremedies.com

The Institute for New Medicine
Located at Georgetown University, the Institute for New Medicine is headed by Candace Pert, Ph.D. The Institute for New Medicine funds research which explores the immune system and its defense. It seeks to elucidate knowledge on cellular communication within the organism. This website contains information describes information about Pert's research with HIV and describes Peptide T, a promising treatment for HIV infection, including the results of clinical trials.
http://www.tinm.org

The Life Extension Foundation
The Life Extension Foundation relies on a scientific board of investigators who study the effects of dietary supplements and prescription medicines on aging, health, and disease. This web site has links to articles published in the organization's journal on a variety of topics, including infectious diseases.
http://www.lef.org

The National Center for Complementary and Alternative Medicine (NCCAM)
This branch of the National Institutes of Health

investigates complementary therapies in clinical trials at various locations throughout the country.
http://www.nccam.nih.gov/

National Institutes of Health. Office of Dietary Supplement
www.dietary-supplements.info.nih.gov/

Hotlines

AIDS Clinical Trials Information Service (ACTIS)
(800) 874-2572
http://www.actis.org

CDC National AIDS Hotline
(800) 342-AIDS
www.cdc.gov/hiv/contactus.htm

CDC National STD Hotline
(800) 227-8922 or (800) 343-2437
En Espanol (800) 344-7432
TTY for the Hearing Impaired (800) 243-7889

Centers for Disease Control and Prevention National Prevention Information Network (CDC NPIN)
(800) 458-5231
http://www.cdcnpin.org

Centers for Disease Control and Prevention National STD and AIDS Hotlines
(800) 342-AIDS (Available 24 hours a day)
Spanish: (800) 344-SIDA Sunday–Saturday 8am–2pm EST
http://www.ashastd.org

Exponents, Inc.
(800) 673-7370

Gay and Lesbian National Hotline
(888) 843-4564

Gay Men's Health Crisis Hotline
(212) 807-6655
(800) AIDS NYC
TTY (212) 645-7470

Hemophilia Association Helpline
(212) 682-5510

HIV Counseling Hotline
(800) 872-2777
http://rpci.med.buffalo.edu/groups/aids/aids1.html

HIV/AIDS Treatment Information Service (ATIS)
(800) 448-0440
http://www.hivatis.org

Hyacinth AIDS Foundation Hotline (New Jersey)
(800) 433-0254

National HIV Telephone Consultation Service (WARMLINE) for physicians and other health professionals
(800) 993-3413
http://www.ucsf.edu/hivcntr/warmline

Office of Minority Health Resource Center (OMHRC)
(800) 444-6472
http://www.omhrc.gov/omhrc/

Rape, Sexual Assault & Incest Hotline of NYC
(212) 227-3300

Low Cost Prescription Drug Programs

http://www.NeedyMeds.com

http://www.themedicineprogram.com

http://www.rxassist.org

Social Security Disability for STDs/HIV

Guide to HIV-AIDS-Related Social Security Benefits
Publication No. 05-10019
http://www.ssa.gov/pubs/10019.html

HIVDent Public Policy News Updates
"AIDS Social Security Rules Studied," May 2003
http://www.hivdnet.org/publicp/ppASSRS062003.htm

Social Security Benefits for People Living with HIV/AIDS.
National Association of Social Workers
http://www.socialworkers.org/practice/hiv_aids/aids_ss.asp

Government Resources

Blood Supply Issues
Food and Drug Administration
http://www.fda.gov/cber/blood.htm

Centers for Disease Control and Prevention (CDC)
CDC Division of STDs and STD Prevention
www.cdc.gov/nchstp/dstd/disease_info.htm

CDC Prevention Guidelines Database
This site is a comprehensive compendium of

all the official guidelines and recommendations published by the U.S. Centers for Disease Control and Prevention.
http://aepo-xdv-www.epo.cdc.gov/wonder/prevguid/prevguid.htm

CDC STD 2002 Treatment Guidelines
This site contains the current treatment guidelines established by the U.S. Centers for Disease Control and Prevention, along with information on symptoms and diagnosis.
http://www.cdc.gov/STD/treatment/4-2002 TG.htm

Government Accountability Office (GAO)
This site includes links to government reports including those on the AIDS pandemic, STD prevalence, occupational safety, federal laws, and syringe exchange programs.
http://www.gao.gov/

Health Resources and Services Administration (HRSA)
HRSA is a division of the U.S. Department of Health & Human Services that directs national health programs which improve the health of the nation by assuring quality health care to underserved, vulnerable, and special-need populations, and by promoting appropriate health professions workforce capacity and practice, particularly in primary care and public health. Among its other functions, HRSA administers the Ryan White CARE Act Titles I, II, III(b), IV, SPNS, and AETCs to provide treatment and services for those affected by HIV/AIDS.
http://www.hrsa.dhhs.gov/

Institute of Medicine
The Hidden Epidemic: Confronting Sexually Transmitted Diseases. Washington, D.C.: National Academy Press, 1997.
http://books.nap.edu/html/epidemic/

Medicaid and Medicare Programs
U.S. Department of Health & Human Services
http://www.cms.hhs.org

National Cancer Institute
This site provides information on the ongoing research projects of the Frederick Cancer Research and Development Center, Developmental Therapeutics Program, and the Office of International Affairs.
http://www.nci.nih.gov

National Institute for Allergy and Infectious Diseases (NIAID)
This site includes information on news releases,

publications, research activities, updated antiretroviral guides, and AIDS vaccines trials sites.
http://www.niaid.nih.gov

Neisseria gonorrhoeae Information/CDC
This site offers information on gonorrhea, including links to reports and guidelines.
http://www.cdc.gov/ncidod/dastlr/gcdir/Gono.html

National Center for Complementary and Alternative Medicine (NCCAM)
(888) 644-3616
http://www.nccam.nih.gov/

National Herpes Hotline
(919) 361-8488

National HPV and Cervical Cancer Hotline
(919) 361-4848
Resource Center www.ashastd.org/hpvccrc/

National Institutes of Health (NIH)
The NIH is a multi-institute agency of The U.S. Department of Health & Human Services that serves as the federal focal point for health research.
http://www.nih.gov

Neisseria Gonorrhoeae
This CDC website offers an array of information regarding identification issues, prevalence, and treatment, and has links to reports and guidelines.
http://www.cdc.gov/ncidod/dastlr/gcdir/Gono.html

NIAID Centers for AIDS Research
This site includes information on the Centers for AIDS Research (CFAR) mission statement and history; includes links to other CFARs nationwide and to the Division of Acquired Immune Deficiency Syndrome (DAIDS).
http://www.niaid.nih.gov/research/cfar

NonProfit Gateway
This site provides a network of links to federal government information and services.
http://www.firstgov.gov/business/nonprofit

Office of AIDS Research (OAR)
OAR is an office within the NIH that is responsible for the scientific, budgetary, legislative, and policy elements of the NIH AIDS research program.
http://www.nih.gov/od/oar/

Planned Parenthood
http://www.plannedparenthood.org/STI/stis_index.html

HIV Center of Excellence; U.S. Department of Health and Human Services, Indian Health Services, Services for American Indians and Alaska Natives
http://www.ihs.gov/medicalPrograms/AIDS/

STDGEN Data Base
This specialized database in an expansion of the HPV project funded by the STD Branch of the Division of Microbiology and Infectious Diseases, NIAID, NIH, Bethesda Maryland. This project includes molecular information pertaining to STD bacteria and viruses, especially molecular sequence data.
http://www.stdgen.lanl.gov

Clinical Trials

Adult AIDS Clinical Trials Group (AACTG)
AACTG is the largest HIV clinical trials organization in the world.
http://aactg.s-3.com

AIDS Clinical Trials Information Service (ACTIS)
Co-sponsored by the FDA, the CDC, and the National Library of Medicine, this site provides quick and easy access to information on federally and privately funded clinical trials that evaluate experimental drugs and therapies for adults and children in all stages of HIV infection.
http://www.actis.org/

Cancer Information Service (virology studies)
http://cancer.gov/clinical_trials

CDC National Immunization Information Hotline
(800) 232-2522

Clinical Trials
http://www.clinicaltrials.gov

Community Programs for Clinical Research on AIDS (CPCRA)
This is a community-based initiative founded by NIAID that aims to serve the population under-represented in earlier clinical trials and focuses on day-to-day living concerns of individuals infected with HIV.
Thhp://www.cpcra.org/

HIV Prevention Trials Network (HPTN)
HPTN is a worldwide collaborative clinical trials network established by the National Institutes of Health to evaluate the safety and the efficacy of non-vaccine prevention interventions, alone or in combination, using HIV incidence as the primary endpoint.
http://www.hptn.org/

HIV Vaccine Trials Network (HVTN)
Formed in 1999 by the DAIDS Division of the NIAID, HVTN's mission is to develop and test HIV prevention vaccines through multi-center clinical trials in a global network of domestic and international sites.
http://www.hvtn.org

The Pediatric AIDS Clinical Trials Group
National Institute of Allergy and Infectious Diseases
National Institutes of Health
http://pactg.s-3.com/

University of Washington Virology Research Clinic
http://www.depts.washington.edu/herpes

Laboratory Tests

Blood Check Laboratory Services
This service offers confidential blood tests.
http://www.blood-check.com
toll-free (877) 256-6324

The College of American Pathologists Web Site
This site has information on most general laboratory tests.
http://www.cap.org

Health-Tests Direct
Blood test information and testing service for STDs.
Division of OHS, Incorporated
1835 Newport Blvd, Suite D-258
Costa Mesa, CA 92627
http://www.health-tests-direct.com/std_sexually_transmitted_disease.htm
(800) 456-4647
(949) 764-9306

National HIV Testing Resources
http://www.hivtest.org/

Quest Diagnostics Web Site offers information about STD tests.
http://www.questdiagnostics.com

University of Virginia Medical School
http://www.healthsystem.virginia.edu/internet/labtests

Laboratory and Pharmaceutical information
http://www.pharma-lexicon.com

Web sites with information on Herpes testing:
http://www.herpeselect.com
http://depts.washington.edu/herpes/
http://www.herpes.com/diagnosis.shtml

Legal Issues

Americans with Disabilities Education Project
ACLE AIDS Project
132 W. 43rd Street
New York, NY 10036

Equal Employment Opportunity Commission
1801 L. Street NW
Washington, DC 20507
(800) 669-3362

Ex-Con Hotline
(212) 206-7070, Ext. 338
This Fortune Society hotline is for ex-offenders
  and youth at risk; offers individual and
  group counseling, HIV/AIDS assistance, substance abuse treatment, inmate assistance,
  peer education training and computer liter-
  acy training. Mon.–Thurs., 10:00 A.M.–4:00
  P.M.

Lambda Legal
Lambda Legal is the nation's oldest and largest
  organization dedicated to the civil rights of
  lesbians, gay men, bisexuals, the transgen-
  dered, and people with HIV or AIDS. Lambda
  Legal has its main offices in New York City
  and branches located throughout the country.
http://www.lambdalegal.org

National Immigration Project
National Association of People with AIDS
1413 K Street, NW, 7th Floor
Washington, DC 20005-3476
(202) 898-0414

The National Institute on Drug Abuse
http://www.nida.nih/gov

The National Library of Medicine's Specialized
  Information Services
http://sis.nlm.nih.gov/HIV/HIVPrison.html

President's Commission on Employment of
  People with Disabilities
1331 F. Street NW
Washington, DC 20004-1107
(202) 376-6200

Prostitutes of New York (PONY)
(212) 713-5678
PONY is an organization of sex workers of all
  kinds in the New York area and is affiliated
  with the International Network of Sex Work
  Projects. Staff members can make referrals
  to attorneys, accountants, and other valuable services.

The U.S. Department of Justice
National Institute of Justice
http://www.ojp.usdoj.gov

HIV/AIDS Resources

Acute HIV Infection and Early Diseases Research Program (AIEDRP)
This program, funded by NIAID, explains how
  HIV-1 causes diseases in adults. Scientists use
  highly active antiretroviral therapy to increase their understanding of the mechanisms and course of HIV disease.
http://www.aiedrp.org

Adult AIDS Clinical Trials Group (AACTG)
AACTG is the largest HIV clinical trials organization in the world.
http://aactg.s-3.com

AIDS Action
The Body: An AIDS and HIV Information Resource
This organization provides current information on AIDS and public policy.
http://www.thebody.com

AIDS Clinical Trials Information Service
National Institutes of Health
http://www.actis.org/clinical_trials

AIDSDRUGS
This is an online database service of the National Library of Medicine with information
  about drugs undergoing testing against HIV
  infection, AIDS, and related opportunistic
  infection.
http://www.actis.org/drugs

AIDS Education Global Information System
An excellent resource for all aspects of HIV infection, including current findings, research
  news, and global initiatives.
http://www.aegis.com

AIDSLINE
An online database service of the National Library of Medicine with citations and ab-
  stracts covering the published scientific and
  medical literature on AIDS and related topics.
http://gateway.nlm.nih.gov/

AIDS Treatment Information Service (ATIS)
This site includes articles, updates, and information about federally approved treatment
  guidelines for HIV and AIDS.
http://www.hivatis.org

National Cancer Institute
Information virology studies.
http://cancer.gov/clinical_trials

CDC National Center for HIV, STD, and TB Prevention
This site provides general information on the CDC, and provides access to featured publications and CDC-sponsored HIV/STD services; it also links to the Elton John AIDS Foundation.
(800) 342-AIDS
http://www.cdc.gov/hiv/dhap.htm

Centers for AIDS research sponsored by the NIH
The following sites list faculty, research courses, and services available:
CFAR at Baylor College of Medicine
http://www.bcm.edu/cfar
CFAR at Case Western Reserve University
http://www.cwru-id.org
CFAR at New York University
http://www.med.nyu.edu/CFR/
CFAR at the University of California, San Diego
http://ari.ucsd.edu
CFAR at the University of California, San Francisco
http://cfar.ucsf.edu
CFAR at the University of Washington
http://depts.washington.edu/cfar

Clinical Care Options for HIV
Provides current information updates, conference coverage, publications and links; provides an e-mail update service.
http://www.healthcg.com/hiv

Critical Path AIDS Project
This site provides information on life-extending or life-saving AIDS prevention, treatment, and referral information; links to other sites.
http://www.critpath.org

Division of Acquired Immunodeficiency Syndrome (DAIDS)
A division of NIAID, DAIDS was formed in 1986 to address the national research needs created by the advent and spread of HIV/AIDS, to increase basic knowledge of the pathogenesis, natural history, and transmission of HIV disease, and to support research to promote HIV detection, treatment, and prevention.
http://www.niaid.nih.gov/daids/

Gay & Lesbian Medical Association
(415) 255-4547
http://www.glma.org

Glossary of HIV/AIDS related terms
San Francisco AIDS Project
http://www.SFAF.org/glossary

Guidelines for Preventing Opportunistic Infections Among HIV-Infected Persons—2002: Recommendations of the U.S. Public Health Service and the Infectious Diseases Society of America.
http://www.cdc.gov/mmwr/

Harvard AIDS Institute
This site provides information about the institute's programs and initiatives; includes resources, laboratory resources, special programs, research information, publications, and training programs.
http://www.hsph.harvard.edu/hai

HIV/AIDS Treatment Guidelines
U.S. Department of Health & Human Services
http://www.hivatis.org/guidelines

HIV InSite (UCSF)
An award winning site with many AIDS resources.
http:HIVinsite.ucsf.edu

HIV Occupational Exposure Hotline
HHS Health Resources and Services Administration (HRSA)
1-888-HIV-4911

HIV Vaccine Development
National Institute of Allergies and Infectious Diseases
http://www.niaid.nih.gov/daids/

Human Rights Campaign (HRC)
HRC acts at the grassroots to ensure that the federal government is committed to HIV/AIDS research, prevention, treatment, and care.
919 18th Street, NW
Washington, DC 20006
http://www.hrc.org

International AIDS Research Strategic Plan
National Institutes of Health
http://www.nih.gov/od/oar

Johns Hopkins AIDS Service
This site provides information regarding research, conferences, and access to the full-text Johns Hopkins HIV Report.
http://www.hopkins-aids.edu

Kaiser Daily HIV/AIDS Report
The Henry J. Kaiser Family Foundation
Daily online newsletter with registration providing latest research and public policy news.
http://www.profile.kff.org/profile

Lesbian and Gay Aging Issues Network of the American Society on Aging (ASA)
http://www.asaging.org/networks/lgain/index.html

Lifelong AIDS Alliance
http://www.lifelongaidsalliance.org

Maternal HIV Consumer Information Project
Http://www.cms.hhs.gov/hiv/maternal.asp

Minority HIV/AIDS Initiative
http://www.hab.hrsa.gov/special/mai.htm

MMWR Reports/Guidelines on HIV/AIDS
This CDC site provides a concise table of various reports and guidelines. Updated regularly, the site provides information on ordering the reports for free or on downloading entire reports.
http://www.cdc.gov/nchstp/od/nchstp.html

The Names Project AIDS Foundation
AIDS Memorial Quilt
101 Kroger St.
Atlanta, GA 30307
(404) 688-5500
http://www.aidsquilt.org

National AIDS Hotline
U.S. Department of Health & Human Services
English (1-800-342-AIDS) and Spanish (1-800-344-7432)
http://www.ashastd.org/nah/.

The National AIDS Treatment Advocacy Project
http://www.natap.org

National Association of HIV Over 50
http://www.hivoverfifty.org

National Alliance for Hispanic Health Community
HIV/AIDS Technical Assistance Network (CHA-TAN)
1501 16th Street, NW
Washington, DC 20036-1401
(800) 772-8312
(202) 387-5000
http://www.hispanichealth.org

National Minority AIDS Council
This site provides NMAC program information and documents the needs of minorities and what is being accomplished. The Update newsletter delivers information on the latest political issues.
http://www.nmac.org

New York City Department of Health & Mental Hygiene
125 Worth Street, Room 207
New York, NY 10013
(800) 277-8922

New York City's Ryan White Care Services
New York City Department of Health & Mental Hygiene

225 Broadway, 23rd Floor
New York, NY 10007
(212) 693-1440
http://www.nyc.gov/html/doh/html/rw/rw.html

NIAID Centers for AIDS Research
This site includes information on the Centers for AIDS Research (CFAR) mission statement and history; includes links to other CFARs nationwide and to the Division of Acquired Immune Deficiency Syndrome (DAIDS).
http://www.niaid.nih.gov

NIH AIDS Research & Reference Reagent Program
www.aidsreagent.org

NIH Division of Acquired Immunodeficiency Syndrome
This site provides information on AIDS therapeutic and prevention clinical trials, vaccine research and trials, conferences, AIDS-related data sets, molecular sequence and HIV compounds; and a resource guide for development of AIDS therapies, repositories, programs, and publications.
http://www.niaid.nih.gov/daids

Prevention Research
National Institutes of Health
http://www.nih.gov/od/oar

Project Inform
This site provides information, inspiration, and advocacy for people living with HIV/AIDS, AIDS drug assistance, hotlines, publications, treatment and outreach programs.
http://www.projinf.org

Ryan White CARE Act
HIV/AIDS Bureau
U.S. Department of Health & Human Services
http://hab.hrsa.gov/history/purpose.htm

San Francisco AIDS Foundation
http://www.sfaf.org

Substance Abuse and Mental Health Services
U.S. Department of Health & Human Services
http://www.samhsa.gov/

UCLA AIDS Institute
This site includes information about this initiative, clinical trials, training opportunities, conferences, symposia, CFAR programs, Multicenter AIDS Cohort program, pediatrics, publications, research, and news releases.
http://www.uclaaidsinstitute.org

Global HIV Initiatives

The British Medical Association
This site provides information on the British Medical Association and its educational projects; includes latest updates on AIDS news and policy issues.
http://www.bma.org.uk

Health Information for International Travel
http://www.cdc.gov/travel/yb/index.htm

The Cochrane Collaboration
This site includes information on clinical trials.
http://www.cochrane.org

Communicable Diseases—Australia
This site provides information from the Australian Department of Health and Family Services as well as other overseas surveillance systems.
http://www.cda.gov/au/index.htm

International AIDS Vaccine Initiative
http://www.iavi.org

International Travel and Health: Vaccination Requirements
http://www.who.int/ith

International Union Against Sexually Transmitted Infections/IUSTI
This site introduces this organization and its objectives.
http://www.iusti.org

Pangaea: The Global AIDS Foundation
An affiliate of the San Francisco AIDS Foundation, the Pangaea Foundation focuses its efforts on the international incidence of AIDS, particularly in developing countries, with Sub-Saharan Africa as its initial focus.
San Francisco AIDS Foundation
http://www.sfaf.org

UNAIDS—The Joint United Nations Programme on HIV/AIDS
This site offers general information, conference information, current reports, press releases, news archives, documents, and links to related websites.
http://www.unaids.org

U.S. Department of Health & Human Services HHS Global AIDS Program
http://www.cdc.gov/nchstp/od/gap

WHO HIV/AIDS Programme
http://www.who.int/hiv/en
Information on Burden of Disease http://www.

who.int/topics/global_burden_of_disease/en

World Bank, AIDS Economics of Prevention and Treatment
This sites provides information on recent publications relevant to the economics of HIV/AIDS, links to selected resources, and a link to the Electronic Newsletter.
http://www.worldbank.org/aids-econ

World Health Organization (WHO)
Avenue Appia 20
1211 Geneva 27
Switzerland
Telephone (+ 41 22)791 21 11
http://www.who.int/en

Resources for STDs/HIV in Children

The Elizabeth Glaser Pediatric AIDS Foundation
A national non-profit dedicated to supporting research for AIDS in children
(31) 314-1459
http://www.pedaids.org/
E-mail: info@pedaids.org

The Pediatric Branch of the National Cancer Institute (NCI)
The NCI conducts clinical trials for HIV-infected children on the NIH campus in Bethesda, MD.
(888) NCI-1937
http://ccr.nci.nih.gov/trials

The National Pediatric & Family HIV Resource Center
Non-profit organization that serves professionals who care for children, adolescents, and families with HIV/AIDS.
(973) 972-0410
(800) 362-0071
http://www.pedhivaids.org

Resources for Adolescents

Advocates for Youth
1025 Vermont Avenue, NW, Suite 200
Washington, DC 20005
(202) 347-5700
http://www.advocatesforyouth.org

American Social Health Association Teen Information
Site sponsored by ASHA geared toward STD education.
http://www.iwannaknow.org

Fazeteen STD articles
www.fazeteen.com/health/articles/std.htm

Go Ask Alice
Internet and bulletin board from Columbia University's Health Education Programs, providing health information for teens from health educators, physicians, and researchers.
http://www.goaskalice.columbia.edu

HIV/AIDS Prevention

HIV Insite
This University of California — San Francisco site deals specifically with HIV/AIDS and children
http://hivinsite.ucsf.edu/

Population Information Program
John Hopkins University
This organization publishes the free AIDS newsletter What's New
111 Market Place, Suite 310
Baltimore, MD 21202
http://www.jhuccp.org/topics/hivaids.shtml

Project Reach Youth, Inc. of Brooklyn
Comic-style pamphlet authored by teens for teens; covers HIV/AIDS
http://www.pry.org/

Sexuality Information and Education Council of the United States (SIECUS)
130 West 42nd St. Suite 350
New York, NY 10036
(212) 819-9770
http://www.siecus.org/

STD Homepage
http://www.teensource.org

TeenGrowth
Provides health information to teens.
http://www.teengrowth.com

Health Insurance

Checkup on Health Insurance Choices
AHCPR Publication No. 93-0018, December 1992
Agency for Health Care Policy and Research
http://www.ahrq.gov/

The Consumer's Guide to Long-Term Care Insurance
Free copy available by writing
Health Insurance Association of America
555 13th St. N.W., Suite 600 East
Washington, D.C. 20004

Medicare Handbook, Publication N1-26-27
Free copy available by writing
Health Care Financing Administration
7500 Security Boulevard
Baltimore, MD 21244-1850
1-800-633-4227
www.medicare.gov/publications/

A Shopper's Guide to Long-Term Care Insurance
Free copy available by writing
National Association of Insurance Commissioners
120 W. 12th Street, Suite 1100
Kansas City, MO 64105

Index

abacivir 5, 20, 23, 186
ABC *see* abacivir
abscess 5, 32, 39, 160, 194
Acer, David 47
acquired immune deficiency
syndrome (AIDS) 1, 2, 5–
36; acute retroviral syn-
drome 10, 11–12, 16; Alaska
natives 50; alternative medicine 27–28, 51, 197, 226;
American Indians 52;
breastfeeding 24, 29, 191;
bug chasers 64–65; child-
birth 8, 28–29, 191; complications 14, 30–35, 97, 150,
217–218, 221; death 6–7, 9,
31, 35, 49; dementia 7, 13,
18, 56, 70; diagnosis 10,
15–18; disease course 10, 11,
12, 14–16, 30, 51; early infection 11, 12, 14, 15, 37; early
intervention services 94–95;
epidemiology 8–9, 148; ethnicity 9, 39–40, 116, 140,
216, 247; etiology 7–8, 112–
113; exposure category 98;
history of 6, 41–48, 163–164,
238, 257–258; housing as-
sistance 47, 148–149; im-
mune system 13, 14, 19, 30;
neonatal 14, 17, 28–29; neoplasms 1, 6, 11, 15, 18, 31–32,
165–167; non-progressors
15, 51, 184; opportunistic
infections 1, 6, 11, 14, 18, 30,
56, 81, 241, 268; pediatric
14, 99, 171–172, 191–193,
270–271; pregnancy 24–25,
28–29, 191; rapid progressors 15; risk factors 9, 24,
26, 27, 29–30, 62, 79, 202,
223, 236; social context 46,

47; social security disability
222; symptoms 10–14, 30,
32, 33, 98–99, 196; treatment 2, 12, 13, 18–25, 34,
38, 226, 264, 267; travel restrictions 46, 47; wasting
syndrome 12, 14, 18, 150,
160, 246, 254–255; women,
considerations in 9–10, 21;
see also AIDS vaccines;
HIV/AIDS; HIV–1; HIV–2;
HIV tests; human immun-
odeficiency virus
ACT UP 36, 46
acupressure 36
acupuncture 36
acute HIV infection 37; *see
also* HIV disease
acute inflammatory demyelinating polyneuropathy 12–
13
acyclovir 34, 37, 134, 135
ADAP *see* AIDS Drug Assistance Program
adult T-cell leukemia/lym-
phoma 38–39, 157–158
Adults AIDS Clinical Trials
Group 38
Africa 6, 9, 39–40, 42, 43;
West 7, 16, 147
AIDS *see* acquired immune
deficiency syndrome
AIDS Clinical Trials Group
40–41, 266
AIDS-defining illness 15,
17–18,
AIDS dementia complex 18,
41
AIDS Drug Assistance Pro-
gram 41
AIDS/HIV disease 50
AIDS quilt 48

AIDS-related complex 48
AIDS-related primary central
nervous system lymphoma
48–49
AIDS Vaccine Evaluation
Group 49
AIDS vaccines 49–50, 51, 166,
266
AIN *see* anal intraepithelial
neoplasia
alkaline phosphatase 50
alpha defensins 50–51, 184
alpha interferon 51, 129, 64
alpha lipoic acid 28, 51, 197
alternative medicine in AIDS
27–28, 51
Alvac-HIV 51
amdoxovir 20
amebiasis 33, 50–51, 189–190
American Red Cross 102
American Social Health Association (ASHA) 52, 224,
263
Americans with Disabilities
Act 47, 95
amniocentesis 52
amniotic fluid 2, 52, 51, 226
Amphotericin B 52
amprenavir 21, 23, 204
Amsler grid 52–53
amyl nitrite 53
anal intraepithelial neoplasia
53
anal sex 8, 9, 53, 106
anergy 53
angiogenesis 53–54
antibiotics 54, 67, 89
antibody 12, 39, 50, 54
antibody tests 15–17, 54,
126–127, 141
anticonvulsant medications
54

273